T0192885

Animal Sourced Foods for Developing Economies

World Food Preservation Center Book Series

Series Editor
Charles L. Wilson

Postharvest Extension and Capacity Building for the Developing World
Majeed Mohammed and Vijay Yadav Tokala

Animal Sourced Foods for Developing Economies: Preservation, Nutrition, and Safety
Edited by Muhammad Issa Khan and Aysha Sameen

For more information about this series please visit:
http://worldfoodpreservationcenter.com/crc-press.html

Animal Sourced Foods for Developing Economies

Preservation, Nutrition, and Safety

Edited by
Muhammad Issa Khan
Aysha Sameen

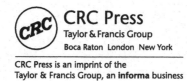

CRC Press
Taylor & Francis Group
Boca Raton London New York

CRC Press is an imprint of the
Taylor & Francis Group, an **informa** business

CRC Press
Taylor & Francis Group
6000 Broken Sound Parkway NW, Suite 300
Boca Raton, FL 33487-2742

First issued in paperback 2021

ISBN 13: 978-1-03-223749-7 (pbk)
ISBN 13: 978-1-4987-7895-4 (hbk)

Library of Congress Cataloging-in-Publication Data

Names: Khan, Muhammad Issa, editor. | Sameen, Aysha, editor.
Title: Animal sourced foods for developing economies : preservation,
nutrition, and safety / editors: Muhammad Issa Khan, Aysha Sameen.
Other titles: World Food Preservation Center book series.
Description: Boca Raton, FL : Taylor & Francis, 2019. | Series: World Food
Preservation Center book series
Identifiers: LCCN 2018036130 | ISBN 9781498778954 (hardback : alk. paper) |
ISBN 9780429676529 (pdf) | ISBN 9780429676512 (epub) | ISBN 9780429676505
(mobi/kindle)
Subjects: LCSH: Food of animal origin--Developing countries.
Classification: LCC TX371 .A557 2019 | DDC 641.3/06--dc23
LC record available at https://lccn.loc.gov/2018036130

Visit the Taylor & Francis Web site at
http://www.taylorandfrancis.com

and the CRC Press Web site at
http://www.crcpress.com

Contents

Series Preface

WORLD FOOD PRESERVATION CENTER® LLC BOOK SERIES

The UN has recently reported that World Hunger is on the rise for the first time in decades. Also, for the first time since the "Green Revolution" crop yields are decreasing rather than increasing. This is in spite of the billions of dollars that are being invested to increase crop production. Compounding this problem is a rapidly exploding world population that is expected to be around 10 billion by 2050. It is apparent that if we remain on our present course we are headed toward a major world food shortage crisis. This food shortage crisis will impact most severely in developing countries where 95% of this new population growth will occur. In order to meet this pending food shortage crisis we need a new strategy—a new agricultural paradigm.

Our present agricultural paradigm is based on the success of the "Green Revolution" during which we were able to increase crop yields by 3%–5% per year in the 1970s and 1980s. This was accomplished by breeding more productive crops, increased use of fertilizers, irrigation, and pesticides. Presently, even with greater investments in the advanced food production technologies of the "Green Revolution" crop yields are decreasing and are below 1% per year. Clearly, we need a new agricultural paradigm.

The World Bank and UNFAO have shown that one-third of the food that is already produced is lost between the time that it is harvested and consumed. This is enough food to feed two billion hungry people annually. Clearly, a new strategy to combat world hunger would be to substantially and sustainably save more of the food that we already produce.

Because, up until now, we have invested so few of our agricultural resources into the postharvest preservation of food (5%) as compared to food production (95%) a substantial postharvest "technology gaps" and "skill gaps" exists, especially in developing countries.

The World Food Preservation Center® LLC was established to help fill these gaps.

The World Food Preservation Center® LLC is accomplishing its mission by (1) promoting the postharvest education (MS and PhD) of young student/scientists from developing countries in the latest technologies for the postharvest preservation of food, (2) the development of postharvest curricula/texts for the secondary education of students in developing countries), (3) the organization of continent-wide postharvest congresses and exhibitions, (4) the publication of a postharvest reference/text book targeted toward the needs of developing countries, and (5) the organization of a Global Mycotoxin Alliance to focus the world's resources on reducing mycotoxin contamination of food in developing countries (http://www.worldfoodpreservationcenter.com/index.html).

The World Food Preservation Center® Book Series is publishing books on such topics as:

Animal Sourced Foods for Developing Economies
People in developing countries currently consume on average on-third the meat and one-quarter of the milk products per capita compared to richer developed economies. But, this is changing rapidly as the economies of developing counties improve. With this increased consumption of animal protein in developing economies comes the need to produce more animal protein in a safe and sustainable manner. *Animal Sourced Foods for Developing Economies* presents the results and experiences of leading scientists in developing economies as they adapt advance technologies and methodologies for the increased production of animal sourced foods.

Charles L. Wilson
Founder, CEO
World Food Preservation Center LLC

Preface

Food is necessity of life as it contains macronutrients that provide energy for livelihood, growth & development and maintenance of human body. Food also provide micronutrients such as minerals and vitamins which regulated biochemical reactions involved in energy production and regulation of body functions. Globally, animal sourced foods make up a considerable portion of a typical diet and demand these products has been escalating in all regions of the world due to the momentous rise in the world population. Meat is, nevertheless, sold as one of the high-priced food commodities particularly in the developing countries. The amount of meat consumed in different countries varies enormously with social, economic and political influences, religious beliefs and geographical differences. It is very high in meat-producing areas such as Uruguay, Argentina, Australia and New Zealand, at 300 g per head per day compared with an average of 10-18 g in Pakistan, India, Indonesia and Sri Lanka. There is a constantly increasing demand for animal sourced foods in the developing countries which can be satisfied by augmented domestic production and imports. It is thought that the major increase in domestic production will come from small producers rather than from creating large production units, but these lack the essential facilities for producing safe and wholesome products. If there is to be a significant increase in animal sourced foods production it will require clear policy decisions with the necessary financial, legislative and technical support. There is considerable potential for increased supplies through better management, selection of animals, avoidance of waste and making use of indigenous species.

Land availability limits the expansion of livestock numbers in extensive production systems in most regions, and the bulk of the increase in livestock production will come from increased productivity through intensification and a wider adoption of existing and new production and marketing technologies. The significant changes in the global consumption and demand for animal source foods, along with increasing pressures on resources, are having some important implications for the principal production systems. Animal sourced food contain high biological value protein and important micronutrients required for optimal body functioning but are regarded as sources of fat that contribute to the intake of total and saturated fatty acids in diet. The quality of protein source has a direct influence on protein digestibility, as a greater proportion of higher quality proteins is absorbed and becomes available for bodily functions. Animal foods has high quantity and quality of protein that includes a full complement of the essential amino acids in the right proportion.

Animal Sourced Foods for Developing Economies addresses five major issues: 1) Food safety and nutritional status in developing world; 2) the contribution of animal origin foods in human health; 3) production processes of animal foods along with their preservation strategies; 4) functional outcomes of animal derived foods; and finally, 5) strategies, issues and polices to promote animal origin food consumption. The contributors critically analyze and describe different aspects of animal's origin foods. Each chapter is dedicated to a specific type of food from animal source, its nutritional significance, preservation techniques, processed products, safety and quality aspects on conceptual framework. Special attention is given to explain current food safety scenario in developing countries and contribution of animal derived food in their dietary intake. Existing challenges regarding production, processing and promotion of animal's origin foods are also addressed with possible solutions and strengthening approaches.

We would like to extend our acknowledgement to our colleagues at National Institute of Food Science and Technology, University of Agriculture, Faisalabad and other universities in Pakistan. We are also thankful to contributors from India, Germany and Gambia for their contributions.

Muhammad Issa Khan & Aysha Sameen
Editors

Editors

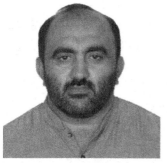

Muhammad Issa Khan is a tenured associate professor at the National Institute of Food Science and Technology, University of Agriculture, Faisalabad, Pakistan. He began his career as a lecturer in 2007 and, after completion of his PhD, he received tenure as an assistant professor in 2010 and tenured associate professor in 2016. He received his PhD from University of Agriculture, Faisalabad in the discipline of food technology with a specialization in functional foods development. His research mainly focuses on the quality and nutritional improvement of meat and meat products. Dr. Khan did his postdoctoral research at the Animal Origin Food Science Laboratory, Seoul National University, South Korea and attended a short professional training session at the Department of Food Science and Human Nutrition, University of Illinois, Urbana–Champaign. He has supervised three PhD and 40 MS students so far, while three doctorate students are under his supervision for their research. Dr. Khan has earned the Research Productivity Award from the Pakistan Council of Science and Technology twice (2014 and 2016) based on his research, scholarly publication, and contribution to science and technology. He also has been categorized as a Productive Scientist of Pakistan in 2016. He has contributed four chapters in books by well reputed publishers and published one text book about meat processing for students of B.Sc. (Hons) food science and technology. He also published 100 peer reviewed research publications in leading journals in the field of food science and technology. He is also a reviewer of more than 15 reputed journals. Dr. Khan offers his services to community organizations for the development of high protein, high energy cookies for emergency conditions and the training of analysts in Public Food Laboratories on quantitative and qualitative analysis of foods. Dr. Khan belongs to a far off village, Haddowali, in District Attock, and his family is engaged in imparting education and research.

Dr. Muhammad Issa Khan
(http://www.uaf.edu.pk/EmployeeDetail.aspx?userid=434)
drkhan@uaf.edu.pk

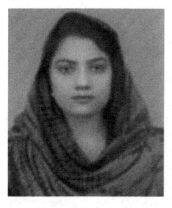

Aysha Sameen is an assistant professor at the National Institute of Food Science and Technology, University of Agriculture, Faisalabad, Pakistan. She started her career as a lecturer in 2005 and was promoted to assistant professor in 2009 after completing her PhD in Food Technology at the University of Agriculture, Faisalabad, Pakistan. Her main research interests lie in the foods of animal origins, especially milk and milk products. She is currently working on the development of a stabilizer for dairy products and different types of cheese, such as Cheddar, Mozzarella, and soft cheeses, dairy spreads, and yoghurt. She has supervised the research of three PhD and 36 M.Sc. (Hons.) students. These students are from different degree disciplines, including food technology, dairy technology, food safety, and human nutrition. She has 41 peer-reviewed research publications in renowned journals in the discipline of food science and technology. She has actively contributed to various international/ national workshops, training sessions, and seminars as an organizer as well as participant. She has contributed chapters in three books by well-reputed publishers. She has offered various advisory, community, and administrative services. She conducted nutritional assessment and awareness camps at different stations in Faisalabad for evaluating the nutritional status of the general public and provided them with counseling accordingly.

Dr. Aysha Sameen
ayshasameen@uaf.edu.pk

Contributors

Mariam Aizad
National Institute of Food Science and
  Technology
Faculty of Food Nutrition and Home Sciences
University of Agriculture Faisalabad
Faisalabad, Pakistan

Sajeela Akram
National Institute of Food Science and
  Technology
Faculty of Food Nutrition and Home Sciences
University of Agriculture Faisalabad
Faisalabad, Pakistan

Faqir Muhammad Anjum
National Institute of Food Science and
  Technology
University of Agriculture Faisalabad
Faisalabad, Pakistan

and

Vice Chancellor, University of Gambia
Gambia, West Africa

Rizwan Arshad
National Institute of Food Science and
  Technology
University of Agriculture Faisalabad
Faisalabad, Pakistan

Nehdia Azhar
National Institute of Food Science and
  Technology
University of Agriculture Faisalabad
Faisalabad, Pakistan

Rituparna Banerjee
ICAR-National Research Centre on Meat
Hyderabad, India

Bernd Hallier
European Retail Academy (ERC)
Roesrath, Germany

Ihsan Ullah
Food and Nutrition Division
Nuclear Institute for Food and Agriculture
Pakistan Atomic Energy Commission
Peshawar, Pakistan

Bushra Ishfaq
National Institute of Food Science and
  Technology
University of Agriculture
Faisalabad, Pakistan

Asghar Ali Kamboh
Department of Veterinary Microbiology
Faculty of Animal Husbandry & Veterinary
  Sciences
Sindh Agriculture University
Tandojam, Pakistan

Muhammad Ammar Khan
Department of Food Science & Technology
University College of Agriculture and
  Environmental Sciences
The Islamia University of Bahawalpur Pakistan
Bahawalpur, Pakistan

Muhammad Issa Khan
National Institute of Food Science and
  Technology
University of Agriculture Faisalabad
Faisalabad, Pakistan

V. V. Kulkarni
ICAR-National Research Centre on Meat
Hyderabad, India

Atif Liaqat
National Institute of Food Science and
  Technology
University of Agriculture Faisalabad
Faisalabad, Pakistan

Sana Mehmood
National Institute of Food Science and
    Technology
University of Agriculture Faisalabad
Faisalabad, Pakistan

Fakiha Mehak
National Institute of Food Science and
    Technology
University of Agriculture Faisalabad
Faisalabad, Pakistan

B. M. Naveena
ICAR-National Research Centre on Meat
Hyderabad, India

Saima Rafiq
Department of Food Science and Technology
The University of Poonch
Rawalakot, Pakistan

Ubaid ur Rahman
National Institute of Food Science and
    Technology
Food Engineering Department
University of Agriculture Faisalabad
Faisalabad, Pakistan

Salim-ur-Rehman
Department of Food Science and Technology
University of Sargodha
Faisalabad, Pakistan

Shaihid-ur-Rehman
University of Agriculture Faisalabad
Toba Tek Singh, Pakistan

Amna Sahar
National Institute of Food Science and
    Technology
Food Engineering Department
University of Agriculture Faisalabad
Faisalabad, Pakistan

Sana Tahira Saleem
Department of Food Science and Human
    Nutrition
University of Veterinary and Animal Sciences
Lahore, Pakistan

Aysha Sameen
National Institute of Food Science and
    Technology
Faculty of Food Nutrition and Home Sciences
University of Agriculture Faisalabad
Faisalabad, Pakistan

Hira Shakoor
National Institute of Food Science and
    Technology
University of Agriculture Faisalabad
Faisalabad, Pakistan

Aamir Shehzad
National Institute of Food Science and
    Technology
Faculty of Food Nutrition and Home Sciences
University of Agriculture Faisalabad
Faisalabad, Pakistan

Mohammad Sohaib
Department of Food Science and Human
    Nutrition
University of Veterinary and Animal Sciences
Lahore, Pakistan

Farwa Tariq
National Institute of Food Science and
    Technology
Faculty of Food Nutrition and Home
    Sciences
University of Agriculture Faisalabad
Faisalabad, Pakistan

Muhammad Rizwan Tariq
Department of Diet & Nutritional Sciences
Faculty of Allied Health Sciences
The University of Lahore
Lahore, Pakistan

Tayyaba Tariq
National Institute of Food Science and
    Technology
Faculty of Food Nutrition and Home Sciences
University of Agriculture Faisalabad
Faisalabad, Pakistan

Aman Ullah
Department of Agronomy
University of Agriculture Faisalabad
Faisalabad, Pakistan

Arun K. Verma
ICAR-Central Institute for Research on Goats
Mathura, India

Huijuan Yang
Department of Food Science
Zhejiang Academy of Agricultural Sciences
Hangzhou, People's Republic of China

Muhammad Yasin
Food and Nutrition Division
Nuclear Institute for Food and Agriculture
Pakistan Atomic Energy Commission
Peshawar, Pakistan

Ayesha Zafar
Department of Food Science and Human
    Nutrition
University of Veterinary and Animal Sciences
Lahore, Pakistan

Asna Zahid
National Institute of Food Science and
    Technology
Faculty of Food Nutrition and Home
    Sciences
University of Agriculture Faisalabad
Faisalabad, Pakistan

Tahir Zahoor
National Institute of Food Science and
    Technology
University of Agriculture Faisalabad
Faisalabad, Pakistan

Aurang Zeb
Food and Nutrition Division
Nuclear Institute for Food and Agriculture
Pakistan Atomic Energy Commission
Peshawar, Pakistan

1 The Role of Food Security and Nutrition to Meet Consumers' Requirements in the Developing World

Mohammad Sohaib, Aman Ullah, Ayesha Zafar, and Sana Tahira Saleem

CONTENTS

1.1 INTRODUCTION

Increase in the prices of food commodities has globally diverted the attention of scientists, policy makers, relevant stakeholders, and the news media towards the issue of food security. The term food security is defined as the availability of quality food to all for an active, healthy life. The supply of food at the national and global level also falls under the food security. According to the Food and Agriculture Organization (FAO), food security "is availability of adequate nutritious food supply at all times for all people, with social and economic access" [1]. The World Food Summit defines food security as "when all people at all times have social, physical and economic access to the enough, nutritious and safe food which keeps them healthy and active" [2]. In 2015, there were approximately 12.7% of US households (42.2 million individuals) that were food insecure.

In recent years, food security has drawn widespread attention due to global food crisis that raised in 2008. That was the year, when food prices reached to their highest levels as compared to past years around the globe. Now practitioners and scientists consider food security in terms of nutrient deficiencies and dietary energy availability, rather than in terms of quality life and nutritional uptake. Micronutrient malnutrition has taken central position in policy discussions about food security. However, food insecurity is the inability to purchase nutritious and safe food for maintaining normal health. Globally, diet-related diseases are increasing due to various, widespread vitamin and micronutrient deficiencies in the food system [3]. The people with food insecurity can have a number of lifelong health effects, ranging from developmental delays to physical and mental health. The deficiency of micronutrients causes low-work productivity, permanent impairment of cognitive ability, and increased rate of mortality and morbidity [4]. The most vulnerable part of society is young children and women of reproductive age. In addition to physical health constraints, the stigma of food insecurity negatively affects a person's self-image, mental well-being, as well as quality of life. Common observed responses to scarce food supplies includes reduced intake of food, adjustments in food budget, and alterations in food stuff. The increase in the consumption of energy-rich foods increases and diversity in the diet decreases. The foods dense in energy contain saturated fats, fortified sugars, and refined grains, and are poor in the nutritional quality and are expensive [5].

Food insecure masses have a diet that contains lower levels of micronutrients, including iron, iodine, zinc, calcium, magnesium, vitamin B complex, and fewer weekly servings of fruits, vegetables, and dairy products. Intake of these types of dietary food stuff causes the development of chronic diseases, such as diabetes, hypertension, and hyperlipidemia. The distribution of the available food depends especially on the individuals within households and on a country, province, region, households. The food access (socio, cultural, and economic access to food), food availability (physical availability through production, import, and aid), and food absorption (food utilization and assimilation) are the broader parameters of food security [6].

1.2   FOOD SECURITY: AN OVERVIEW

Ensuring food security has become the biggest challenge in the face of situations, such as limited arable land, changing climate, physical isolation, difficult terrain, and limited market access. Furthermore, the increasing rate of out-migration is causing labor shortages in agriculture and leading to underutilization of agriculture potential. The decrease in the agriculture production is further aggregating the condition of food security due to fluctuations in market prices of imported food items as people have to rely on imported food [7].

It is difficult to afford nutritious foods on a limited budget, which exacerbates chronic disease risk for low-income populations. The least expensive forms of food energy are foods in the fats category, grains, and other carbohydrates. Conversely, fruits and vegetables are the most expensive in terms of calories, whereas meat, poultry, and fish are the most expensive per serving. Individuals who are food insecure often rely on low-cost, energy-dense, but nutrient-poor foods to satisfy hunger. To address the health risks associated with food insecurity and provide competent counsel, dietetics students and future health practitioners must understand the consequences of hunger and the stigma associated with both nutrition assistance and obesity; for the sake of better health outcomes. They must also have empathy when working with clients who struggle to afford nutritious diets [8].

Food security is a measure of welfare at the household level. A food secure household is one that has the ability to meet the food demands of its members. The difference between permanent and transitory food insecurity is in the duration; in the former, no-access to the sufficient food is on a long-term basis, and, in the latter, food shortage is for a short period of time (periodic food insecurity), such as seasonal food insecurity. The reasons associated with household food security may not assure food for all members, because household preferences may not prioritize food purchases over acquisition of other goods and services (such as health, school fees, and housing). Additionally, intra-household allocation of food may not be based on the needs of each individual member. A case in point is many households exist with both obese and undernourished members. Moreover, the factors responsible for good nutrition, apart from the food factors, include water quality, access to primary health care, sanitary conditions, and infectious diseases preventions. Thus, food security is not nutritional security [9].

Food and nutrition security is based on four key pillars including the availability of food that can be produced in a given region and sold by grocery stores. Improvements in the means of agriculture are directly related to the increase in food availability, which affects the amount of food that can be produced; "availability" is linked with the supply side of food security. The availability of sufficient quality food is more related to supply side of food security and determined by food production and trade. Availability of food can be measured indirectly by food balance sheets, national income as well as consumer expenditure data [10]. The second pillar involves access to the ability of individuals to get food, as well as the absence or presence of safeguards for those who cannot get food by licit means. For example, the level of access to food available to individuals is related to the number of grocery stores in a given region. The actual global or regional distribution of food resources reflects the food access and the inequalities embedded therein, associated with the demand side of food security. It is about individuals and households having ample resources for their getting hands on the appropriate foods to attain a nutritious diet. Income and food poverty factors are closely linked to the food access [11].

Third parameter of food security is food utilization that involves how an individual ingest and metabolize available food on the basis of knowledge, feeding practices, access to adequate and safe water, sanitation, as well as health care practices. It also shows whether households and a single individual make proper use of the food to which they have access. Either the individual are provided with affordable or balanced food having all essential nutrients or with lower quality or less nutritious diet. Is the food properly prepared under safe, sanitary conditions to deliver their full nutritional value? Can their bodies metabolize and absorb essential nutrients? Utilization's core focus is diversity of dietary quality, as micronutrient deficiencies are associated with the inadequate intake of essential minerals and vitamins in the diet. Finally, the availability as well as access to food at all times throughout the month, year, and in the future, affects the stability of food items. The involvement of risk factors such as poverty, socioeconomic and political instability as well as peoples skills make it difficult for individual/community for provision of safe, nutritious and healthy food.

The economy of Pakistan is based on agriculture being an agricultural country. Currently, agriculture sector is facing serious concerns, such as irrigation issues because of water shortages and less rainfall due to climate change. Certain crops like rice, vegetables, cereals, spices, and other grains are climate dependent and are facing the biggest threats. The rising temperature and changing rainfall is also causing a shortage of water that further escalates the problem of food security resulting lower productivity in food sector. Food insecurity is considered a central hindrance towards economic development of a country. In many low-income countries, to cope with the issue of under nutrition, particularly among the poor, consumer food subsidies are an important policy instrument. In promoting greater nutrient intake and overall nutrition, social protection measures, such as food assistance programs, play a crucial role [12].

The provision of staple food at subsidized prices is important in this concern. The food availability at the subsidized price not only increases access to food to the beneficiaries, but also provides an implicit income transfer which is the basic difference between the open market and subsidized price for every unit of the food item purchased. This gain in income would result into consumption of a nutritious basket of food items has been a much debated issue due to limited empirical evidence. Theoretically, price subsidies would have a positive impact if the income gain is spent on the consumption of more nutritious food.

1.3 THE IMPORTANCE AND ROLE OF NUTRITION: FACTS AND ARTIFACTS

The science that explores the interaction of nutrients and other substances in food (e.g. anthocyanin's, phytonutrients, and tannins) in relation to growth, maintenance, reproduction, diseases, and health of an organism is called nutrition. Nutrition also investigates the ways through which diseases, problems, and issues can be cured with a nutrition rich diet or can be lessened to some extent. Additionally, it also helps to identify diseases, conditions, or problems associated with a poor diet (malnutrition), food allergies, metabolic diseases, and so forth that can be rectified by dietary interventions. For the physical and cognitive development of the body, behavioral and scholastic performance, better health and productivity, improved quality of life, and socio-economic development of the country, optimal nutrition is essential (Figure 1.1).

With the growing food demands, increases in the supply chain production of food faces three main problems. Firstly, the increase in agriculture crop production is not enough to meet the future or long term goals. Therefore, innovations and skills are required to increase the yield of crops without

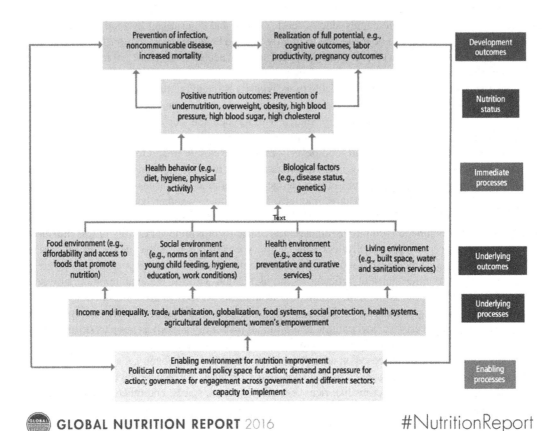

FIGURE 1.1 The underlying drivers leading towards improved nutrition status of humans.

using more land. Secondly, natural resources have been closely linked in order to increase crop production ultimately contributing towards food security. However, some of the factors such as global warming, urbanization, excessive use of natural resources and environmental degradation are serious threats to natural resources ultimately reduce crop production. Agricultural land is used for making biofuels and other non-food products being converted into urban infrastructure. In order to create land for agricultural purposes, deforestation leads to an unbalance the natural environment (e.g. biodiversity loss, greenhouse gas emissions). Thirdly, this all impacts weather and gradually leads to climate change. Climatic change affects all kinds of creatures on land including human, plants, animals, along with aquatic life. All challenges contribute to a globalized world where trading in food is growing day by day. Trading creates networks between all stakeholders across the world, or separate production from consumption leads to efficient distribution of resources and leading towards price stability of the food commodities [13]. Pakistan is challenged by food insecurity, under-nutrition and over-nutrition, and a growing epidemic of preventable chronic and infectious diseases that have put a severe burden on health services, resulting in avoidable disabilities and premature deaths. Good nutrition is essential for the prevention, control, and treatment of these diseases. A synergistic relationship between nutrition and disease exists. Appropriate dietary practices and lifestyle modifications are required to prevent the rising prevalence of malnutrition, chronic diseases, and premature deaths [14].

Changes in the lifestyle and nutrition transition have led to an increased occurrence of overweight and obesity and a plague of non-communicable diseases (NCDs), such as diabetes, cardiovascular disease, hypertension, and cancer. NCDs are the leading causes of premature deaths in both the developed and developing countries accounting for 38 million of the world's 58 million deaths in 2012 [15]. Expenditure on the treatment of NCDs amounts to billions of dollars annually adversely affecting

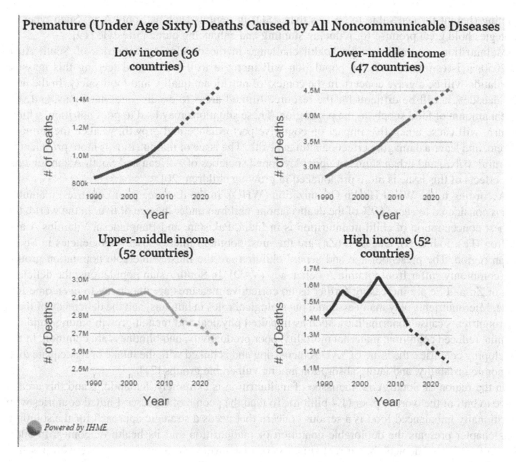

FIGURE 1.2 Underlying data source: Institute for Health Metrics and Evaluation, Global Burden of Disease Study 2013.

the economy of countries, causing an increase in disabilities, premature deaths, and impaired physical productivity and economic outputs. NCDs are responsible for a higher prevalence of disability adjusted life years (DALYs) and cause innumerable sufferings for families and societies. In Pakistan, an estimated 10%–10.8% of the adult population (aged 25 years and above) is suffering from diabetes [16] and the numbers are expected to increase to 14.5 million by the year 2025 [17].

Worldwide, the leading causes of disability and premature deaths in adults are cardiovascular diseases (CVDs). Low-income to middle-income countries bear the brunt by accounting for over 80% of the global disease burden and the overwhelming health expenditures amounting to billions of dollars annually. Among adult deaths (aged 30–70 years old) CVDs account for 19% of all the deaths occurring in Pakistan [18] (Figure 1.2).

1.4 MALNUTRITION IN SOUTH ASIA

Meeting nutrient needs of people living in regions like South Asia is a big challenge mainly because of their diet habit. Their diets are dominated with staple foods with low nutrients as well as poor bioavailability of the minerals. In such populations, the gaps in nutritional suitability date back to agricultural revolution ~10,000 years ago. The prenatal and post-natal nutrition strategies can have a positive impact on the growth of children. Furthermore, intervention packages, which include improved nutrition in diet during pregnancy and post-natal periods, prevention and control of prenatal and post-natal infection, and subclinical conditions, decreases the issues of malnutrition and stunting (height for age value to be less than 2SD) in regions such as South Asia. Such types of strategies hold great promise for reducing stunting and enhancing human lifestyle [19].

Malnutrition is a major public health challenge in the developing countries of South Asia. In 2050, it is estimated that the population will increase to 9 billion and feeding this massive population will be a grave concern in the context of nutritional quality and food safety. In the next few decades, it will be difficult for the resource limited areas to ensure safe, nutritious, and sufficient amount of food supply to the population. These situations may lead to poor nutrition, which, in turn, will cause a negative impact on cognitive performance and growth, weaken the immune system, and leave a damaging effect on human health. The issue of malnutrition is more prevalent in the rural, tribal, and urban slums of underdeveloped societies of African and South Asian regions. The effects of this issue is more pronounced in growing children [20].

According to the World Health Organization (WHO), in the resource poor countries, malnutrition is considered to cause 60% of the deaths among children under the age of five. In the world, the highest concentration of child malnutrition is in India, Pakistan, and Bangladesh. Vitamins A and D, Iron (Fe), Iodine (I), and Zinc (Zn) are the most common micronutrient deficiencies in South Asian region. The preschool-age and school children are the most vulnerable population groups that commonly suffer from vitamin A deficiency (VAD). In South Asian populations, the deficiencies of Zn and Fe are increasing further as no corrective measures are underway to overcome this issue. Micronutrients play many essential physiological roles in humans, and the deficiency of these micronutrients cause abnormalities, such as impaired physical and mental growth among children, anemia, reduced cognition, maternal mortality, poor productivity, and blindness are common. In the developing countries, the issue of VAD is increasing and is linked with the intake of inadequate diet, economic instability, and faulty absorption among vulnerable groups [21].

In the region of South Asia, the issue of malnutrition is extremely demanding, and this area is home to half of the world's poor (1.4 billion). To feed the people of resource-limited countries with nutritionally imbalanced food is a serious concern that needs a strategic approach for the solution. This chapter presents the deplorable condition of malnutrition and its health outcomes. In addition to this, it also depicts the current situation of malnutrition in South Asia along with possible approaches to mitigate this issue of public concern (Figure 1.3).

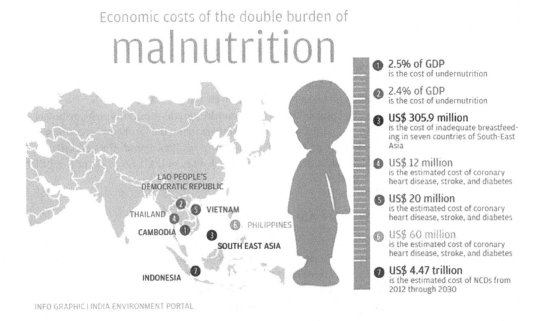

FIGURE 1.3 Economic costs of the double burden of malnutrition.

1.5 MALNUTRITION IN PAKISTAN

Malnutrition is a condition that arises from taking a diet in which nutrients are deficient or in limited access, and consumption of such type of diet results in health problems. There are two extreme, one is called **under nutrition** in which diet is deficient of the recommended nutrients (calories, carbohydrates, protein, minerals, or vitamins), while the other is **over nutrition**, over-consumption of nutrients that exceeds the limit required for normal growth, development and metabolism, both can leads to serious health issues. The risk of infectious diseases increases, and the immune system weakens because of malnourishment. The susceptibility to infection, as well as other associated risks, increase under micronutrient (including iron, zinc, and vitamins) deficiencies. The factors behind malnutrition include high food prices, poverty, conventional dietary practices, and agricultural productivity are the main reasons along with individual preferences [22].

Malnutrition in All Its Forms	
Child stunting	Low height for age
Child wasting	Low weight
Child overweight	High weight for height
Adult overweight	Carrying excess body fat with body mass index >25
Micronutrient deficiency	Iron, folic acid, vitamin A, zinc, iodine below healthy threshold
Adult obesity	Carrying excess body fat with a Body Mass Index (BMI) >30
Non-communicable diseases	Diabetes, heart diseases, and some cancers

Pakistan is an agricultural country blessed with natural resources. Despite its huge natural resources and vast agricultural lands for food production, malnutrition is still prevalent in a large segment of the Pakistani population. The nutritional insufficiency is mainly associated with low socioeconomic position as well as insufficient economic capability of the people to regularly consume valuable foods, especially milk, eggs, meat, and other dairy products. According to the National Nutrition Survey (NNS) of Pakistan, 45.3 million people (28% of population) are prone to food insecurity. It also further depicts stunting, wasting, and micronutrient malnutrition as endemic in the country. The survey reported little change over the last decade in terms of core maternal and childhood nutrition. The micronutrient deficiencies are widespread in children, specifically under the age of 5 years (61.9% anemia, 43.8% iron deficiency, 54% vitamin A deficiency, 39.2% zinc deficiency, and 40% vitamin D deficiency), and amongst mothers (vitamin A deficiency 17.2%, anemia 50.4%, Zn deficiency 42.1%, calcium deficiency 52.9%, and vitamin D deficiency 23.2%) [23]. Several studies reported the prevalence of malnutrition in Pakistani community. The stunting of growth is commonly prevalent amongst children 25–36 months of age. Anemia (78%) is the most common micronutrient deficiency, whereas stunted patients (44%) had coexisting rickets. Accordingly, a study was carried out to determine micronutrient deficiencies as well as stunting frequency among children in hospital. According to the WHO classification of malnutrition mild (weight for height ratio between -1 standard deviation (SD) to -2SD), moderate (-2SD to -3SD) and severe (less than -3SD of National center for health statistics (NCHS)/WHO reference values), patients (aged 6–60 months) admitted to hospital were assessed for nutritional status and stunting. For the confirmation of the clinical diagnosis of Fe deficiency (anemia and rickets), laboratory investigations were done and they found that 44 patients (29%) had moderate stunting, 27 patients (18%) had mild stunting, 63 (44%) patients were severely stunted, whereas 16 patients (10.7%) had normal stature. Furthermore, the most common micronutrient deficiency diagnosed in 117 (78%) patients was anemia [24] (Figure 1.4).

Malnutrition is also the leading contributor for increased mortality and hospitalization, further enhancing the risk of nutritional decline. A study was carried to evaluate the prevalence of

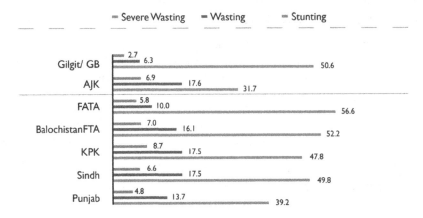

FIGURE 1.4 Nutritional status of children under 5 years of age. (From Pakistan National Nutrition Survey—2011.)

malnutrition along with a nutritional risk assessment among hospitalized children. Accordingly, a nutritional risk score (NRS) and anthropometry measurements were done on 157 children, and the results indicated stunted, wasted, obese, and overweight children frequency as 8.9%, 4.5%, 10.4%, and 15.1%, respectively. Further, it was reported that 48% of obese or overweight children were among students aged (10–18 years). The NRS reported that 47.8% children were at high risk regarding nutritional deterioration. However, children with higher nutritional risk scores had a lower weight for their age, and a longer hospitalization as well as lower BMI percentiles ($p = 0.001$) than children at no risk [25].

A study was conducted in the Dadu district to evaluate the influence of cash-based interventions to improve the nutritional status of children less than 5 years of age. Data were obtained at baseline and after 6 and 12 months of study. Parameters of study included household food security, women's empowerment, expenditures and social capital, morbidity, health seeking, nutrition behaviors, hygiene, dietary diversity, and hemoglobin concentration. The results showed that cash-based interventions improve nutritional status as well as food security at the household level [26,27].

1.6 FOOD SECURITY AND CLIMATE CHANGE

Food systems are constantly changing markedly with human settlement also because of agriculture, industrialization, trade, migration, and, now, due to the digital age. During these transitions, there has been a progressive population explosion resulting in net ecosystem loss and degradation. Climate change now gathers pace, caused by ecological dysfunction. Across the globe, the impact of climate changes on human well-being is not uniform and varies with the ecological conditions, geographic location, and with the level of economic development of the country. The countries with low economic levels and increasing poverty and poor living conditions suffer more due to climate change, rather than those countries that have better living conditions. Pakistan is at the edge of vulnerability to the adverse impacts of climate change due to rising temperatures, melting of glaciers (Himalayan), extremes in the monsoon rains, and the increasing intensity and frequency of extreme weather events that cause natural disasters (flood, drought). The vulnerability of Pakistan to climate change is based on many factors. Firstly, it is a country highly dependent upon agriculture in terms of ensuring the availability of food along with a source of revenue and employment. Secondly, there is no advanced level monitoring system in Pakistan to predict the occurrence of extreme weather events in a timely manner. Lastly, the majority of the country's population has no capacity to cope with the risks associated with climate change due to deplorable socio-economic conditions [28].

In this context, a study was conducted to categorize agro-ecological zones of Pakistan on the basis of vulnerability towards climate change, as well as to identify potential health consequences with references to Pakistan. Accordingly, the vulnerability index of climate change was constructed with three sub-indices: (a) exposure on ecological basis, (b) population sensitivity, and (c) the capacity of the population to adapt to the climate change. With high sensitivity and lower adaptive capacity to climate change, Balochistan is the most vulnerable region followed by low-intensity Punjab and Sindh. The health risks of the region including Baluchistan, Punjab and Sindh are linked with the threat from climate change. Due to climate variability, the flooding causes the risks of diarrhea and gastroenteritis, skin and eye infections, malaria, and acute respiratory infections. In the same way, exposure to drought poses health risks (anemia, night blindness, and scurvy) in the form of malnutrition and food insecurity. Health risks, such as heat stroke, malaria, dengue, respiratory diseases, and cardiovascular diseases, are the consequence of increases in temperature. There is a need at the government level to improve the socio-economic status of the lagging regions to reduce the vulnerability due to climate change [29] (Figures 1.5 and 1.6).

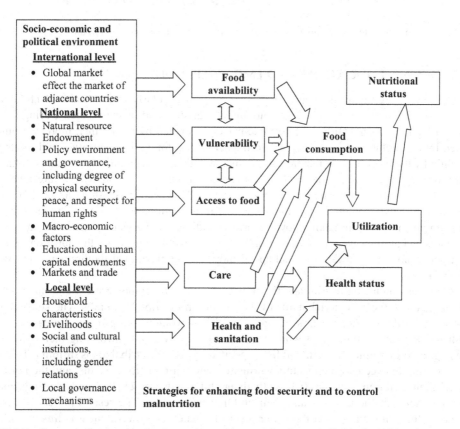

FIGURE 1.5 Framework related to food security and its contribution to individual nutritional status.

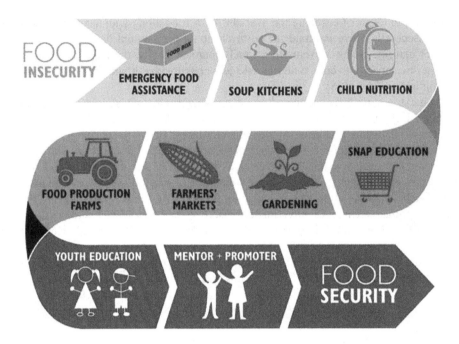

FIGURE 1.6   Role of different factors that can lead to increase food security in human.

1.7   WOMEN'S EDUCATION AND EMPOWERMENT

Malnutrition is a big threat all around the globe, most particularly to the health of children and women; about 2 billion people worldwide are undernourished and facing hunger. During the early stages of life, a child's nutrition is almost exclusively provided by the mother, moreover nutrition provided by the mother to child has positive impact on the child's life. Nutrition and foods given to the child by the mother (as principal care) coincide with the family nutritional status. It has been reported that women's literacy levels (education) and an unbiased social system are meaningful tools that can be used to mitigate the threat to nutrition. However, in South Asia, these conditions are reversed because women do not much interest in education, are less mobile, and have poor social strength and decision making power. Various studies indicate that women, who have a better social status and an improved level of education, have a positive impact on the nutrition of a child; as educated women have awareness and spend more on the nutritional requirements and food of family than men.

A study was conducted to evaluate the impact of women's empowerment and maternal malnutrition status on the nutritional status of their children aged 6–24 months. The study reported that 46% of children under 5 years of age and 47% of women living in rural areas were malnourished. This was assumed that women's empowerment was a contributing factor toward the increasing trend of malnutrition in children, specifically living in tribal areas of India. To explore the relationship between women's empowerment, maternal nutritional status, and the nutritional status of their children, 820 mothers with their children were selected and the anthropometric measurements of the mothers and their children were taken. The results indicated that poor maternal malnutrition status and the lower level of women empowerment was linked with high rates of malnutrition among the children. Hence, it was concluded that improving women's nutrition status along with their empowerment can reduce the prevalence of malnutrition in children under 5 years of age [30].

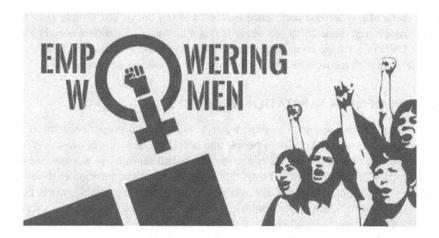

About one-third of people around the world have no access to proper or improved sanitation facilities around the globe. A quarter of the 1.5 million people die from diarrheal disease every year. The study conducted in India evaluated the effectiveness of a rural sanitation intervention to prevent diarrhea, child malnutrition, and soil transmitted helminth infection. Researchers randomly assigned 50 villages to the intervention group and 50 villages to the control group. This intervention elevated mean-level village latrine coverage from 9% of households to 63%, compared with an increase from 8% to 12% in control villages. The nutritional status was not as improved as expected before the initiation of study. These efforts improved the sanitation facilities and reduced the prevalence of diarrheal diseases; hence, efforts should be done in this regard to combat the poor nutritional status related to diseases that spread through improper sanitation facilities [31].

Child health and nutrition status is strongly linked with maternal education. This hypothesis was tested by [32] who stated that mother's education is very vital to affect positively her own and children's health and nutrition in developing economies. Child health and nutrition status is strongly linked with maternal education. As we know that a mother's education directly impacts the health status of her own as well as on her child health. The researchers estimated a Linear structural relations (LISREL) system of production functions for documenting the maternal and child health and reduced form associations for nutrition, household water and sanitation, medical care usage and with underlying variable illustrations of these dependent variables and of community and maternal endowments. If the maternal endowment is omitted, then the mother's schooling is a very strong indicator of a child's health. An educated mother seems to have strong, positive impacts on health and nutrition status of both herself and the child. But only a mother's education cannot be indicated as a separate standard to assess health status because when the maternal endowment (i.e., abilities, health status, habits, and family background) is involved, the results may change. Thus, this factor raises the doubts about standard evaluations of the impact of maternal schooling on nutrition and health.

A study was done on peri-menopausal women to check the effect of nutrition education intervention to stabilize their incident menopause. For this purpose, their body mass index (BMI), plasma lipid profile, fasting plasma glucose and prevalence of metabolic syndrome were determined. A village and small town nutritional education system was planned to reduce the risk of cardiovascular diseases. Investigation of previous study before nutrition indicated that blood pressure, BMI, low and high density of triglycerides, cholesterol (lipoprotein) and systolic blood pressure increase in females experiencing menopause. Whereas, after nutritional treatments, triglycerides plasma status substantially reduced. Dominance of syndrome (metabolic) after and before menopause was (99 and 73) out of 301 sample size, respectively, as observed in the pre-intervention cluster. However, after post-intervention, the cluster of metabolic syndrome prevalence was (66 and 68) out of 262 sample size, respectively. Moreover, the conclusion made about this study is that a nutrition educational agenda for the reduction of risk of CVD in a village coincided with a deterrence in the escalation of BMI and metabolic syndrome in relation with menopause, cholestrolemia, and systolic blood pressure [33].

1.8   IMPROVEMENT IN SANITATION FACILITIES

Fulfillment of basic necessities, such as pure water to humans and proper removal of human and household garbage, improves the health of people and decreases incidents of disease. Village conditions, in respect to the provision of good education and health services, is worse when observed in developing countries. In addition, proper attention is not given to malnutrition in developing countries because few physicians and nurses are available in hospitals. Regrettably, worse conditions of malnutrition are found in South Asian countries; malnutrition points toward more serious issues, such as poverty and unlimited social constraints and problems. One thing that also needs attention is physicians should treat people at the individual level, rather than a collective just to make more money, and they also should be more concerned about health of people.

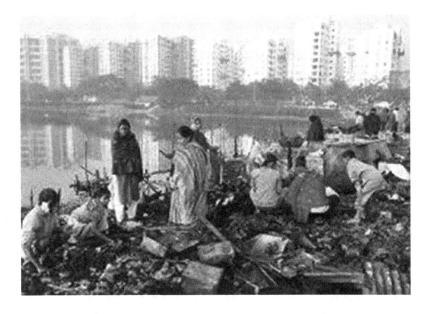

There is a small but measurable impact of sanitation and hygiene interventions on stunting but not on wasting. The objective of this study was to evaluate the effectiveness of a household water, sanitation and hygiene (WASH) package on the performance of an Outpatient Therapeutic feeding Program (OTP) for severe acute malnutrition (SAM). Researchers conducted a cluster, randomized controlled trial embedded in a routine OTP. The intervention members received an additional household WASH package consisting of chlorine, a water storage container, and soap. The study was conducted for about one year. The results indicated that by adding a household WASH package did not decrease the prevalence of post-recovery relapse, but it did increase the recovery rate among children admitted in OTP [34].

This study examined the sanitation-related psychosocial stressors during routine sanitation practices and its relationship with malnutrition in Odisha, India. During one year of the study, interviews were conducted with 56 women in four life stages: adolescent, newly married, pregnant, and established adult women in three settings: urban slums, rural villages, and indigenous villages. Researchers indicated that sanitation practices included more than urination and defecation. These practices also indicated some other sanitation-related issues such as carrying water, bathing, washing, changing clothes, and menstrual management. The study concluded that poor sanitation practices were related to the poor nutritional status of the women [35].

The study reviewed the implications of inadequate facilities for sanitation and water in regard to the health of children and the general development in urban areas. Researchers indicated that rates of child morbidity and mortality are very poor in urban areas and, in some cases, the prevalence of child mortality is even high in urban areas as compared with rural ones. This review summarizes the possible factors that contribute to increased child mortality and morbidity. One of the most important factors is the lack of sanitation facilities that directly cause sanitation-related illnesses, such as diarrhea and vomiting. This not only effects nutrition and the health status of the child, but also delays cognitive development in the early stages of life. Poor sanitation practices, thus, cause malnutrition and other complications [36].

1.9   FOOD FORTIFICATION PROGRAMS

Protein, vitamins, carbohydrates, and minerals are necessary for the human body for growth and development. In most developing countries, diets with insufficient levels of iodine, iron, vitamin A, and zinc are more dominant and considered the main reason for the marginal health of people. Deficiency of these nutrients lead to goiter, anemia, and metabolic syndrome. To overcome these problems, food fortification is considered a good approach for the improvement of nutrition of humans in most of these developing regions. Moreover, fortification also has the potential to reduce the micronutrient deficiencies in targeted populations. Fortified wheat consumed by people of developing countries of world also helps to mitigate the iron insufficiency. Fortification of flours in addition with other food items is a good approach to reduce the risk of hidden hunger prevalent in South Asian countries. In Khyber Pakhtunkhwa, a province of Pakistan, the flour fortification program has been magnificently executed. This could also be advantageous for other South Asian countries.

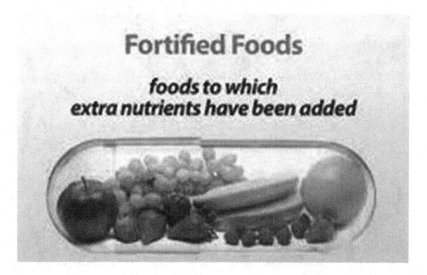

Malnutrition poses serious threat to human life, including micronutrient malnutrition, which affects more than half of the population of the world, mainly in developing nations of the world. National and international food fortification programs aim to prevent and treat micronutrient deficiencies. These programs show a positive impact on the nutritional status of the targeted individuals, but unfortunately the deficiencies cannot be eliminated. Biofortification is the delivery of micronutrients through micronutrient dense crops. It offers a sustainable and cost-effective approach, complementing these efforts by reaching rural populations. Bioavailable micronutrients in the edible parts of staple crops at concentrations high enough to impact on human health can be obtained through breeding, provided that sufficient genetic variation for a given trait exists, or through transgenic approaches. Research is being conducted to enrich the major food staples in developing countries with the most important micronutrients: iron, provitamin A, zinc, and folate [37].

There are certain measures taken in several countries to improve the nutritional status of the individuals in the targeted population. Although, these practices are slow in most of the needy, unindustrialized countries of the world where nutritional deficiencies effecting health is a major health concern. It occurs due to lack of nutrition policies or their ineffective implementation. Narrowly focused control programs including homestead production, plant breeding, fortification, and supplementation are in effect, but in general, they have not been holistically planned and integrated into overall development programs. Such incorporation is vital to certify sustainability into the next century. Thus, there is a need of a new program that includes an innovative way of thinking by nutrition experts and policy planners to cover all the aspects related to the planning and implementation of the policies [38].

Economic analysis has indicated that the next generation can greatly benefit from the fortification approach. The most important goal of fortification is to broaden the food horizon in addition to fulfilling food requirements. Conversely, micronutrient deficiencies cannot be cured through fortification alone, as women undergoing pregnancy have need of iron, which cannot be safely applied through fortification. So the neediest people still must have some additional options. Furthermore, fortification gives good results if iron is widely deficient because it is not expensive, its cost will be high for vitamin C and calcium. Fortification becomes more attractive and beneficial if the deficiency exist in a large domain, because it is sometimes difficult to access a targeted group of people in a remote geographical areas for folic acid and iodine. Moreover, it is also very difficult to access the needy people who cannot afford high priced food and must purchase low-grade food, which is less likely to be fortified, such as iodized salt [39].

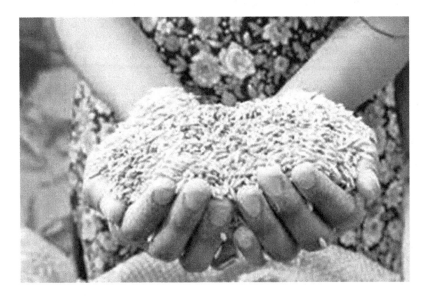

Pakistan joined the global scaling up nutrition (SUN) Movement in 2013 to overcome malnutrition issues in the country. The Vision 2025 initiated by the Government of Pakistan envisages a hunger-free Pakistan by adopting innovative and cost-effective strategies. Accordingly, the plan aims for the provision of safe food and adequate nutrition at all levels along with a communication strategy for awareness and behavior changes. Micronutrient Initiatives (MI) is the leading organization working exclusively to eliminate micronutrient deficiencies in the world's most vulnerable populations. This organization works in partnership with governments, civil society organizations, and the private sector to address hidden hunger.

The National Food Fortification Alliance has been re-established at the Ministry of National Health Services, Regulation and Coordination to restart a fortification program, which was abandoned due to devolution in Pakistan. The wheat flour fortification with iron and folic acid is being revitalized to overcome micronutrient deficiency disorders with the support of the Food Fortification Program (FFP). In Pakistan, the government, donors, the UN, and the Civil Society Alliance (CSA) are functioning. Both the SUN Academia & Research (SUNAR) as well as the Sun Business Network (SBN) is established. Considering the nutritional situation in South Asia, there is a dire need to launch new fortification programs as dietary interventions to combat malnutrition, especially in Pakistan. However, investments must be made to strictly monitor and evaluate the process of these programs to ensure they obtain the targeted results. The supplementation of foods with iron, folates, as well as multiple micronutrients is a pragmatic choice to combat early pregnancy and to ensure infant and young child nutrition. Additionally, training for imparting nutritional education along with research to quantify the obtained results will be a right step to reach adequate nutrition in peoples [40].

1.10   PROMOTION OF URBAN AGRICULTURE AND KITCHEN GARDENING

Food security is much more than the food production, distribution, and its consumption. From birth, food is the top most priority of human being as it gives energy to live and grow stronger. Food has a cultural value apart from dietary needs. Different cultures have different food preferences and food taboos. Culture is also defined by dietary choices and plays role in religion as in Islam only halal foods are allowed, in Judaism kosher foods are permitted, and in Hinduism beef is restricted. In addition to this, the different countries' or regions' dietary choices have different characteristics, and this is highly linked to a culture's cuisine.

Urban agriculture (UA) is the production of crops and the rearing livestock animals within urban areas, town, and cities. This modern concept of agriculture can play a crucial role to address urban food insecurity problems, and is bound to become increasingly important due to growing urbanization in the developing regions. The food security inferences of urban agriculture is mainly unavailability of authentic and reliable data; however, survey data exist for major cities that can be used to promote the urban agriculture in coming days. The promotion of this agriculture will facilitate the production of fresh fruits and vegetables ultimately increasing the availability of food in the food chain. This will not only enhance food availability, but will also enhance nutritional security [41].

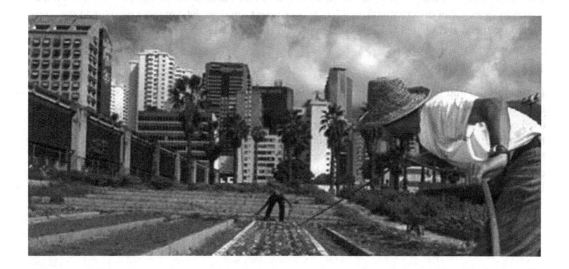

Food security contains the sufficiency, availability, access, and stability of the food. Adequacy is the overall supply that covers all nutritional desires, both quantitatively and qualitatively. Additionally, it should not contain toxins, should have good taste and texture, and should be culturally accepted. Stability is the supply of food at all the times, and access means that a community has the resources to get the desired food. These imply that there should be effective markets and distributions of income.

1.11 GLOBALIZATION, URBANIZATION, AND NUTRITIONAL CHANGE IN THE DEVELOPING WORLD

Globalization and urbanization may improve access as a result of improvements in production practices and prices, as well as marketing and trade practices of non-traditional foods. Throughout the developing world, the dietary patterns have been changing due to these forces. A longitudinal study from China indicated that with the changes in food availability, the consumption patterns have changed. With large changes in rural areas due to high levels of urban infrastructure and resources, potentially obesogenic dietary patterns are emerging. Recent data on women from 36 developing countries illustrate that the shifts in the dietary patterns may have implications for obesity or overweight in rural and urban settings. The data emphasize the importance of policies adapted by the developing countries that includes preventive measures to minimize further adverse shifts in diet and activity, and risks associated with it.

The modern world is undergoing rapid modifications in dietary patterns and structures along with impacts on body composition, consequently having effects on health profiles. This chapter gives an overview of the shifts in dietary patterns and its impacts on health in low- and moderate-income countries. Broad shifts have and continue to occur around the world in population size and age composition, disease patterns, and dietary and physical activity patterns. The former two sets of dynamic shifts are termed the demographic and epidemiological transitions. The latter, whose changes are under the category of nutritional outcomes, including variations in average height and body composition, is termed as nutrition transitions. The developing world is more prone toward seeing the most rapid and abrupt changes in dietary and physical activity patterns and rates of obesity. These changes give us an overview as to which steps are important to address the problems related to poor health and nutrition status [42].

1.12 MULTI-SECTORIAL NUTRITIONAL STRATEGY OF PUNJAB

The strategies are developed in order to improve nutritional status and food insecurity in the Punjab region by combining different stakeholders (government, civil society organizations, and developmental partners) and sectors (health, education, population, and social protection) (Table 1.1).

1.13 CONCLUSION

Ensuring food and nutritional security is to improve the well beings of human and the development of the country as the development and growth of a country is depicted by the living standard of the people. However, in the developing regions like South Asia the interaction between food security and nutritional interventions is useful approach to alleviate the cause of hidden hunger. The intake of sufficient food along with the required nutrients in the diet can prevent development of many complications, which may range from temporary (low work capacity, learning disabilities) problems to permanent issues, such as permanent cognition abnormalities and fertility issue.

TABLE 1.1
Sectorial Strategies

Sectors	Strategy
Health Sector	• Mainstreaming nutrition in health • Equitable access to nutrition services for poor and marginalized people • Strengthening capacity of provincial and local governments to provide basic nutrition services in an inclusive and equitable manner
Housing, Urban Development, and Public Health Engineering Sector	• Equitable access to safe and clean water • Promote best practices and behavioral change regarding hygiene practices • Equitable access to total sanitation services • Development and implementation of policies and strategies
Population Sector	• Improving access to family planning services with Public Private Partnership (PPP) • Reducing unmet needs by ensuring availability of quality FP products and developing a social marketing and branding mechanism • Integrating Nutrition in Population Welfare department by promoting birth spacing, counselling of Pregnant Lactating Women (PLW), adolescent girls and family members especially husbands • Formulation of a multi-sectoral Population policy for an integrated approach with other sectors • Holistic communication strategy for behavior change based on research into consumer behavior to develop targeted strategies • Counselling and improving access to family planning information and raising awareness about benefits of birth spacing on family and society
Food Sector	• Physical access to food throughout the year for all target groups • Ensure and improve food quality from farm to fork • Provision of safe food • Ensure economic access to food • Reduce micronutrient deficiency in adolescent girls, pregnant and lactating women, and children through fortification
Social Protection Sector	• Strengthen social protection sector to scale up nutrition sensitive interventions • Improving economic access to address nutritional needs through poverty alleviation and social protection • Promote nutrition awareness for healthy and safe dietary practices
Agriculture Sector: Crops	• Mainstreaming nutrition in agriculture • Increase productivity of nutritious food by developing and promoting high yield varieties of grains and pulses • Equitable access to vegetables and fruits • Addressing malnutrition through bio-fortification • Scaling up kitchen gardening
Agriculture Sector: Livestock	• Increasing accessibility of animal protein sources at household level • Increase productivity through sustainable livestock farming and capacity development to combat protein energy malnutrition • Reduce nutrient deficiency in targeted groups by increasing physical access to livestock-based products
Education Sector	• Equitable access to education • Improve quality of education and integrate nutrition in school curriculum • Provide and promote quality hygiene and sanitation practices within school premises • Capacity development to introduce and promote nutrition as a profession • Improvement of nutritional status among school going children

REFERENCES

1. FAO (2016) World food security: A reappraisal of the concepts and approaches. Director General's Report.
2. World Food Programme (2009) *Emergency Food Security Assessment Handbook (EFSA)*, 2nd ed. Rome, Italy.
3. WHO/FAO (2003) *Diet, Nutrition and the Prevention of Chronic Diseases.* Geneva, Switzerland.
4. WHO (2006) *Working Together For Health.* Geneva, Switzerland.
5. Vozoris NT, Tarasuk VS (2003) Household food insufficiency is associated with poorer health. *J Nutri* **133**(1): 120–126.
6. Koren O, Bagozzi BE (2016) From global to local, food insecurity is associated with contemporary armed conflicts. *Food Sec* **8**(5): 999–1010.
7. Rasul G, Hussain A, Khan MA, Ahmad F, Jasra AW (2014) Towards a framework for achieving food security in the mountains of Pakistan. ICIMOD working paper (2014/5).
8. Seligman HK, Laraia BA, Kushel MB (2009) Food insecurity is associated with chronic disease among low-income NHANES participants. *J Nutri* **140**(2): 304–310.
9. Pinstrup-Andersen P (2009) Food security: Definition and measurement. *Food Sec* **1**(1): 5–7.
10. Hendrix CS, Haggard S (2015) Global food prices, regime type, and urban unrest in the developing world. *J Peace Res* **52**(2): 143–157.
11. Barrett CB (2010) Measuring food insecurity. *Science* **327**(5967): 825–828.
12. Lentz EC, Barrett CB (2013) The economics and nutritional impacts of food assistance policies and programs. *Food Policy* **42**: 151–163.
13. Fischler F, Wilkinson D, Benton T, Daniel H, Darcy-Vrillon B, Hedlund K, Heffernan P et al. (2015) The role of research in global food and nutrition security-Discussion paper. EU-Scientific Steering Committee.
14. Layman DK, Clifton P, Gannon MC, Krauss RM, Nuttall FQ (2008) Protein in optimal health: Heart disease and type 2 diabetes. *Am J Clin Nutri* **87**(5): 1571–1575.
15. Mensink, RP (2016) Effects of saturated fatty acids on serum lipids and lipoproteins: A systematic review and regression analysis. World Health Organization, Geneva, Switzerland.
16. Achadi E, Ahuja A, Bendech MA, Bhutta ZA, De-Regil LM, Fanzo J, Fracassi P et al. (2016) Global nutrition report 2016: From promise to impact: Ending malnutrition by 2030. International Food Policy Research Institute, Washington, DC.
17. Rafique G, Azam SI, White F (2006) Diabetes knowledge, beliefs and practices among people with diabetes attending a university hospital in Karachi, Pakistan. *East Med Health J* **12**(5): 590–598.
18. Mensah GA, Brown DW (2007) An overview of cardiovascular disease burden in the United States. *Health Affairs* **26**(1): 38–48.
19. Dewey KG (2016) Reducing stunting by improving maternal, infant and young child nutrition in regions such as South Asia: Evidence, challenges and opportunities. *Matern Child Nutri* **12**(1): 27–38.
20. Buttriss J, Riley H (2013) Sustainable diets: Harnessing the nutrition agenda. *Food Chem* **140**(3): 402–407.
21. Akhtar S, Ahmed A, Randhawa MA, Atukorala S, Arlappa N, Ismail T, Ali Z (2013) Prevalence of vitamin A deficiency in South Asia: Causes, outcomes, and possible remedies. *J Health Pop Nutri* **31**(4): 413.
22. Akhtar S (2016) Malnutrition in South Asia—A critical reappraisal. *Crit Rev Food Sci Nutri* **56**(14): 2320–2330.
23. National Nutrition Survey. 2011. Planning Commission Planning and Development Division Government of Pakistan.
24. Ejaz MS, Latif N (2010) Stunting and micronutrient deficiencies in malnourished children. *J Pak Med Assoc* **60**(7): 543–547.
25. Aurangzeb B, Whitten KE, Harrison B, Mitchell M, Kepreotes H, Sidler M, Lemberg DA, Day AS (2012) Prevalence of malnutrition and risk of under-nutrition in hospitalized children. *Clin Nutri* **31**(1): 35–40.
26. ACF International Network (2007) Implementing cash-based interventions: A guideline for aid workers, ACF food security guideline. http://www.actionagainsthunger.org.uk/resource-centre/online-library/detail/media/implementing-cash-based-interventions-a-guideline-for-aid-workers.
27. Fenn B, Sangrasi GM, Puett C, Trenouth L, Pietzsch S (2015) The REFANI Pakistan study—A cluster randomised controlled trial of the effectiveness and cost-effectiveness of cash-based transfer programmes on child nutrition status: Study protocol. *BMC Public Health* **15**(1): 1044.
28. Wheeler T, Braun JV (2013) Climate change impacts on global food security. *Science* **341**(6145): 508–513.

29. Malik SM, Awan H, Khan N (2012) Mapping vulnerability to climate change and its repercussions on human health in Pakistan. *Glob Health* **8**(1): 31–36.

30. Sethuraman K, Lansdown R, Sullivan K (2006) Women's empowerment and domestic violence: The role of sociocultural determinants in maternal and child undernutrition in tribal and rural communities in South India. *Food Nutr Bull* **27**(2): 128–143.

31. Clasen T, Boisson S, Routray P, Torondel B, Bell M, Cumming O, Ensink J, Freeman M, Jenkins M, Odagiri M, Ray S (2014) Effectiveness of a rural sanitation programme on diarrhea, soil-transmitted helminth infection, and child malnutrition in Odisha, India: A cluster-randomised trial. *Lancet Glob Health* **2**(11): e645–e653.

32. Behrman JR, Wolfe BL (1987) How does mother's schooling affect family health, nutrition, medical care usage, and household sanitation? *J Economet* **36**(1): 185–204.

33. Cicero AF, Dormi A, D'Addato S, Gaddi AV, Borghi C (2010) Long-term effect of a dietary education program on postmenopausal cardiovascular risk and metabolic syndrome: The Brisighella Heart Study. *J Women's Health* **19**(1): 133–137.

34. Altmann M, Altare C, van der Spek N, Barbiche JC, Dodos J, Bechir M, Aissa MA, Kolsteren P (2018) Effectiveness of a household water, sanitation and hygiene package on an outpatient program for severe acute malnutrition: A pragmatic cluster-randomized controlled trial in Chad. *Am J Trop Med Hyg* **98**(4): 1005–1012.

35. Sahoo KC, Hulland KR, Caruso BA, Swain R, Freeman MC, Panigrahi P, Dreibelbis R (2015) Sanitation-related psychosocial stress: A grounded theory study of women across the life-course in Odisha, India. *Soc Sci Med* **139**: 80–89.

36. Bartlett S (2013) Water, sanitation and urban children: The need to go beyond "improved" provision. *Environ Urban* **15**(2): 57–70.

37. Mayer JE, Pfeiffer WH, Beyer P (2008) Biofortified crops to alleviate micronutrient malnutrition. *Cur Opin Plant Biol* **11**(2): 166–170.

38. Underwood BA, Smitasiri S (1999) Micronutrient malnutrition: Policies and programs for control and their implications. *Annu Rev Nutri* **19**: 303–324.

39. Horton S (2006) The economics of food fortification. *J Nutri* **136**(4): 1068–1071.

40. Mason JB, Saldanha LS, Ramakrishnan U, Lowe A, Noznesky EA, Girard AW, McFarland DA, Martorell R (2012) Opportunities for improving maternal nutrition and birth outcomes: Synthesis of country experiences. *Food Nutri Bull* **33**(2): S104–S137.

41. Zezza A, Tasciotti L (2010) Urban agriculture, poverty, and food security: Empirical evidence from a sample of developing countries. *Food Policy* **35**(4): 265–273.

42. Popkin B, Ng SW (2007) The nutrition transition in high- and low-income countries: What are the policy lessons? *Agri Econ* **37**(1): 199–211.

2 Contribution of Animal Origin Foods in the Human Diet

Amna Sahar and Ubaid ur Rahman

CONTENTS

2.1   INTRODUCTION

Animal source foods (ASF) are foods that are obtained from animal sources and mainly include eggs, cheese, meat, yogurt, and milk [1]. ASFs present a variety of nutrients that are very difficult to obtain in significant amounts from those that are obtained from plant sources alone [2]. If we take the example of animal source nutrient including energy and animal source protein intake, both match exactly to the retinol (Vitamin A), riboflavin (Vitamin B2), and cyanocobalamin (Vitamin B12). Proteins obtained from ASF are rich in energy that can be digested easily by human body and they are of good quality [1]. As these proteins contain almost all essential amino acids, and some non-essential amino acids, they are considered high-quality food proteins [3]. Effective and low in calories, certain micronutrients can also obtain from ASF. Plentiful and bioactive micronutrients that can be obtained from ASFs are B12, calcium (in milk), and iron and retinol (in meat and offal) [1].

Products that are obtained from animal source especially dairy products are enrich with dietary B12 and retinal (Vitamin A). The amount of zinc obtained from meat is 10 times greater than the amount of zinc obtained from beans and maize. A child needs 1.7–2.0 kg of maize or beans to fulfill the daily energy requirement, which is obviously not possible for a child to eat daily, while the same energy requirement can be fulfilled by using 60 gm meat only. Similarly, milk products are a good source of calcium. Drinking milk for calcium intake is a good option as calcium through cereals need to intake 345 mg/day, which is not an efficient approach. Nutritional value obtained from meat, poultry, and fish are in the form of long-chain fatty acids, (pentanoic and hexanoic acids), selenium, and taurine that are quite important for the human body.

That's the major health benefit of ASF that are particularly present in meat. For example, heme protein is found only in meat, and it is absorbed and utilized by body in significant amounts.

Even a great number of micronutrients can be obtained from plants like calcium, zinc and iron are also found in high amount on spinach and legumes, but adsorption rate is comparatively less. Moreover, some plant-based foods viz. uncooked and unfermented seeds, nuts and cereal grains possess considerable quantities of phytates which bound the nutrients such as zinc, iron and calcium and reduce their absorption in body after consumption [3]. Polycyclic amines, like tannins, present in high levels in coffee, rhubarb, red wine, spinach, and tea leaves [1]. These compounds also prevent adsorption of calcium (Ca), iron (Fe), and zinc (Zn) [4]. Iron and zinc adsorption is also hindered by tea and coffee. On the other hand, heme protein, present in meat, bounds Fe and Zn which enhances the absorption of these minerals in body after consumption of animal-based foods [1].

In meat and milk, dosage and bioavailability of the minerals are not equal. Meat contains iron, zinc, protein, and the B group vitamins, especially vitamin B12, while milk contains calcium, vitamin A (retinol), and vitamin B12 [3]. Milk and meat eaten at a time decrease the minerals bio-availability as calcium and casein (iron and zinc) are present in insoluble form.

However, more nutritional value is provided by animal resources, but, in poor countries, people cannot afford the food from animal sources [2]. Less accessibility and purchasing ability of the foods of animal sources can also reduce their use in daily consumption [2]. When people cannot afford food products from animal sources, they prefer to use foods with cheap prices like legumes, cereals, and starchy roots. By not choosing these costly foods and eating foods of low nutritional value, this significantly affects the nutritional status of everyone [1].

Religion and social customs can also stop some people using the foods from animal sources. In poor countries, it is the perception that although foods from animal origins have significant nutritional value, they are costly [2]. Animals are kept by people on a small scale only for the purposes of security and money.

Consumption of meat-based products provides more energy and protein as compared to milk and plant-based food products. In Europe and North America, although milk consumption is not great, the use of meat is 30%–40% greater than the other countries of the Indian subcontinent [1]. The Food and Agriculture Organization (FAO) in the US reported that 115.5 kg meat and 247 kg of milk is consumed by a person per year, while in Europe the amount varies at 71.6–83.1 kg of meat and 228.7–232.7 kg of milk. Foods from animal origins can provide energy up to 1.9 MJ/day and 28 g/day of protein to a person. That could refer to the 34% of an adult's protein use and 16% of the caloric value. Food from animal resources can provide 7% of energy and 15% of protein in India, while for the US values are 28% and 64%, respectively.

Foods from animal resources mainly provide protein, which is one of the essential nutrients. Foods from animal resources provide 28–50 g/day of protein in Europe, while for Africa the value decreases to 10 g/day [4]. Ranges vary from country to country, for example Mozambique and Burundi the amount is 3.4 g/day and for France the value is 75.1 g/day.

Human population is a more important factor that decides the consumption of animal protein [2]. Religious faiths and social factors are affected by the addition of other sources of proteins [3]. Mostly human populations in areas, like deserts and the Arctic, where crops production is not suitable, also depend on animal source protein. In arctic regions, people mostly fulfil their protein and energy requirements from animal sources particularly sea food [2]. Likewise, people of deserts region mostly consume camel's meat.

In developed countries, consumption of animal's products is varied due to religious issues and health concerns. Vegetarian people do not eat consume and fulfil their energy requirements only from plant sources. Similarly, some people consume a very little quantity of meat and have a limited choice e.g., they only consume chicken meat and avoid consuming beef or pork [1].

Protein contents of meat usually range from 15–23% depending upon the source and type of meat which describes its high nutritive value. Meat also contains fat contents ranged from 0.8 to 47% fat contents in different types of animals. A fat layer is formed around an organ and stored in adipose tissue when the animal is fully fed. Sometimes fat that is present in the form of muscle fibers bundles and that is known as marbling. Cholesterol contents in meat are also ranged from 63 mg to 389 mg per 100 g of meat [1]. Mostly phospholipids are present in the cell membrane and ranged from 0.5 to 1% present in lean meat. Small amount of carbohydrates is also present in meat. Two most common types of carbohydrates present in meat are glycogen and glucose. The best source of iron and phosphorus is meat, and it is also an important source of vitamin B complex. Cathepsins enzymes are also found in meat during ageing. Hydrolyzing of meat protein also occurs due to these enzymes. The softness of animal meat occurs due to these [3]. The red color of meat is due to the presence of myoglobin.

Due to the high amount of fat contents, meat has a −ve health impact. Cancer is also promoted by red meat according to some research [4]. For prevention of obesity, cancer and metabolic syndrome it is very necessary to intake low quantity of red meat [1]. No doubt, meat provide most of the minerals and various types of vitamins that are not present in plant-based foods and their bioavailability is not good [2]. Foods having low glycemic index, low carbohydrates, and protein rich meat products are important in obesity case. Consumption of meat is also reported to cause other complications such as diabetes and cancer [5]. Various important or essential nutrients are present in meat that is essential for human development. Meat is a main part of the diet and provides many amino acids and micronutrients (minerals and vitamins). Micronutrients help to control energy metabolism.

Due to their functionality, eggs have gained a great interest because they are a good source of calories, almost 1.5 kcal/g. Eggs are also a good source of proteins and are not costly. Eggs are a rich source of fat soluble substances [3]. They are an essential part of the diets of all ages of people in every step of life. The role of eggs is multipurpose in every stage of people's diet. They are also an essential part of diet of children. Furthermore, there are many useful functions of eggs in the world because they have no issues of religious basis or no limitation [5].

One large egg contains 6.5 g protein, which is found in the yolk and white albumin. Egg whites are an ideal source of protein because all the essential amino acids are present in it [4]. Every year many food-borne illness occur from consuming eggs because they are source of *Salmonella*. Due to their easily handling, low cost, and easily storage, eggs have gained more interests for manufacturers.

In the total fat of eggs, half of the fat present is in unsaturated form. They are an essential source of many vitamins like cyanocobalamin, vitamin D, folate riboflavin, and mineral iron. The bioavailability of eggs is high and a good iron source, like meat. They are good source of food for those people who are iron deficient [1]. Egg yolk is a good source of minerals and fat-soluble vitamins. Vitamin C is the only vitamin that is not found in eggs.

In 2012, almost 21.2 billion chickens are present in Asia, Africa, Europe, America, and Oceania in the range of 12, 1.79, 2.01, 5.28, and 0.13 respectively [3]. Globally, greater than 90% production of eggs occurs in these countries. Moreover, 66.4 million tons productions of shelled eggs has been reported in these five countries in 2012 in which mostly eggs are produced in the range of 57.8%. Globally, yearly egg production was increased to 2.3% from 2000-2010. According to United Nations and Food and Agriculture Organization, the eggs production has raised 70.4 million tons in 2015 while they will be raised to 89 million tones in 2030. China is ranked first in egg production [4]. It produced 23.9 million tons of eggs in 2011 and almost 28.3 million metric tons of eggs produced in 2012 [5]. Recently, China has produced 45% of the total world eggs production.

Milk is a vital source for dietary fat, energy, and protein. In 2009, milk contributed to almost 134 kcal, per capita in 24 hours. Milk provides 8 g of protein and 7.3 g fat per capita in a day (FAOSTAT, 2012) [2]. Milk provides just 3% of the dietary energy in Asia and Africa, while 8%–9% in Europe and Oceania. In Asia and Africa, protein is provided almost 6%–7% as compared to Europe is 19%. Dietary fat is supplied 6%–8% in Asia and Africa while 11%–14% in Europe, America, and Oceania [1].

Milk is provided macronutrients and micronutrients so globally it is consumed in the form of beverages [3]. Due to its proper composition milk is mostly consumed by children and adults [4]. Mostly cardiovascular diseases occur due to saturated fats present in milk. A major component of milk is water, which is almost 68% in reindeer milk while in donkey milk is 91%. A main carbohydrate of milk is lactose [5]. The adsorption of minerals (magnesium, calcium, and phosphorus) and vitamin D in the intestine occurs due to the lactose. Milk is very important for every stage of life because micronutrients are required for the development of muscle, the skeleton, and neurological system.

2.2   NUTRITIONAL BENEFITS OF ANIMAL ORIGIN FOOD

2.2.1   MACRONUTRIENTS IN MEAT

The composition of meat is water, protein, fat, and soluble non-protein substances in the range of 75%, 20%, 3%, and 2%, respectively. In smaller quantities, carbohydrates and micronutrients, like vitamins and minerals, are also present in meat, and they are very essential for metabolism.

2.2.1.1   Water

Water is an important part of body and is essential to carry out metabolic activities. Water contents of meat are ranged from 4% (beef fat) to 76% (lean veal meat). The texture, color, and flavor of meat are affected by its moisture content. In muscle fiber, mostly water present in free form while in connective tissue less water is present [3]. Due to the structure of fiber, water retained in small quantities during curing, storage, and heat treatment. When disruption of muscle cell occurs, then the water holding capacity will be decreased [4]. Acidity will be changed due to the application of chemicals and organic acids.

2.2.1.2   Protein

Protein is an essential component of the dry matter of lean meat [5]. There are nine amino acids present in meat that are essential and semi-essential [4]. These amino acids are not produced by the human body [2]. So, these are gained by food sources. During digestion, when protein is degraded into amino acids and absorbed, it can be utilized for the biosynthesis of endogenous proteins [1]. Proteins have many functions in the human body. It can be utilized for the repairing of damaged tissue, growth, antibodies, and the regulating of enzymes and hormones.

2.2.1.3   Fat

The main dietary source of energy is fat [3]. It is also carried out through essential fatty acids. It can also help fat soluble vitamins [4]. In fatty tissues, animals fat mostly occurs and found in adipose tissues. Fat deposits in various forms like intramuscular, intramuscular and subcutaneous fatty tissues form. Mostly unsaturated fatty acids almost ≤50%–70% occur in meat lipids. In this quantity, beef consists of 50%–52%, chicken contains 70%, and lamb has 50%–52% fat. Genetics and diet are factors that affect the composition of fat [5]. When the content of saturated and mono-unsaturated fatty acidy increases, then poly unsaturated fatty acids decrease.

Phospholipids are also present in muscle lipids. In cell membranes, polar lipids are also found. Most saturated and unsaturated fatty acids are also provided by diet. Omega-3 fatty acids consist of eicosapentanoic aid and docosahexanoic acids [3]. These have a good impact on human health (Figure 2.1).

2.2.2   MAJOR MICRONUTRIENTS IN MEAT

Chief macronutrients that are present in meat are proteins and fats, and they possess major compositional analysis [4]. Furthermore, micronutrients, such as minerals and vitamins, implicated in the vital metabolic processes are also a main part of meat composition.

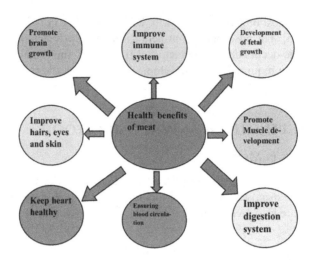

FIGURE 2.1   Health benefits of meat.

2.2.2.1   Iron

Iron deficiency is a common endemic deficiency in both developed and developing countries. Due to iron deficiency, about 20%–50% of the world's population suffers losses. Heme iron or non-heme iron is classified as a food grade iron [3]. Hemoglobin and myoglobin are heme-iron derivatives. The main food source is meat, and non-heme iron is mainly derived from grains, fruits, and vegetables. Meat contains iron, heme in 50%–60% and non-heme. The bioavailability of non-heme iron is influenced by meat. Vitamin C and meat are the only two nutritional factors that increase the bioavailability of non-heme iron [5]. Non-blood iron intake from meat is usually 15%–25% and 1%–7% from plant sources. Iron intake of meat and meat products is 14%, while carcasses and meat products account for 12.5% of total iron intake. Meat-enhanced non-heme iron bioavailability is often referred to as "meat factor." The human iron pool (serum ferritin) has a strong correlation with heme iron [1].

2.2.2.2   Zinc

Zinc obtained from diet can be also obtained through all meats, but specifically beef is an excellent sources. Meat and products made from meat account for a third of the total zinc intake in the world. Oxalates and phytates are zinc inhibitors, which are packed in plant foods. Meat helps absorption of zinc by 20%–40%. Zinc is required for the cognitive development as well as growth, reproductive, healing of wounds, and development of a well-built immune system [4]. Zinc deficiency is becoming more common, particularly amongst young people. Iron and zinc absence often occur concurrently [3]. A meat developed diet of adolescents can assist in explaining both iron and zinc deficiencies. Absorbance of minerals present in meat is very easy.

2.2.2.3   Selenium

Meat contains about 10 mg of selenium per 100 g, which equates to 25% of our daily needs [2]. Herbal foods are considered to be richer in bioavailability of selenium than animal feed. Recent data show that meat (raw and cooked) provides a significantly higher bio-available source of selenium. Selenium, as an antioxidant, is said to prevent certain types of cancer (prostate) and coronary heart disease [3]. Because of their age, beef and pork contain more selenium than lambs, as selenium can accumulate in the meat over time.

2.2.2.4 Other Minerals

Meat is supplemented in providing purposeful amounts of copper, minute amount of iron, iodine, chloride, and the magnesium [4]. Meat contains phosphorus, approximately of 20%–25% of an adult requirement of phosphorus [1]. Phosphorus is significant for biochemical functions in major nutrients, especially in carbohydrates metabolism [5].

2.2.2.5 Vitamins

Meat is an excellent source of vitamin B_{12} which provides over two thirds of the daily requirement of healthy individual. Vitamin D % in meat is reasonably low, and it is difficult to measure. The B-vitamins that are present in meat are thiamin, riboflavin, biotin, B5, niacin, vitamin B_6, and vitamin B_{12}. Riboflavin and thiamine are found in enough amounts in meat. Lean meat (without fat) contains more water-soluble vitamins (vitamin B and C) than non-lean meat. Pork has 5–10 times more thiamine percentage than beef or lamb. Meat is enhanced with niacin. Vitamin B_6 is essential cofactor for 100 cellular enzyme or more reactions, above all related to amino acid metabolism and the inter-conversion. Liver and kidney are the main source of pantothenic acid [1]. It also assists in normal functioning of the nervous system [3]. Riboflavin also gives support in supplying energy and supporting healthy skin, eyes, and vision. Liver is an excellent source of vitamin A, but in fat containing meat tissue levels are near to the ground. Older animals possess higher concentrations of all vitamins, as a result the levels in beef are typically higher than those in veal, and mutton has more compared to lamb [5].

2.2.3 MACRONUTRIENTS IN MILK

Milk is made by a female's secretary cells; it is a white color food. It is formed by a lactation procedure [2]. It is a main important property of animals [2]. The milk is collected in an animal's udder and formed by the memory glands [4]. After birth of a baby, the first day of milk is known as colostrum. The main compositions of milk include water, protein, fat, and lactose. Other vitamins and minerals also present in milk.

2.2.3.1 Water

Water is a main component of milk because it is present in large amounts as compared to other components [1]. Almost 88.6% water present in milk [3]. This amount is regulated by the quantity of lactose of the glands. In milk water contribute principal share. This amount of water is carried out solvent properties and it is best for exogenous and endogenous milk part.

2.2.3.2 Carbohydrate

The main carbohydrate of milk is lactose. It consists of a D-glucose molecule and a D-galactose molecule. The absorption of calcium, magnesium and phosphorus and utilization of vitamin D is occurred by the help of lactose. The lactose sweetness level is almost 0.3 times as compared to the solution of sucrose of same concentration [4]. Milk sweetness level is masked by casein protein. For milk fermentation Lactobacillus is utilized. The fermented dairy products are cheese and yogurt. Lactobacillus plays a vital role in milk fermentation. Lactic acid bacteria make lactic acid that is used in milk fermentation [3]. It is produced in the lactose cellulose Golgi vesicles. This is occurred due to alpha-lactalbumin, which is the major important milk protein. Lactose can be removed from milk or crystallized by lactose in industrial practice. Crystalline lactose production is great, especially for pharmaceuticals and foods; almost all pills contain lactose as filler.

2.2.3.3 Protein

In most quantity milk proteins are present. They consist of all essential amino acids. These amino acids are not produced in our body. Amino acids are building blocks of proteins. Milk proteins are similar to egg proteins [4]. Cysteine and methionine are present in less quantity. Sulfur containing amino acids are also present. There are two types of milk protein like casein and whey [1]. Casein consists of 80% of total quantity of milk protein [2]. The complex structure of milk protein is casein that comprises of major component of amino acids that are important for nutrition [5]. Milk proteins consist of 95% of crude protein and other remaining protein 5% of non-protein nitrogen and small peptides.

There are four types of casein protein i.e., $\alpha s1$, $\alpha s2$, β, and the k caseins. Kepa casein is most important type of casein as compared to other types of it. It is important for dairy processing and it is utilized in micelles' constancy [2]. Casein micelles are produced by calcium phosphate. In whey protein, soluble proteins are also present. Mostly branched chain amino acids like leucine, valine, and isoleucine are present in whey protein as compared to casein. Casein comprises many amino acids like valine, histidine, methionine, and phenylalanine [4]. It also consists of non-essential amino acids containing arginine, tyrosine, proline, and glutamic acid.

The essential amino acids are carried out by milk proteins and 100% digestibility of milk proteins. When heat is applied to milk, then digestibility of milk is slightly lower. Casein has a capability to bind phosphate and calcium [3]. These two nutrients are important for growth. Insulin is used to stop the release of hormone sensitive enzyme lipase

T and B cell mitogens are controlled by K-casein. Spreading of lymphocytes occurs due to whey protein. Dairy protein has an impact on human metabolism. It helps to control appetite and body weight [5].

2.2.3.4 Fat

The main source of energy is milk fat. More polyunsaturated fatty acids are present in goat and milk that are essential for metabolism. In milk, fat is present in emulsion form. In milk, fat is present in small cells that are dispersed in water. These fat contents vary in breed and food. Unsaturated fatty acids of milk contain one double bond, which plays a role to form a structure to lipid formation [1]. Goats' milk has more fat content as compared to other species of animals. Goats' milk has 95% triglycerides of whole lipid. Phospholipids of 30–40 mg/100 mL present in milk that contains 8–10 mg lipids. Cholesterol presents in free form in 10–20 mg/100 mL.

Milk fat provides 9 kcal/g [3]. It has a role in body building. Fats cause many health risks. These risks occur due to more consumption of fat [4]. It mostly causes cardiovascular diseases. Essential vitamins, like vitamin A and vitamin D, is also provided by milk fat [2]. For epithelial cells, vitamin A is necessary. It also plays a vital role in vision and reproduction. Vitamin D is very important for bone growth [2]. Due to the high energy level milk fat, it has an important part in human diet. Consumption of high doses of milk fat is harmful due to the saturated fatty acids and cholesterol.

Phosphorus and nitrogen are also components of some lipids. Phospholipids are also present in butterball membranes. Milk fat is a main source of phospholipids.

2.2.3.5 Minerals

Structural organization is made by minerals. When contents of minerals increased from 0.1 g also contains less amount of calcium and some salts potassium, sodium, and magnesium can also be differentiated [2]. The important salt is calcium phosphate. It has many advantages and it is very important for development of bones. Solubility of this salt is very poor. Milk has high amount of calcium phosphate that is required for the formation of casein micelles [3]. For humans, the important source of calcium is milk and dairy products [4]. Milk is also essential source of other minerals like zinc. Iron is present in less quantity in milk.

2.2.3.6 Vitamins

The levels of vitamins A, D, and E vary according to the season, such as the significant increase in vitamin concentrations during the grazing season [4]. During the extraction process, these vitamins are lost as these vitamins are lipo-soluble and other vitamins are present in the serum and are water-soluble. In fresh milk, the vitamin C content is very low and can be lost during pasteurization and when contact with air [6].

2.2.3.7 Enzymes

The enzyme consists of a protein with a specific globular structure and living cells. These enzymes play an important role in the processing and storage stability of milk. Among these enzymes, lipases and proteases affect protein stability, and the taste of milk and oxidoreductase affects lipids and alters taste [3]. Each enzyme has its isoelectric point and can be denatured by various reagents with denaturing effects such as temperature, pH change, organic solvent and ionic strength.

The main protease in milk is protease. Plasmin is the main protease in milk, which is the same as blood protein of the same name. The plasma concentration of plasmin varies depending on the amount of blood components that enter the milk [3]. The enzyme is very stable at pH of the milk and retains its enzymatic activity even after pasteurization.

2.2.4 MACRONUTRIENTS IN EGG

Protein is the chief and most important constituent of egg tailed by fat [4]. The other significant components of egg are micronutrients e.g. iron, choline, iodine, folate, biotin, riboflavin, selenium, phosphorus, vitamins that are soluble in fat like E, D, A, and B12 that are essential for the basic sustenance, physical and mental wellbeing [1].

2.2.4.1 Calories

Due to high nutrient value and low caloric content eggs are termed as nutrient dense food. The food which gives high amount of essential nutrients and low calories to fulfill daily requirements of a person is called nutrient dense food [2]. Nutrient dense foods are very essential for human health and should be the part of person's daily diet to provide essential nutrients to body [2]. An egg of average medium size delivers 76–78 kcal to the body that is around 4% of grown up female daily requirement and 3% of grownup man.

2.2.4.2 Fat

Egg comprises approximately 4.7–5.8 g fat, out of which 196 mg is cholesterol; saturated fat is 1.6 g, and 2.3 g monounsaturated [4]. Cholesterol and lecithin (fat like stuffs) are very important for proper functioning and for the structure of cells within the body [2]. The cholesterol is essential for flexibility, penetrability, and maintenance of the cell membranes and bile fabrication, cortisol, sex hormones, and vitamin D [1]. Cholesterol keeps skin flexible and elastic as it is the raw component for the fatty lubricates. Eggs are enriched in cholesterol, nonetheless they deliver squat energy to the body [3]. The role of lecithin is the transference of cholesterol absorption in the blood. Nutrients bioavailability, for example lutein and zeaxanthin, is enhanced by the lipid milieu of egg yolk [6].

2.2.4.3 Protein

Eggs are vital and fulfill the 12% of daily dietary requirements by providing 6.5 g of protein. Eggs are an incredible and important source of high quality protein having high biological value. Protein is approximately 12.5% of the egg weight and is present in both the egg yolk and egg white (albumen); but is more concerted in albumen [4]. Egg protein is an excellent cradle of the necessary amino acids that are requisite to form the muscles and endure the development in children, adolescents, and adults [1]. High quality protein helps prevent the collapse of skeletal muscles and prevent health menaces linked to ageing in older people [4]. Eggs are vital source of good quality protein for the consumers who do not drink milk.

2.3 MICRONUTRIENTS

2.3.1 Vitamin A

Vitamin A is a fat-soluble vitamin and is present in are milk, butter, egg yolk, liver fatty fish, and fortified margarine. In egg yolk, the amount of vitamin A is 95 µg, which is nearly 14% of the daily requirement of the body. This vitamin is necessary for the skin maintenance of membrane, normal growth, and for visualization in faint light. Lack of vitamin A can cause loss of vision, night impaired vision, and subordinate the confrontation to infections [3]. In liver, high amounts of vitamin A are stored and not excreted with urine, which leads to high toxicity in body.

2.3.2 Vitamin D

Vitamin D is found in egg yolk, sunshine, oily fish, breakfast cereals, and fortified margarine. Egg yolk contains 0.9 µg of this vitamin [4]. It aids the absorption of potassium and calcium from food, which is good for the strong teeth and bones development. Vitamin D likewise offers advantages to avert CVD, autoimmune sicknesses, cancer, diabetes, and depressed the maturity [3]. A dearth of vitamin D will cause rickets in children, and osteomalacia in the young because of the disaster of the bones calcification [1]. A spare amount of this vitamin can be poisonous [6].

2.3.3 Vitamin E

Egg yolk, vegetables, nuts, and cereals are sources of vitamin E. In egg yolk, 0.56 mg of vitamin E is present. It is an antioxidant and guards the cell membranes from damage by oxidation in the body. Malabsorption from food leads to deficiency of this vitamin [6]. The effects of undue amount are not known.

2.3.4 Vitamin B12

Meat, offal, egg, and milk are good sources of vitamin B12. It is near 1.25 µg in egg yolk that is 90% of human daily requirement [4]. It is needed for the apt growth of blood cells and nerve strands. Vitamin B12 is also imperative to guard against Alzheimer's disease and help with the postponement of the cognitive decline. Shortage of this vitamin will basis the pernicious anemia, and deadly possessions of too much quantity are unknown.

2.3.5 Vitamin B6

Vitamin B6 is also known as pyridoxine. It is found in various foods like fish, beef, eggs, and poultry. About 8% of the daily requirement of vitamin B6 for a person comes from egg yolk, which contain 0.6 mg of this [4]. B6 is imperative for protein digestion. Deficits in vitamin B6 can occur as a result of medications or impediment of disease.

2.3.6 Vitamin B1

B1 is also known as thiamine, and found in fruits, nuts, green vegetables, pluses, eggs, and fortified cereals. An egg can fulfill 5% of the daily requirement of body as it contains 0.05 mg thiamine.

Thiamine is involved in the discharge of energy from carbohydrates [3]. The brain uses the glucose as an energy source, so this vitamin helps in proper functioning and working of nerve cells and brain. Alcohol intake leads to a deficit of this vitamin, and its absence will result in beriberi disease.

2.3.7 FOLATE

Good sources of folate are liver, orange juice, and dark green vegetables, but eggs, relativity, have less amount of this. Folate in eggs is about 25 µg, which brings about 8% of the daily requirement [6]. Folate is needed for the development of red blood cells. To avoid neural tube defects in newborns, folate is necessary for mothers at the early stages of pregnancy [4]. It also prevents CVD, and by improving endothelial working, reduces the risk of stroke. In common inhabitants, its dearth can cause megaloblastic anemia and possibly depression.

2.3.8 RIBOFLAVIN

Riboflavin is present in a good amount in eggs, cheese, yogurt, yeast extract, liver, milk, and green vegetables. Egg has 0.24 mg of riboflavin that satisfies 15% of a person's daily necessity [6]. Riboflavin, also recognized as B2, is indispensable for the breakdown of fat and protein and extract energy for body use [3]. Their insufficiencies will result in instabilities in the skin around the mouth, nose, and mucous skin. B2 is excessively excreted from the body and adverse effects are unidentified.

2.3.9 IRON

There are two forms of iron, heme iron and non-heme iron. Heme can be simply engrossed but other cannot. Heme iron is present in eggs and meat. Eggs hold 0.95 mg, that is 10% of the daily requirement [1]. This mineral is the chief element of hemoglobin in bodily fluid cells and carrying oxygen all over the body [4]. Its scarcity will lead to anemia.

2.3.10 SELENIUM

Selenium in eggs is 0.55 µg in amount, that is 1% body's daily requirement. This is an antioxidant and it averts the oxidative impairment inside the body. It reduces the threat of cardiovascular disease, and colonic, prostate, and lung cancers [4]. In early and later stages of cancer, the expansion selenium has defensive effects [7].

2.3.11 ZINC

Zinc is mainly found in pulses, eggs, milk, wholegrain cereals, meat, fish, and cheese. Egg comprises 0.65 mg of Zinc, that is 7% of the daily human necessity [8]. Zinc is imperative for regular growth, fighting infection, enzyme activity, and wound healing also sexual maturation. Scarcity is occasional, but it can affect the arrested improvement and deferment of adolescence.

2.3.12 CHOLINE

Choline is the basic constituent of egg and about 280 mg of egg [3]. Choline is necessary for normal functions of the body's cells. An adequate amount of choline is required during reproduction. Foremost support of methyl group in the diet is by choline, and it directly affects the lipid metabolism/transportation as well as cell and nerve signaling [4]. A sufficient supply of choline inhibits breast cancer and DNA damage [7]. Choline is critical for brain and memory development in early stage because it can cause the hyper-methylation of adenosine and cytosine residues in DNA which is harmful to the fitness.

2.3.13 LUTEIN AND ZEAXANTHIN

In egg yolk, zeaxanthin and lutein are served as antioxidants and carotenoids [4]. These amass in the macular area of the retina of the human eye and assist the optical task by providing shield from light [6]. The scarcity of these components in food will result in a deficit in the macular region, which will eventually cause macules collapse.

2.4 PRODUCTION OF ANIMAL PRODUCTS AND THEIR HEALTH PRIVILEGES

The inclination of consumers for animal-based food is considered on the bases of their higher nutritional value but is most likely clarified by organoleptic properties, such as their texture and taste [3]. Rather than getting major nutritional advantages entirely from plants, they are partly taken from animal sources to meet the basic nutrient requirements. The nutrients taken from animal products are nearer to those, which are needed by humans [8]. Hence, animal proteins are esteemed for accompanying the proteins of indispensable foods, such as cereals, by providing critical amino acids and lysine. This is principally essential for rising children, for whom amino acid necessities are utmost dire.

2.4.1 MEAT-BASED PRODUCTS

Meat is an excellent source of valuable nutrients, such as protein, indispensable amino acids, vitamins, and minerals [4]. Currently, the use and appeal of functional ingredients in meat have been augmented [6]. There has been an increasing trend of consumers demanding meat foods that have extra nourishment, such as less cholesterol and salt content, and improved fatty acid outline for better health and fitness welfares [8]. Studies have shown that definite bioactive peptides, which have prospective well-being paybacks, are made during treatment of meat [7].

2.4.2 SAUSAGES

Sausages are formed by accumulating materials in precise amounts with meat in a structural design and organized process [4]. For sausage preparation, fresh and high value meat of lamb, beef, mutton, poultry, beef, or pork are used [4]. There are several other things also used in sausage making like salt, binder, spices, curing and extender agents, and water ice [3]. The use of salt is to boost the relish and taste and has the capability to minimize microbial deterioration and improve water holding capacity [6]. Water ice succors salt to extract or solubilize the meat protein besides assisting during the mixing process. The flavor and color of sausages can be enhanced by using curing agents in sausages [7]. Also, curing agents impede the microbial rising. The first phase for sausage making is the meat grating, then add salt for preserving tenacity plus to endorse the proper dispersion, mechanical mixer for mixing [1]. The salting practice is done in a chiller for the whole night at 1°C–4°C and can be performed after the ultimate chopping during smoking. For easy extraction of protein, mincing of meat in very fine particles after grinding should be done [4]. The function of proteins is to bind the H_2O that around the precipitations of fat and retain them circulated [4]. Grinding should be performed in range of 6–8 minutes [3]. For covering purposes, animal intestine is used in which the mixture is packed.

Fresh meat use for making fresh sausages and no handling is an intricate process. Such sausages are not fermented, smoked, salted, or cooked [8]. Before eating, user heats the fresh sausages, and these must be stored in a cool environment. In some sausages, cured meat is used, and these are smoked and precooked sausages. The shelf life of fresh sausages can be improved by decreasing the moisture content by cooking. Emulsion-type sausages are another sort of sausages, which are ready to eat and can made from homogenized and dried meat, seasoning, water, and fatty tissues. These sausages, also called scalded sausages, as they are not completely cooked and are pasteurized [4].

To improve the product stability, cultures are added to make fermented sausages. They are classified as semi-dry and dry fermented sausages [6]. By adding cultures, activity of unwanted microorganisms can be reduced, and it boosts the safety and quality of the meat products [8]. Probiotics, when taken in adequate amounts, promote beneficial bacteria, which provide a lot of well-being benefits to humans. Meat products play a key role in the transferal of probiotic cells to the human digestive system [1]. Sausages also transfer probiotics, as these are enclosed by fat. Sustainability of probiotic cultures are exaggerated by numerous aspects, such as pH, acidity, H_2O_2, temperature, sugar, oxygen and moisture content, salt, additives, organic acid concentration, and existence of microorganisms [4]. Fermented sausages have very low pH, so feasibility of probiotic organisms is badly pretentious in these sausages. Growth of probiotic bacteria is inhibited by acidic pH, which adversely affects their stability [4].

2.4.3 MILK-BASED PRODUCT

2.4.3.1 Cheese

Cheese is one of the most important dairy products having significant health benefits with long shelf life and prepared form milk by concentrating the milk [3]. It has a vital role in human diet having essential nutrients, which are beneficial for human fitness [6]. It has a high percentage value of fat and protein that make it nutritive and an energy-full nutriment. Also, cheese is a very good form of necessary nutrients, like as fatty acids, amino acids, protein, fat, minerals, bioactive peptides, and vitamins [7]. Cheese developed for lactose intolerant people serves as a nutritive food because it is free from lactose [4]. It has been ascertained that two bioactive tri-peptides that exist in sour milk fermented with *Lactobacillus helveticus* have the capability to decrease blood pressure. Amino acids are richly present in cheese and play a central part in the improvement and development of human body [8]. Cheese also comprises of a high extent of saturated and trans-fatty acids, nonetheless no ailment has been found associated to the intake of cheese [6]. Cheese has anticarcinogenic properties due to the presence of conjugated linoleic acid (CLA) and Sphingo lipids. Cheese is also a good source of Calcium (Ca), which shows an imperative part to the upkeep and development of strong teeth and bones. Calcium, together with a low-calorie diet, has optimistic consequences on lowering blood pressure and contributes in reducing weight. In modern times, diverse ailments, such as diabetes, obesity, osteoporosis, cancer, and cardiovascular sicknesses, are related to the intake of food, because of this nutritionists are directing people to those food materials that are good for human wellbeing [4]. Currently, cheese is not used up for avoidance of starvation, but as well offer crucial amino acids that are essential for social wellbeing [7] (Figure 2.2).

On the basis of milk used, manufacturing processes, consistency, fat constituents, and fermentation, cheese can be categorized into several types [6]. During cheese maturing, a certain quantity of lactose is eroded away and the remaining lactose is altered in lactic acid. Except in some varieties of fresh and soft cheese, all types of cheese have no lactose [4]. Cheese contains protein, essential amino acids, and fat content, which vary in ranges amid 20%–35% of parched mass. In cheese, the common saturated fatty acids are myristic, palmitic and stearic acid, and oleic acid as unsaturated fatty acid [3]. Saturated fatty acids increase the occurrence of coronary heart disease due to having negative effect on blood lipids, and also harmful to the health [8]. All dairy products have different quantities of minerals and vitamins; principally Ca is the most vital mineral in cheese. Cheese, moreover, provides zinc, phosphorus, and magnesium, also vitamins such as those in the B group and vitamin A [7].

Dental cavities take place due to the elimination of tooth coating by acids that are made during sugar and starch fermentation by microbes [3]. Sugar is also present in milk as lactose, but it is not toxic in nature and likewise lessens the risks of teeth decay if supplemented in daily diet. Consistent consumption of dairy products such as yogurt, whole milk, cheese, or sour milk has opposite relation with weight gain [6]. Calcium ingestion from 400 to 1000 mg reduces fat in the body owing

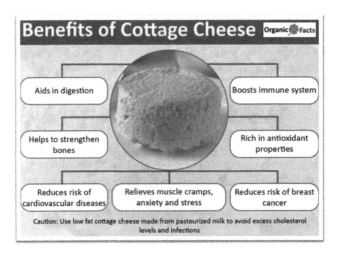

FIGURE 2.2 Health benefits of cottage cheese.

to the formation of calcium and fatty acid retarding the absorption in gut and decreasing the blood pressure [1]. Other bioactive complexes, such as conjugated linoleic acid (CLA), also perform essential role in weight control [9].

The threat for heart disease increases due to insufficient consumption of dairy products [4]. In cheese, high concentrations of bioactive peptides are present; the most investigated biological job of such peptides is to inhibit the influence of angiotensin converting enzyme, which is crucial enzyme in blood regulation [3]. Cheese constituents, like vitamin D, Mg, Ca, and other bioactive peptides, have an affirmative influence in edifice of bone density and diminish the bone damage [10].

2.4.3.2 Yogurt

The most popular fermented dairy product is yogurt, which is consumed all over the world because it has beneficial nutrition bioavailability, good health effects, as well as high digestibility [8]. It contains a high value of calcium that provides substantial quantity of calcium in bio-available state [11]. Protein of good biological worth and indispensable amino acids, such as glycine and proline, are present in yogurt and play a vital role in nutrition and for good health. Minerals and vitamins are also found in yogurt in bioavailable form [6]. Yogurt contains a high amount of carbohydrates, vitamins (such as niacin, thiamin, riboflavin, folate, and cobalamin), protein, and minerals (such as P and Ca) [10]. According to the FDA, yogurt is a fermented item that is manufactured by expending bacterial culture in one or more dairy foods, such as cream, milk, and skim milk and also includes variety of ingredients, such as sweeteners, stabilizers, flavors, and fruits [12]. The nutritional composition of yogurt is influenced by milk type, flavors, starter culture, sweeteners, fermentation time, and all other elements. *Lactobacillus bulgaricus* and *Streptococcus thermophiles* cultures are used and have ability to produced lactic acid [4]. Yogurt entails milk solids not fat 8.25%, milk fat 3.25%, and 0.9% acidity, which is said as lactic acid. In many countries, the standards of commercial yogurt are that, content of milk solid varies from 14%–15% to 8.2%–8.6% for solid not fat [9]. Yogurt compositions are diverse depending on the milk origin either from cow, sheep, buffalo and goat is conventionally used likewise camel and mare milk in some areas of world is also used for yogurt production [6]. Yogurt is an excellent nutrient source for lactose intolerant peoples, gastrointestinal disease like inflammatory and irritable bowel disorders, and it also helps in losing weight and is good for immune functions [13] (Figure 2.3).

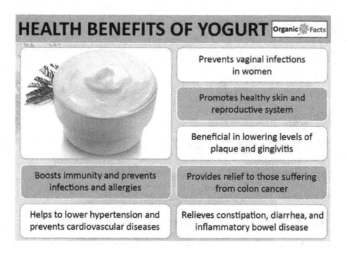

FIGURE 2.3 Health benefits of yoghurt.

Food markets offer different types and varieties of yogurt, such as plain yogurt, frozen yogurt, flavored, drinking type, dried powder yogurt, as well UHT and pasteurized yogurt [8]. By using whole milk, full fat or regular yogurt has been prepared, low or no fat yogurt is made by taking skimmed milk [6]. In yogurt solid content increase by taking skim milk powder and whey protein concentrate likewise fat by using cream or butter. To upturn the yogurt firmness, stabilizers, mostly pectin and gelatin, are added that develop the texture as well as provide assistance on the even spreading of ingredients and constrain whey split-up to get desirable characteristics [2].

Yogurt is known as probiotic carrier because it has capability to transfer probiotic bacteria to the human body in a specific amount and has a lot of beneficial health effects [4]. Probiotic yogurt also called bio-yogurt is a very popular type of yogurt and is made by using beneficial microorganism cultures that have a good role to provide health benefit when consumed [14]. *Lactobacillus acidophilus* and *Bifid* bacteria are the most commonly used probiotics [9]. Because of the creamy and acidity flavor bio-yogurt is more prevalent than standard yogurt. It also aids in digestion [11]. It has been perceived that the daily consumption of bio-yogurt delivers therapeutic benefits, as well as it has anticarcinogenic and antimicrobial properties and helps lower the cholesterol and increase lactose intolerance. Gastrointestinal disorders and irritable bowel syndrome can be treated with yogurt and other fermented dairy products [2]. Immunological activity by producing cytokine, improving natural killer cell activity, and T-cell function can be enhanced by using yogurt [10].

2.5 EGG CONCENTRATE

2.5.1 INTRODUCTION

Egg is that the wonderful common wellspring of excellent value protein, vitamins, lipids and minerals [4]. Protein is needed for simplest potential structure/muscle advancement in persons as well in animals [6]. For the foremost half we depend on the vegetable and animal hotspots for protein since they maybe provide the specified basic amino acids and minerals, such as iron, potassium, phosphorus, Ca, and zinc to the body [3]. Eggs are a wealthy wellspring of folic

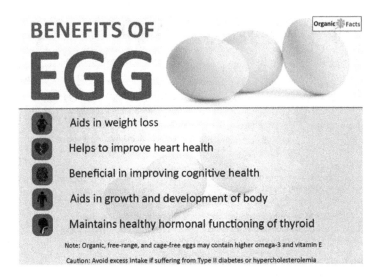

FIGURE 2.4   Health benefits of egg.

acid, B-complex vitamin (cyanocobalamin), lactoflavin (riboflavin), and fat dissoluble vitamins (A, E, and D) [2]. Currently eggs are utilized in various products particularly in the baking industry.

Additionally, eggs have also been consumed in the form of hard-cooked hacked eggs, crepes, scrambles egg blends, prepared egg patties, prepared deep-fried eggs, quiches and omelets [8]. Egg powder is another important product having vast applications in food industry. Egg powder is used in cake mix and some types of bread kitchens and is also eaten up in eateries, military foundation, doctor's facilities and hotels [3]. Dried egg whites are utilized in cake mix generation, sweet toffee, and candy manufacturing and meringue precipitate fabricate [9] (Figure 2.4).

2.5.2   Whole Egg Composition

Whole egg covers of two sections: the albumin and egg yolk. Albumin is around 67% of the total weight of egg yolk [4]. The egg white contains of 87.8% (w/w) of water, 9.7%–10.6% (w/w) protein and 0.5%–0.6% (w/w) sugars [5]. Vital little bit of minerals, chlorine, sulfur, riboflavin, sodium, potassium; metallic element aboard 56 of the mixture egg protein is obtainable in egg whites [2]. In egg whites, carbohydrates area unit discovered either in conjugated or free form with protein and 98% of egg whites sugars is glucose [8]. In egg whites, lipids area unit on the market in unimportant total that is 0.01% and extremely nearly seventeen calories area unit contributed by egg whites of associate expansive egg [3]. The ingredient is 33% of combination weight of fluid egg and contains of 440 yards of its protein [8]. An enormous ingredient provides 5 g of fat; of that 0.7 g area unit unsaturated, 1.6 g saturated fat and 1.9 g monounsaturated fat [10]. In basic words ingredient subsidizes 8% total fat and % of unsaturated fat of each day mention esteems [11].

An entire substantial egg delivers 213 mg of cholesterin. In people, dietary cholesterin expands the body fluid combination and cholesterol focus that is accountable for CVD [4]. The amount of cholesterin in human body fluid is not influenced by the intake of two eggs in a single day and utilization of four eggs have virtually no impact. Egg also contains some additional minerals (iodine, manganese, copper, selenium, calcium, phosphorus, zinc) and vitamins (D, E, A). Egg yolk adds 59 calories (West and Zhou, 1989).

2.5.3 Technology to Produce Egg Powder

By using a spray dryer, eggs are transformed into dried powder form for long duration conservation [2]. The essential piece of this innovation is to shower fluid sustain material into hot desiccating state for the vanishing of water [5]. During this procedure heat ranges from 100°C to 300°C and this procedure will likewise be referred to as the core of the strategy. The ultimate item is as agglomerates and parched powder has the high reposition security, easy to take care of and carriage [2]. The state of the last results of spray drying be influenced by physical, compound characteristics of nourish material, arrange and activity of appliance. Amid spray drying vanishing through the beads is inspired by the warmness and gas exchange [3].

2.5.4 Phases of Spray Drying Technology

1. Feed concentration.
2. Feed atomization is vital to form sensible circumstances for vanishing from sustain and to induced ultimate item with enticing qualities.
3. Air bead interaction within the compartment, the connection of atomized fluid with the new gases vanishes ninety fifth of water from beads in an exceedingly few moments seconds.
4. Drying and dissipation of damp from droplets, it happens in a pair of organizes (a) in 1st stage vanishing rate stays consistent thanks to the closeness of adequate damp within the drop to come after the nonexistent damp from its surface and (b) once at the drop surface there's no soaked condition thanks to less damp at that time second vanishing stage starts and it'll give birth to the arrangement of casing at the drop surface [9].
5. Concluding step is the split-up phase; in these juncture cyclones, electrostatic precipitators and bag strainers are used (Figure 2.5).

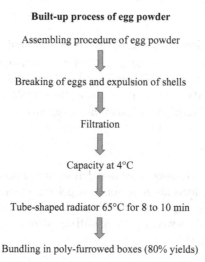

Built-up process of egg powder

Assembling procedure of egg powder

⬇

Breaking of eggs and expulsion of shells

⬇

Filtration

⬇

Capacity at 4°C

⬇

Tube-shaped radiator 65°C for 8 to 10 min

⬇

Bundling in poly-furrowed boxes (80% yields)

FIGURE 2.5   Flow line for egg powder.

In a conventional egg breach system to remove the shell and discharge after breaching, the mixture is poured into the separator for clarification where the liquid egg and shells of egg are parted [8]. After separation, the liquid egg is moved to a storing tank and is cooled down up to 4°C by means of chilled water casings and sluggish speed agitation [9]. At that time mix is nourished to the tubular radiator by positive uprooting pump and warmed up to 65°C for six minutes through high temperature water [2]. This warming can offer the adequate purification of mix. Mix is tense through high weight lines to the atomizing spouts. A tube-shaped spray dryer contains two tapered openings; one for powder and one for air [3]. Vapor is used to warm the separated parching air. Exceptionally planned venture comprising of atomizing fountain spears area unit used to acquaint the air with the drying compartment [4]. The egg mix is atomized within the sizzling air and hotness of the air decreases quickly attributable to the flash drying that is responsible of the less hurt to the item [2]. Dehydrated air and, therefore, the desiccated powder area unit changed to the violent wind from base of the slot and powder is isolated from air. Dry powder should comprise 95% mixture egg solids [5]. The powder is filled in compartment subsequently to the cooling [11].

2.5.5   OTHER DRYING APPROACHES

2.5.5.1   Pan Driers

Pan drying, like the previous technique, nevertheless at identical time used for drying egg. A pan drier contains of take with egg whites belt on that fluid egg is unfold as skinny film [3]. This belt travels over warm air, and moisture is expelled up to the amount about 12%–16%. This item is named flake category and an artifact finer than flake is named a coarse item [2]. At the purpose, once the egg is beaten into a foam and unfolded on the moving belt, this is referred to as foam/lighten drying [9].

2.5.5.2   Foam Spray Drying

This technique is used for dehydrating dairy and egg things [3]. The egg things dried out by this strategy have numerous qualities and mass thickness than overall splash parched things [8]. Desiccated egg products may be place away for extensive day and age than fluid egg even at warmth e.g. egg whites may place away for sixty days at 54°C. The required moisture contents in desiccated eggs are in the range from 6.5%–8.0% [15].

2.5.5.3   The Warmth Handling Wants of Spray and Pan Dried Egg Whites
- *Spray dried* egg whites need to be warm at 130°F for 7 days until the purpose that it progresses toward turning into enterobacteria (*Salmonella*) negative
- *Pan dried* egg whites need to be warm systematically at 125°F for 5 days until the purpose once it progresses toward turning into *Salmonella* negative

2.5.6   USES OF EGG POWDER

Parched egg things may be used to strengthen and deliver mayonnaise, pasta, salad dressings, and bakery products [2]. Dried products are used for their gelling, coloring, emulsifying and foaming characteristic and are easy to transport and handle [5]. The properties of egg are connected with heat (temperature) and atomization weight and by utilizing legitimate mix stowage lifetime of egg item may enlarge than fluid egg [12].

- Stable oil-based mostly emulsions may be created by utilizing egg white powder.
- Powder of egg albumin increment the emulsion limit of mayo and sauce.

- Egg powder is that the key part for emulsion, which will face up to extraordinary temperature and not breakdown during processing.
- Albumin powder has the additional immense proscribing capability than the fluid egg.
- Egg powder is that the key fixing in green goods lover things and meat things (hams, burger, wieners).

2.6 CONSUMPTION PATTERNS AND TRENDS

In developing countries, utilization of animal-based products as a source of nourishment is influenced on the regular income and urbanization [8]. These are promptly changing the final utilization of food and adjustment in structure of consumption program [2]. Per capita utilization of results of animals' start line has been enlarged from 1861 to 2651 kcal in 1961 to 2007 severally. In the developing countries 14% per capita utilization isn't the maximum amount as developed nations. In countries like Pakistan, India and China etc. the ingesting of milk has become doubled, meat intake has become tripled and consumption of eggs has enhanced to fivefold (Steinfeld, 2006) [1].

2.6.1 MEAT AND MEAT PRODUCTS

From last 50 years, the use of meat has enlarged from 23.1 kg to 42.20 kg per unit for each individual once a year from 1961 to 2011, separately [12]. Developed nations have non-inheritable traditional level of animal-based proteins (ABP) as per their requirements. Utilization of meat mainly depends upon income. ABP has an unprecedented supply in consumption routine of developed countries but supply and consumption of ABP mainly depends upon income of people in developing countries [2]. From past 20 years, developing nations have rehearsed to devour domesticated animals exceptionally mono gastric animals like poultry [12].

2.6.2 MILK AND DAIRY PRODUCTS

Dietary patterns and intake levels of milk and farm products of developing and developed nations are connected [3]. In developing nations, level of combination of dietary energy has enlarged from 3.4 to 4.4% from 1961 to 2007, severally of farm products [8]. Dairy foods play a remarkable role to expand the combination dietary energy consumption in South Asia in 1960s–2007. As indicated by per capita utilization of milk and dairy foods, there is a substantial distinction amongst developing and developed nations (Figure 2.6).

2.6.3 EGGS AND EGGS PRODUCTS

Universally, utilizations of eggs can impact human fitness and limit the danger of various human ailments because of its straightforward accessibility and affordability [3]. The healthful esteem has been increased for man and children with developing personalities by upgrade of egg production and intake in developing and developed nations [5]. The simplest wellspring of a solid consumption program and life is eggs that are elementary for mental improvement and development of youngsters [1]. For past 40 years, utilization of eggs has progressed extensively throughout the World. In countries like Pakistan, China and India per capita utilization of eggs is increasing perpetually [12].

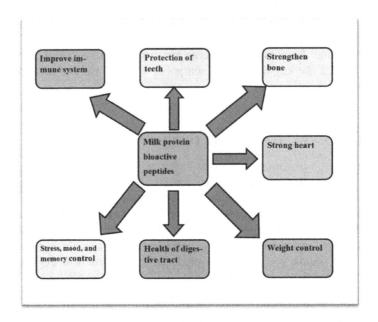

FIGURE 2.6 Health benefits of milk protein.

2.7 BENEFITS, CONCERNS, AND CHALLENGES TO ANIMAL ORIGIN FOODS

2.7.1 MILK AND DAIRY PRODUCTS

Obesity and heart diseases are main factors to reduce fat intake in developed and developing countries [5]. To address these medical issues, manufacturers need to be compelled to produce systems for the modification of milk fat substances [8]. Diminishing dairy fat substances can often limit the danger of these infections in developing countries [2]. Many developing countries confront various difficulties of increasing fat utilization in populaces with low-fat and general low-consumption of energy [15].

2.7.2 MEAT AND MEAT PRODUCTS

Meat can potentially eradicate the skin diseases, mend the immune system, promote muscle growth, repair of body tissues, and provide a rich source of long-term energy, as well as help in the hemoglobin production [13].

2.7.3 EGG AND EGG PRODUCTS

Eggs are a most vital wellspring of protein and nutrients. As per their wholesome quality, eggs have additional successful health advancing characteristics [5]. They have great therapeutic potential [15]. They will like outside intervention to boost development, muscle tissues, and metabolic exercises [13]. Consumption of eggs can reduce the danger of heart illness (CVD), nervous system-related disorders (CNS), enhance psychological and mental well-being, inflammation and immune infection. Eggs also play significant role in reducing the deformities of neural tubes in new borne infants [14].

2.8 CONCLUSION

Animal source foods such as meat, milk, cheese, yogurt or egg constitutes are consumed to enhance the heath status of an individual. However, a continuous increase in the cost of animal products is the major issue in the developing countries which results in low consumption of these products. For instance, meat has plenty of nutrients including vitamins and minerals, but it also contains significant quantity of fat which may cause many disorders particularly cardiovascular diseases. Conclusively, consumption of animal-based products is mainly dependent on the income of people and promoting the use of animal-based products is the major challenge for developing economies. Hence, policy-making authorities of developing countries should develop new strategies to increase the consumption of animal-based food products for improving the health status of people.

REFERENCES

1. WHO. 2013. *Country Cooperation Strategy at a Glance-Pakistan.* Geneva, Switzerland.
2. Sinha, N. 2007. *Handbook of food products manufacturing*, 2 volume set. John Wiley & Sons.
3. Owens, C.M., Sams, A.R. and Alvarado, C., 2000. *Poultry meat processing.* CRC Press.
4. Mitchell, M.A. and Kettlewell, P.J., 2009, May. Welfare of poultry during transport–a review. In *Poultry Welfare Symposium.* Cervia: Association Proceeding.
5. West, B. and Zhou, B.X., 1989. Did chickens go north? New evidence for domestication. *World's Poultry Science Journal*, 45(3), pp.205–218.
6. Steinfeld, H., Wassenaar, T. and Jutzi, S., 2006. Livestock production systems in developing countries: status, drivers, trends. *Rev Sci Tech*, 25(2), pp.505–516.
7. Yusop, S.M., O'Sullivan, M.G., Preuß, M., Weber, H., Kerry, J.F. and Kerry, J.P., 2012. Assessment of nanoparticle paprika oleoresin on marinating performance and sensory acceptance of poultry meat. *LWT-Food Science and Technology*, 46(1), pp.349–355.
8. Rehman, A., Jingdong, L., Chandio, A.A. and Hussain, I., 2017. Livestock production and population census in Pakistan: Determining their relationship with agricultural GDP using econometric analysis. *Information Processing in Agriculture*, 4(2), pp.168–177.
9. Yang, C., Du, H., Li, X., Li, Q., Zhang, Z., Li, W. and Jiang, X., 2011. Evaluation for meat quality performance of broiler chicken. *Journal of Animal and Veterinary Advances*, 10(8), pp.949–954.
10. Anjum, M.A., Sahota, A.W., Akram, M., Javed, K. and Mehmood, S., 2012. Effect of selection on productive performance of Desi chicken for four Generations. *The J. Anim. and Plant Sciences*, 22(1), pp.1–5.
11. Arain, M.A., Khaskheli, M., Rajput, I.R., Faraz, S., Rao, S., Umer, M. and Devrajani, K., 2010. Effect of slaughtering age on chemical composition of goat meat. *Pakistan Journal of Nutrition*, 9(4), pp.404–408.
12. Berri, C., Wacrenier, N., Millet, N. and Le Bihan-Duval, E., 2001. Effect of selection for improved body composition on muscle and meat characteristics of broilers from experimental and commercial lines. *Poultry Science*, 80(7), pp.833–838.
13. Brandao, M.P., Neto, M.G., dos Anjos, V.D.C. and Bell, M.J.V., 2017. Detection of adulteration of goat milk powder with bovine milk powder by front-face and time resolved fluorescence. *Food Control*, 81, pp.168–172.
14. FAO. 2011. *Dairy Development in Pakistan.* Rome, Italy.
15. Fletcher, D.L., 2002. Poultry meat quality. *World's Poultry Science Journal* 58(2), pp.131–145.

3 Animal Tracing
A Basis for Branding Animal Origin Foods in the Market

Bernd Hallier

CONTENTS

3.1 INTRODUCTION

Tracing of food products is a prerequisite in the modern times as people are very conscious about the product what they are consuming due to increasing the awareness about food safety issues. Traceability is a mechanism that creates a link among producers, firms, retailers, and consumers. The prime objective of traceability systems is to provide a precise history and origin of the food products as consumers want to know it due to traditional and religious compulsions. It has become very crucial in the meat processing industry to know about the total supply chain to combat food safety problems, which arise due to mishandling at any stage of production, processing, and distribution. Due to advancements in technologies, different traceability systems are being developed that aim to reduce the costs of traceability management. Different methods like branding, ear notches, and paint marks were being used to identify and monitoring of the animals in the farm. However, in modern supermarkets, the first tracing activities had been the introduction of barcode systems at the point of sale (POS) in Europe and the United States (US) in the beginning of the 1970s. The idea was to control the stock and the sales per item via a system with electronic devices. To gain efficiency for such new business administration within an outlet, the pioneers of retail started cooperation contracts with the producing industry to get from the producers ordered items with a code printed on each item already as a part of the product-packaging design. In Germany, retail and manufacturers founded a 50/50 joint venture called Centrale fuer Coorganisation (CCG) [1], which established a number-system for Germany—and within a second step helped to organize the European unit for this called European Article Numbering (EAN). Nowadays, the system is organized globally by the GS1 (Global Standard) [1], which is shared by all the international organizations and has been established on the national level within 20 years after the first pioneers.

Nevertheless, it must be stated that the process still is going on in the less developed markets, which even in the second decade of the new century, still have wet-markets with no information technology (IT) infrastructure in the back-store or do not have fixed prices. Therefore, the advantages of barcoding must be summarized for modern supermarkets again:

- A fixed price allows changing from a service-type store to self-service store. This is decreasing the personnel costs tremendously. The competitive improvement can be seen by the increase of self-service chain stores versus traditional stores.
- The growing number of stores within each chain store company is decreasing its overheads, and by this leads to competitive advantages due to the electronic data control of each store via the system.
- The industrial barcode saves costs via an in-store article pricing: the scanner at the cash-zone is identifying the product and, by this, its price.
- In Europe, in some chain stores, prices are flexible by hours: during low-frequency times, the price for certain items is lower to attract pensioners, for example, or other low-income customers. This lowers the work-peaks for personnel, which again is decreasing the cost for personnel.
- While the above-mentioned advantages are wins for the retail side, the win for the manufacturers is the electronic control of the penetration and sales of his products either in form of lists or in advanced cooperation even electronically.

Of course, such an implementation of a system takes money, time, and learning. The following Chart 1 [2] shows that in Germany the market penetration of scanners took about 25 years (Figure 3.1).

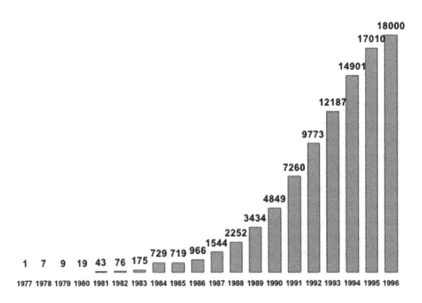

FIGURE 3.1   Taken from lecture Prof. Dr. B. Hallier.

FREQUENT SHOPPER PROFILE

Store Number:	000123	
Card Number:	654321	

JANE Q. SHOPALOT
67 ATLANTIC AVENUE
MANASQUAN   NJ   08736

SSN: 999-99-9999

ISSUE DATE 09/10/90
ISSUE STATUS   INITIAL

People in houshold	= 4
People under age 18	= 2
Owner of any pets	= dog
Marital Status	= married
Age of person	= 34

DATE FIRST SHOPPED :	09/11/90	
DATE LAST SHOPPED :	04/11/91	

Month:	APR	MAR	FEB
Purchases			
GROCERY	42.76	146.23	213.82
DAIRY	7.25	31.97	39.99
MEAT	17.35	81.60	88.79
PRODUCE	20.20	50.62	76.24
DELI	13.45	26.47	43.86
SEAFOOD	30.75	.00	.00
FROZEN	12.60	26.88	33.04
LIQUOR	.00	.00	.00
FLORAL	12.50	.00	36.94
Total $	156.86	363.77	532.68
TOTAL TRIPS	2	5	6

FIGURE 3.2   Taken from lecture Prof. Dr. B. Hallier.

Combined with a loyalty-card for the customer, the retailer can track the sales of his items towards the shopping basket as can be seen from Chart 2 [2], which was prepared from a data collection in 1990/91 from a US retailer (Figure 3.2).

In this case, the retailer knows the name of his customer, that she is married, and that she has a dog. Month by month (in this case, in a comparison of 3 months) the retailer can analyze the purchases of his customer by each category. In the context of animals, the retailer could use this instrument with variations to see if the customer prefers local meat, organic grown-ups, imports, or specific meat brands.

3.2   TRACING/TRACKING FOR ANTI-CRISIS MEASURES

The history of the technical development of barcoding has to be understood, in general, and, in the case of the first tracing/tracking of cows in Germany and Europe, the fact that the EHI Retail Institute is in Germany owning 50% of the retail shares of GS1 Germany.

In 1994 in the UK, the Mad Cow Disease (BSE) epidemic started, and, in Germany, the sales of beef declined between 25% and 30%. Retailers realized that they did not know for their mass-distribution from where the beef was coming from, and if they could guarantee to the customers that no British beef was among the meat for sale [3]. The EHI was asked to help as a think-tank, and a Round Table was established [1, p. 14] (Figure 3.3).

On the one hand side, the German retailers sat, and on the other side the main suppliers were represented by national organizations. For the first time for the Total Meat Supply Chain, a flow-chart

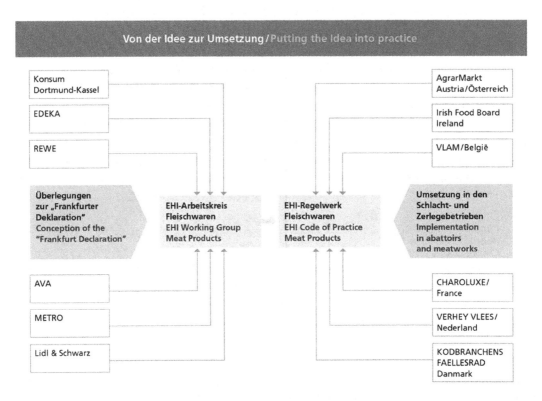

FIGURE 3.3 From crisis to competence. (From Hallier, B. et alia, *From Crisis to Competence*, Bonn, Germany, 2011, p. 14.)

was developed to follow in an abstract way the birth of the calves already from its sperm via the growing-up, the slaughtering, the cutting, the distribution via wholesale to retail, and the sales in self-service or via the counter [1, p. 18] (Figure 3.4).

Based on those discussions, a rather simple first label (EHI-Label) was created [1, p. 13] with the following content (Figure 3.5):

- Slaughtering/cutting house with address and EU-number
- Category of the beef
- Item/article
- Country/region of origin
- Identification number

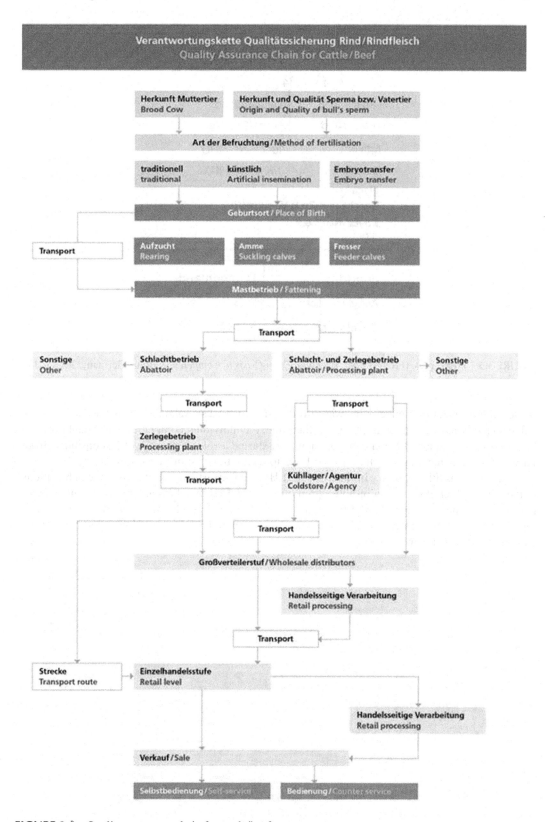

FIGURE 3.4 Quality assurance chain for cattle/beef.

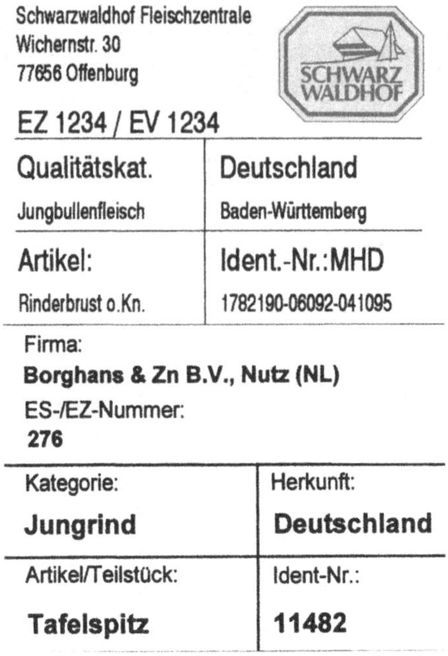

Schwarzwaldhof Fleischzentrale Wichernstr. 30 77656 Offenburg	
EZ 1234 / EV 1234	
Qualitätskat.	Deutschland
Jungbullenfleisch	Baden-Württemberg
Artikel:	Ident.-Nr.: MHD
Rinderbrust o.Kn.	1782190-06092-041095
Firma: **Borghans & Zn B.V., Nutz (NL)** ES-/EZ-Nummer: **276**	
Kategorie:	Herkunft:
Jungrind	**Deutschland**
Artikel/Teilstück:	Ident-Nr.:
Tafelspitz	**11482**

FIGURE 3.5   From crisis. (From Hallier, B. et alia, *From Crisis to Competence*, Bonn, Germany, 2011, p. 13.)

In December 1995, this pioneer-label was introduced in the first six retail chains in Germany also as a first step of a new way of thinking. Until that time, the individual companies had thought only to be responsible for their own company, but now they started a voluntary chain of responsibility from farm to fork! The main task at that time still was to regain the trust of the consumer.

Supported was this voluntary initiative of the EHI by an advertising campaign in the publications of the meat and retail sector, by in-house promotion of the EHI members and by special magazines developed for the documentation of the status quo of technical development for tracing and tracking and for dissemination even to all members of the German Parliament and to experts within the EU-organizations [1, p. 63, 66, 39].

International gemeinsam für gläserne Produktion und Distribution

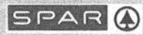

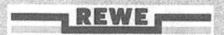

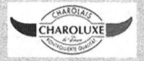

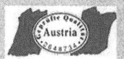

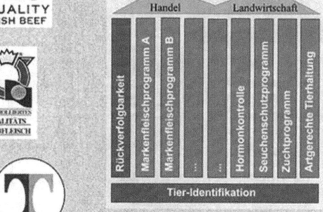

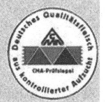

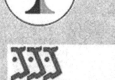

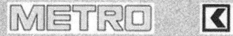

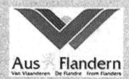

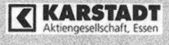

EHI
Internationale Kompetenz im Handel
Fax: 02 21 / 5 79 93 45

Spotlight

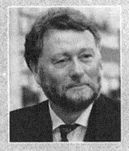

Dr. Bernd Hallier
Geschäftsführer
EuroHandelsinstitut e.V.
Aufsichtsratsvorsitzender
ORGAINVENT GmbH

Vom EHI-Etikett zur EU-Verordnung

„Entscheidend für die Rentabilität der
Fleischabteilung ist die Rückgewinnung des
öffentlichen Vertrauens. Voraussetzung hierfür
ist ein langfristiges, anerkannt positives Verhalten.
Die Umsetzung der EU-Verordnung 820/97 ist
hierbei ein wichtiger Meilenstein. Sie schreibt ab
01.07.1998 für freiwillige Etikettierungssysteme
eine europaweite Standardisierung der
Anmeldungs- und Überprüfungsverfahren vor.
Koordinationsstelle für den deutschen
Lebensmittelhandel ist die ORGAINVENT GmbH."

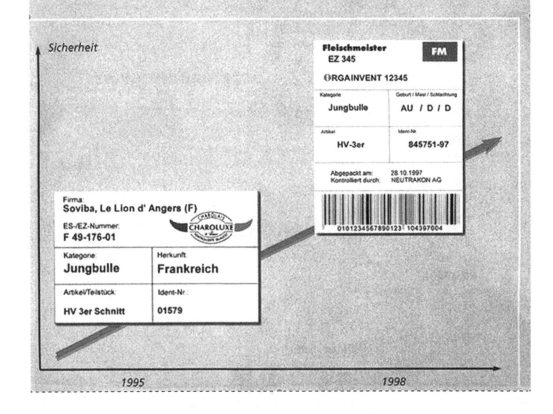

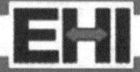

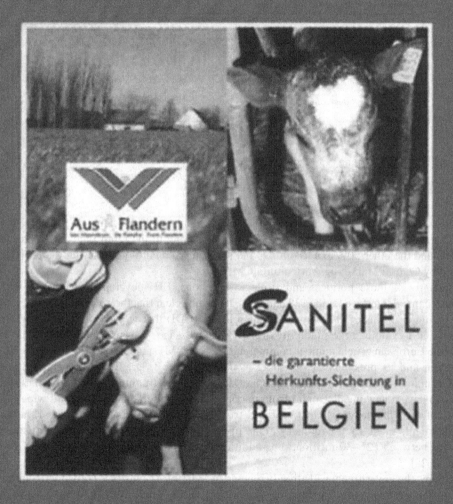

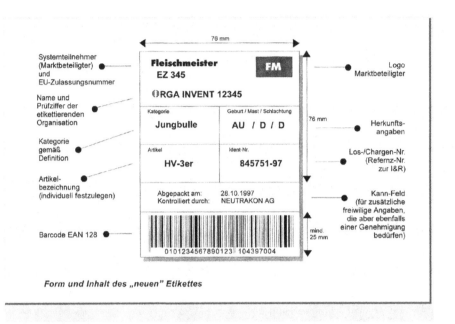

FIGURE 3.6   Handelsbiatt, 2000.

To institutionalize this chain of responsibility, a joint venture with the name of Orgainvent was founded in 1997 [1, p. 159]. Fifty percent of the shares belong to the retail industry (represented by the EHI) and the other 50% to agriculture, and slaughter and cutting houses (at the initial start represented by Central Marketing Agriculture [CMA]).

Independently of those political and strategic decisions, EHI developed together with GS1 Germany a technical interface for the 128 barcodes. It became clear that the efficient tracing/tracking needed a common means of electronic data interchange (EDI) that would span every stage from farm to fork. GS1 examined the suitability of individual message types and incorporated the catalogue into the European article number commercial (EANCOM) standard [1, p. 21] (Figure 3.6).

Orgainvent and its president of the supervisory board, Prof. Dr. B. Hallier, pushed politicians in Germany [4] and in the EU to prepare an obligatory tracing/tracing system, as there were fears to have a new meat scandal from uncontrolled suppliers who then could wipe off all the efforts of the voluntary system to rebuild trust. According to expert estimates, the value of the investments made by the industry alone in Germany in the period of 1995 until the end of 2000 was between €25–30 million, plus additional investment by exporters for the German market [1, p. 28].

In Germany, the government had already reacted by starting a Livestock Transport Regulation with one of the first ear tag identification systems for cattle, and the EU Commission reacted with a draft for cattle tagging and beef labeling Reg. (EC) 820/97 as well as later with Reg. (EC) 1760/2000. It was no surprise that the EU sample label corresponded 1:1 with the EHI label.

This obligatory labelling then became mandatory for all EU countries and was further developed step by step [1, p. 87f].

Tracing and tracking systems as anti-crisis instruments are a kind of insurance against an unlimited stop of products of a whole category within a food scandal. If a wrong product appears in the market now, with tracing and tracking established the source can quickly be found, and the area of sourcing be supervised by counteractions.

3.3 TECHNICAL AND MARKETING DEVELOPMENTS

The second technical generation is the change from earmarks/barcodes towards chips or, as it is at the moment, the inclusion of chips into the earmark of the cows. A chip enables much more info to be stored than the traditional tools. In the end, even the medical treatment of an animal during its total lifetime can be stored and traced by chip technology.

The third technical generation is the QR-Code, which can be used on the packaging and can be read by distributors, or even end-consumers, via terminals or mobile phones. In Germany, such a system was first tested by the name of FLEISCH/Meat-trace (F-trace) in 2011 by the retail chains ALDI and EDEKA [5].

Tactically, the retailer wants to position either his chain store or the meat product as a brand. The focus has changed from anti-crisis to pro-active! The retailer communicates with the consumer beyond the level of security: now the message is quality of the supply-chain or advice for the processing/cooking [1, p. 118] (Figure 3.7).

This system also allows regional campaigns, which, for example, can promote the criterion of livestock transport (time, radius) as a distinguished criterion for quality or distinctions according to animal welfare [6].

But, of course, the application is also no longer limited to animals and meat but could be used for any agricultural product as a part of good agricultural practice. The only limitation is the price for the product; the value of a cow allows higher investment than for a chicken or for a mango. But watching the demand for information at the level of consumers and realizing the power behind ordering systems of retail, it becomes obvious that tracing/tracking is a tool of competition.

3.4 RETAIL AND CONSUMERS

Retail constitutes the final stage in the food value chain, which delivers goods to consumers and provides the information requested by the market. Transparency, therefore, always needs the interface with both: retail and consumers. The consumer perspective on transparency is primarily characterized by pull situations. Various technology developments, for example smartphones, support these initiatives. In developed countries, a consumer may enter a shop or approach product displays with a communication device that may guide him through the shop to find the product that matches his profile.

Retail wants to have all the information at hand that the customer might want ask for. The strength of a good retailer is the ability to deliver both the product and the information about the

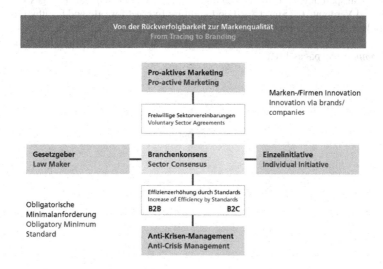

FIGURE 3.7   From tracing to branding.

product—even about preparing meals with that product. Within the Total Supply Chain, the retail's interest is the assurance of food safety and quality through business procurement agreements specified at the time of the order [7].

Within the Total Supply Chain from farm to fork in future public-private partnerships (PPP), the Internet will enhance applications of public and social relevance and through competition [8]. It will allow more real-time data processing for real-time applications. Within the European Union (EU), such innovations of the information and communication technology (ICT) are promoted and funded under the title SmartAgriFood (EU FP7) programs. They cover smart farming on sensors and traceability; smart agri-logistics on real-time virtualization, connectivity, and logistics intelligence; smart food awareness focusing on transparency of data and knowledge representation.

Important for the efficiency for transparency is a common understanding of the meaning of data items allowing for correct interpretation within the IT systems of all stakeholders involved nationally and internationally [9]. Currently, a number of data dictionaries, thesauri, ontologies, and encoding systems exist in the food and agricultural sector that each focus on certain subdomains. Methods to achieve semantic interoperability are required to be able to transfer information systems and to convert existing data to human readable and understandable signals.

In short, food traceability solutions in the market place must be adopted by the meat processors and importer to ensure safety and quality for the end consumers. It will not only win the consumer trust and confidence but also lead towards the competitive advantage and profitability to remain active in the market place.

REFERENCES

1. Hallier, B. et alia, *From Crisis to Competence*, Bonn, Germany, 2011, page 159.
2. Hallier, B., chart from lecture material.
3. EHI, Press Release, From the Frankfurt Declaration towards an EHI-label, Cologne, 20.02.1995; Beef will get a passport, Lebensmittel Zeitung, 24.02.1995; "Green Light" for Frankfurt Declaration, Lebensmittel Praxis, 5/1995.
4. See for example copy of letter to the German Federal Chancellor Gerhard Schroeder, at Hallier, B. et alia, *From Crisis...*, page 30.
5. Hallier, B., Smartphones and QR-codes, in: Hallier, B. et alia, *From Crisis to Competence*, pages 148ff.
6. Giesen, H., Westfleisch – Constant improvement, in: Hallier, B. et alia, *From Crisis to Competence*, pages 126ff; Rouchy, S., Beef marketing within an international competition, in: Hallier, B. et alia, *From Crisis to Competence*, pages 132f.
7. Schiefer, G., Transparency, in: Hallier, B. et alia, *From Crisis to Competence*, pages 122f.
8. Wolfert, S. and Verdouw, C., SmartAgriFood – Future Internet for safe and healthy food from farm to fork, in: Hallier, B. et alia, *From Crisis to Competence*, page 124.
9. Martini, D., A backbone infrastructure to tracking and tracing systems, in: Hallier, B. et alia, *From Crisis to Competence*, pages 141ff.

4 Processing, Storage, and Transportation of Milk Products

Farwa Tariq, Aysha Sameen, Tayyaba Tariq, and Mariam Aizad

CONTENTS

4.1   INTRODUCTION

Technology is the science and the application of scientific, economic, as well as sociological, knowledge and legal rules to produce raw materials and their further processing into semi-finished and finished good. Technology reflects the relationship between the object, the means, and the labor in a process, as well as the individual unit operations in the production process. During the development of a technology into an independent branch of science, a further categorization takes place. We distinguish between the technology of material processing (mechanical technology) and the technology of material conversion (chemical and biological technology). Specialized areas have been developed, such as biotechnology and food technology, wherein you can find dairy technology.

4.1.1   DAIRY TECHNOLOGY

Dairy technology can be defined as a combination of theoretical and practical knowledge based on a scientific background, and the control of processes for the treatment and conversion of milk into milk products. With the increasing variety of milk products, as well as the innovations in machinery and plant design, the basic technologies for dairy processing are constantly being modified. The movement toward electronic data processing, modern separation techniques (like ultrafiltration, reverse osmosis or electro dialysis), aseptic filling technology or biotechnology, and the constantly changing consumer requirements with regard to product quality and safety are controlling the development of the dairy industry [1].

4.1.2   DAIRY TECHNOLOGY AND PAKISTAN

The current energy crisis in Pakistan effects different sectors of the business community including the dairy business. The Food and Agriculture Organization's (FAO) published data of 2010 increased the interest regarding the composition of milk, especially buffalo milk, by revealing that it has a 63% contribution in national milk production. It's far more essential to know for the maximum value the additions in the dairy food chain as the nutrients now most effective determine the nutritional cost of milk for human consumption, but also help to define marketplace strategies for different age groups, like toddlers and adolescents, lactating mothers, young adults engaged in tough jobs, or elderly human beings. In Pakistan and around the world, buffaloes are the most important source of milk for human consumption. Its popularity and high consumption is due to their rich sources of lipids, protein, lactose, and minerals, and easy availability.

Nutritional value and suitability in preparation of traditional and industrial dairy products has secured the important value of buffalo milk for long time.

Annual milk production in Pakistan is 35.5 billion liters, making it amongst the leading top ten milk producers in the world [2]. Pakistan is considered the second largest goat and buffalo milk producer worldwide with 0.7 and 22.3 billion liters production, respectively. Shares of buffalo milk are the highest (62.8%), followed by goat (2.0%), cow (34.9%), sheep (0.1%), and camel (0.2%). As far as the dairy industry is concerned in Pakistan, it is an unrecognized sector where the share of formal sector for industrial processing is only 3%–4% of the total national milk production processed by very few national and multinational companies, such as Haleeb, Nestle, Engro, Gourmet, Noon, Halla, and Shakargaj [2].

The dairy technology sector remained under developed and ignored for several decades while among the domains of agriculture, but now the situation is changing due to increased internal mobility of investors with great interest and it is becoming a priority area in food technology. The Ministry of Livestock and Dairy Development was also created to show the enhanced recognition of the importance of this sector. The businesses community of different sectors of Pakistan has been badly affected by the current energy crisis (electricity and gas), particularly textiles industries, and has started to shift towards dairy business [3].

4.2 BUFFALO MILK COMPOSITION

According to the definition from the The United States Department of Agriculture (USDA) [4], water buffalo milk is the normal lacteal secretion practically free of colostrum, obtained by the complete milking of one or more healthy water buffalo. It is one of richest natural products from a compositional point of view, since it is characterized by high fat, ash, proteins, caseins, total solids, and lactose contents as compared to goat, camel, cow, and human milk. The high solid content of buffalo milk not only makes it ideal for dairy product's processing, but also saves energy in conducting that process. Cheeses and yogurts made from buffalo milk are naturally thick-set without recourse to adding additional gelling agents and milk proteins. Dairies love to work with buffalo milk as it makes the best mozzarella. The richness and smooth texture of buffalo milk helps to convert it in a truly wonderful range of multiple award-winning products [4].

4.2.1 PROTEINS

Buffalo milk contains higher protein content as compared to cow milk [3,5]. Total protein consists of higher caseins content (~80%) as compared to whey proteins (~20%) with traces of minor proteins [6,7]. Whey and minor protein content is higher in colostrum as compared to mature milk. Cow milk and buffalo milk contains equal proportions of whey proteins, and the amino acid composition of buffalo α-lactoglobulin (α-Lg) is similar to that of cow milk [8]. Buffalo milk contains higher lactoferrin content than cow milk [9].

4.2.2 FAT

Buffalo milk is almost twice as rich in fat than cow milk and is responsible or higher nutritive and energy value. It has an average value of 8.3% but can increase up to 15% under normal conditions [10]. Kundi buffalo contain significantly low-quantity saturated fatty acid content (66.96 g·100 g^{-1}) than Nili-Ravi buffaloes (69.09 g·100 g^{-1}), higher monounsaturated fatty acid content (27.62 and 25.20 g·100 g) and total *trans* fatty acids (3.48 vs. 2.48) [11]. Buffalo milk fat has a higher density, melting point, saponification value, and specific gravity but lower refractive index, iodine, and acid values than cow milk fat, although they are affected by season, thermal oxidation, and stage of lactation [12]. Buffalo milk and ghee made from buffalos contain less free fatty acids than milk and ghee from cows [13,14].

4.2.3 LACTOSE

Lactose is also called milk sugar. Lactose is a disaccharide composed of galactose and glucose bonded together by glycosidic linkage. It is present in buffalo milk in a higher amount as compared to goat, cow, camel, and sheep milk. The lactase enzyme is present in the small intestine that breaks the bond to convert it into simple sugar, then it can be used by the body. Decreased activity of the lactase enzyme in the small intestine can lead to the problem of lactose digestion, also called lactose intolerance.

Complex oligosaccharides constitute a large portion of lactose in milk and perform biological functions that are closely related to their structural conformation. They are beneficial for postnatal stimulation of the immune system and gut microflora present in colon. They provide defense against viral and bacterial infections by acting as competitive inhibitors for binding sites on the intestinal epithelial surface [15,16]. Oligosaccharides level of sheep, goat, and cow are lower as compared to buffalo milk [17,18] (Table 4.1).

4.2.4 MINERALS AND VITAMINS

Buffalo milk has been reported to contain more mineral content as compared to cow milk. It is characterized by higher calcium content than in goat, camel and cow milk. Buffalo milk is also rich in phosphorous contents. Traces of carotene are buffalo milk along with higher amounts of vitamin A [23]. However, a reduction in vitamin A content is observed due to heating [24]. Many studies reported that higher vitamin C (ascorbic acid) content is present in buffalo milk than cow milk [25,26] (Table 4.2).

TABLE 4.1
General Composition of Buffalo Milk (g·kg^{-1})

Protein	Fat	Lactose	Ash	Total Solids	References
43	77	47	8	175	[19]
44	71	52	8	175	[20]
46	73	56	—	176	[21]
50	71	46	9	177	[22]

Source: Sahai, D., *Buffalo Milk: Chemistry and Processing Technology*, Shalini International (SI) Publications, Karnal, India, 1996.

TABLE 4.2
Vitamins Concentrations of Buffalo Milk

Vitamins	Concentrations
Vitamin A (IU·mL^{-1})	340
Vitamin C (ascorbic acid) (mg·L^{-1})	0.67
Riboflavin (mg·L^{-1})	1.59
Pyridoxine (mg·L^{-1})	3.25
Thiamine (mg·L^{-1})	0.2–0.5
Tocopherol (μg·g^{-1})	334.2

Source: Sahai, D., *Buffalo Milk: Chemistry and Processing Technology*, Shalini International (SI) Publications, Karnal, India, 1996.

TABLE 4.3

Concentrations of Major Enzymes in Buffalo Milk

Enzymes	Concentration
Lysozyme ($\mu g \cdot mL^{-1}$)	0.2
Xanthine oxidase (Units$\cdot mL^{-1}$)	0.1
Lactoperoxidase (Units$\cdot mL^{-1}$)	5.2–9.8
Lipase (Units$\cdot mL^{-1}$)	0.2–1.1
Ribonuclease ($\mu g \cdot mL^{-1}$)	9.8
Alkaline phosphatase (Units$\cdot mL^{-1}$)	0.1–0.2
Protease (Units$\cdot mL^{-1}$)	0.8

Source: Sahai, D., *Buffalo Milk: Chemistry and Processing Technology*, Shalini International (SI) Publications, Karnal, India, 1996.

4.2.5 ENZYMES

Buffalo milk contains numerous minor proteins having physiological functions. These minor proteins include metal-binding proteins, enzymes, vitamin-binding proteins, numerous growth factors, and enzyme inhibitors [27]. Carotene and vitamin A in different seasons are 3.0 and 67.1, 2.9 and 73.3, 1.8 and 48.1, 2.2 and 48.4 $\mu g \cdot 100$ mL^{-1} in winter, spring, summer, and autumn, respectively [28,29] (Table 4.3).

4.3 YOGURT

Yogurt is a dairy product that is widely used in many countries. Man has used this product for many centuries. Presently, yogurt is considered as a very popular dairy product in the world. According to the Code of Federal Regulations (CFR) of the United States Food and Drug Administration (US FDA), yogurt is defined as a coagulation of milk produced by culturing several dairy ingredients with a starter culture that contains lactic acid producing bacteria, such as *Streptococcus thermophilus* and *Lactobacillus bulgaricus* [30].

In India, approximately 7% of the milk production is used for yogurt making, and similarly in Bangladesh and Pakistan 4% of milk produced is used for yogurt production [31,32]. There are various types of yogurt that depend on the methods of production, flavors, and post-incubation processes. Based on fat content, there are three major types of yogurt, which according to legal standards, are full fat, medium, and low-fat yogurt [33].

According to the physical structure of coagulum and method of production, yogurt is classified into two types, set and stirred types [34]. The set type of yogurt is formed by coagulation of milk in retail containers, and, in this way, a continuous semi-solid product is formed. While a stirred type of yogurt is formed by coagulation of milk, then its gel structure is broken down before cooling and packaging. Low viscosity is produced in stirred yogurt, which can be considered a fluid yoghurt [35]. Health conscious consumers prefer to use low-calorie yogurt, which is also a type of yogurt, and its viscosity is improved by adding thickening agents, such as gelatin, carrageenan, and stabilizers. Natural yogurt (plain type) is a well-known traditional product and has sharp nutty flavor, which is a main characteristic of this type of yogurt. Fruit yogurts are prepared by adding fruits in the form of puree, fruit preserves, or jam when sugar, sweetening agents, colors, and synthetic flavors are added into natural or plain yogurt. In this way, flavored yogurts are prepared [36].

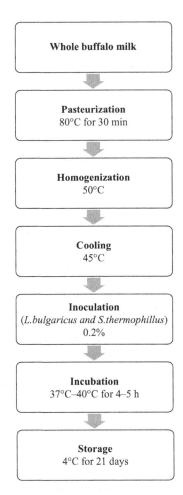

FIGURE 4.1 Flow diagram for yogurt production. (From Hashim, I.B. et al., *J. Dairy Sci.*, 92, 5403–5407, 2009.)

4.3.1 Yogurt Production

Milk sugar lactose is broken down into a lactic acid, which maintains the pH below 5 and causes casein micelles (hydrophobic protein) to lose its tertiary structure due to the protonation of its amino acid residues. The semi-solid texture of yogurt is formed by reassembling denatured proteins with hydrophobic molecules and intermolecular interaction of caseins [37] (Figure 4.1).

4.3.2 Storage and Transportation

Incubation is carried out at 43°C for 4 hours after packing in plastic cups. After the yogurt is prepared, it is stored at 4°C for further analysis [38]. Transportation is carried out in containers with low temperatures.

4.4 CHEESE

Pakistan is the fifth largest milk producer in the world. The traditional cheese of Pakistan is known as "Paneer" (acid cheese), which is unprocessed and mostly used in Pakistani cuisine and sweets. After Paneer, the second most produced cheese is Cheddar cheese. The manufacturing of Mozzarella was started few years ago and its main consumption is as a pizza topping. All cheeses are mainly produced from cow milk, buffalo milk, or a mixture of both. A combination of Mozzarella and Cheddar cheeses as pizza topping ingredients is preferred by the pizza lovers of Pakistan.

Cheese is another concentrated and fermented dairy product obtained from curd, which is produced after casein coagulation in the presence of lactic acid producing bacteria and enzyme [39]. This product is made either from goat milk, bovine milk, sheep milk, camel milk, or mixture of two types of milk [40]. Vitamins, protein, minerals, fat, and essential amino acids are present in an abundance in cheese. But cow milk and camel milk cheese has low cholesterol levels and lactose while their vitamin contents are high. Allergic people prefer to eat fermented dairy products as compared to raw milk sources [41]. Harmful disease-causing microbes are prevented by a process called fermentation. In addition, fermented milk products have more nutrition and health benefits as compared to fresh raw milks. Many dairy products are preserved by lactic acid fermentation [42–44]. The pH of the milk is reduced by a process called acidification during dairy products manufacturing. Chemical composition of cow milk and camel milk are different, therefore lactic fermentation of both shows different behavior at microbiological, biochemical, and structural levels [45].

The variety of cheese determines the shelf life of cheese, which is 4–5 days to 5 years [40]. For the production of cheese, one third of the total world milk production is used and available in different qualities and flavors [46]. From camel milk, the production of cheese is difficult because of its weak clotting ability, weak curd formation, and longer coagulation time as total solid contents of camel milk are low as compared to bovine milk. Solution of this problem is achieved either by the addition of calcium chloride to strengthen curd formation or by the addition of bacterial culture with rennet or by the addition of camel gastric enzyme [47–50]. Low concentration of kappa casein and large casein micelles mask the functions of rennet in camel milk as compared to bovine, therefore the coagulation problem is encountered [51]. The function of kappa casein is to enhance the coagulation of milk and stabilize the casein micelles structure. Only 3% concentration of kappa casein is present in camel milk, while in cow milk its concentration is about 13% of the total milk protein [52] (Figure 4.2).

4.4.1 Types of Cheeses

According to International Dairy Federation, around 500 varieties of cheese are known [52]. These varieties are categorized based on different standards, such as country or region of origin, source of milk, fat content, techniques of preparation, texture, and length of aging. Globally, combinations are preferred, and no single method of preparation is used, mostly [53]. The most familiar and frequently used approach is based on moisture content, that's then in addition to distinguished through fat content material and curing or ripening techniques [54]. The following are types of cheeses:

4.4.1.1 Moisture Content (Soft to Hard)

Categorizing cheeses by firmness is a common but inexact practice. The lines between "soft," "semi-soft," "semi-hard," and "hard" are arbitrary, and many types of cheese are made in softer or firmer variations. The main factor that controls cheese hardness is moisture content, which depends largely on the pressure with which it is packed into molds, and on its aging time [55].

4.4.1.2 Fresh, Whey, and Stretched Curd Cheeses

The main factor in the categorization of these cheeses is their age. Fresh cheeses without additional preservatives can spoil in a matter of days.

4.4.1.3 Content (Double Cream, Goat, Ewe, and Water Buffalo)

Some cheeses are classified by the source of the milk used to prepare them or by the additional fat content of the milk from which they are produced. While a large portion of the world's commercially available cheese is produced using cow's milk, numerous parts of the world also make cheese

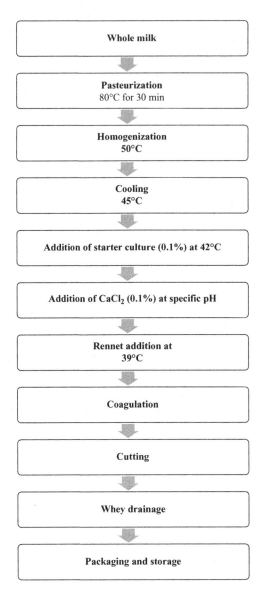

FIGURE 4.2 Flow diagram for cheese preparation. (From Ye, R. and Harte, F., *J. Dairy Sci.*, 96, 799–805, 2013.)

from goats and sheep. Double cream cheeses are soft cheeses of cow's milk enriched with cream, so their fat content is 60% or, in the case of triple creams, 75%. The utilization of the expressions "double" or "triple" is not intended to give a quantitative reference to the alteration in fat substance, since the fat content of whole cow's milk is 3%–4% [56].

4.4.1.4 Soft-Ripened and Blue-Vein

There are at least three main categories of cheese in which the presence of mold is a significant feature:

- Washed rind cheeses
- Soft ripened cheeses
- Blue cheeses [57]

4.4.1.5 Processed Cheese

Processed cheese is made from traditional cheeses of various ages and degrees of maturity in the presence of emulsifying salts, often with the addition of preservatives, more salt, food colors, and other dairy and non-dairy ingredients followed by heating and constant blending to shape a consistent product with a broadened time span of usability. This type of cheese is low-cost, reliable, and melts smoothly. It is available in many varieties and it is sold either sliced or unsliced in packages. It is also available in aerosol cans in some countries. The processed cheese originated in the early twentieth century [58–61].

In the United States, processed cheese is a broad term used to describe several categories of cheese as defined by the Code of Federal Regulations (CFR). According to the CFR, the difference between these categories is due to different requirement of minimum moisture content, minimum final pH, and the number and quality of optional ingredients that can be used [62]. Pasteurized processed cheese spread (PCS), pasteurized processed cheese food (PCF), and pasteurized processed cheese (PC) are the three main categories defined by CFR [63].

The versatility of processed cheese can be ascribed to its distinctive functional properties (when added in a specific food), which indicate the performance of the cheese amid all phases of preparation and consumption of the food and would ultimately contribute to the taste as well as the aesthetic appeal of that prepared-food [64] (Figure 4.3).

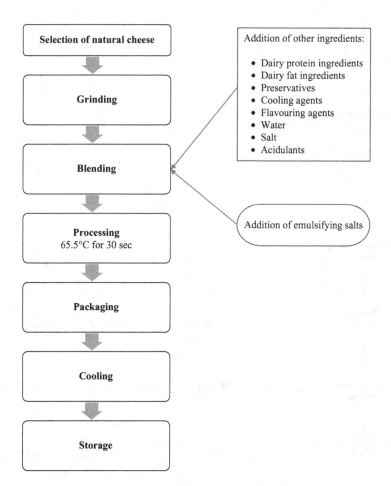

FIGURE 4.3 Flow diagram for process cheese preparation. (From Kapoor, R. and Metzger, L.E., *Compr. Rev. Food Sci. Food Saf.*, 7, 194–214, 2008.)

4.4.1.6 Cheddar Cheese

Cheddar cheese was conventionally produced as large cylindrical-shaped loaves with a weight of around 30 kg, but, nowadays, cheese is produced in rectangular blocks in the modern industrial process to facilitate the handling of the cheese. Cheddar is classified as a hard cheese because it has approximately 55% of moisture on a fat-free basis (MFFB). It has a closed structure due to the absence of any gas holes because it uses homo-fermentative starter cultures. The consistency of Cheddar cheese is stiff and powdery due to its firm and short texture. Its color ranges from white or ivory to light yellow or orange and has a long shelf life [65] (Figure 4.4).

4.4.1.7 Mozzarella Cheese

Mozzarella cheese is a soft, unripened cheese variety of the Pasta-filata family, which had its origin in the Battipaglia region of Italy [67]. Conventionally, Mozzarella cheese was prepared from buffalo

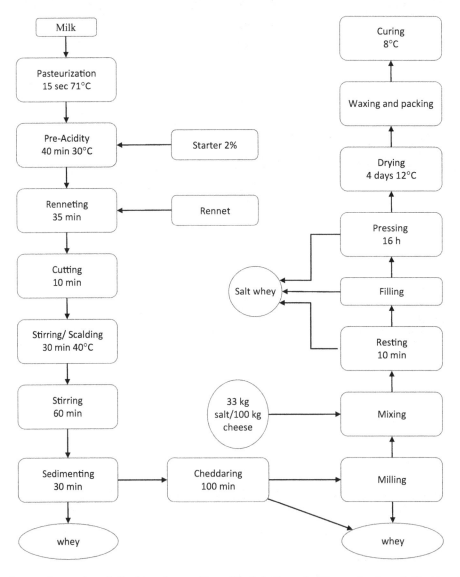

FIGURE 4.4 Processing of Cheddar cheese. (From Khaled, N. et al., The production of Cheddar cheese, 2015.)

milk but, nowadays, with appropriate modifications it is produced from cow milk in the US, Italy, and other European countries [68]. Mozzarella cheese is appreciated for its stretch property and it has white, soft with a glossy surface, which makes it suitable for the preparation of lasagna, veal cutlet alla Parmigiana, and as a topping on pizza [69,70]. Owing to its stretching property, Mozzarella cheese is used as a topping on pizza pie. The production of Mozzarella cheese has greatly increased due to the popularity of the pizza parlor, especially amongst youngsters. In Italy, the contribution of Mozzarella and pizza cheeses accounts for 78% of the total Italian cheese product [71] (Figure 4.5).

4.4.1.8 Pizza Cheese

Any type of cheese suitable for use on pizza can be referred as pizza cheese. This type includes many varieties of cheeses that are specifically manufactured and designed for pizza toppings. Due to an increase in pizza consumption globally, large varieties of cheeses produced in the US and other countries are used as ingredients on pizza [73]. The most popular varieties are natural Mozzarella. Cheddar, Mozzarella alternatives, and processed and modified cheeses (Figure 4.6).

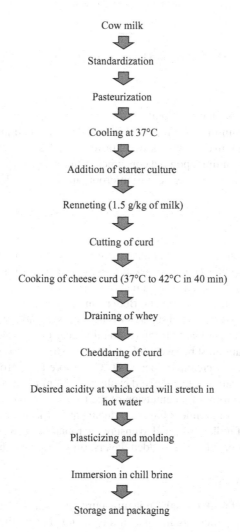

Cow milk

⬇

Standardization

⬇

Pasteurization

⬇

Cooling at 37°C

⬇

Addition of starter culture

⬇

Renneting (1.5 g/kg of milk)

⬇

Cutting of curd

⬇

Cooking of cheese curd (37°C to 42°C in 40 min)

⬇

Draining of whey

⬇

Cheddaring of curd

⬇

Desired acidity at which curd will stretch in
hot water

⬇

Plasticizing and molding

⬇

Immersion in chill brine

⬇

Storage and packaging

FIGURE 4.5 Processing of Mozzarella cheese. (From Jana, A.H. and Mandal, P.K., *Int. J. Dairy Sci.*, 6, 199–226, 2011.)

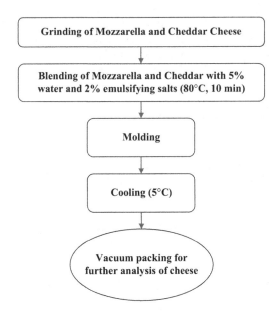

FIGURE 4.6 Processing of pizza cheese. (From Govindasamy, L. et al., *J. Texture Stud.*, 36, 190–212, 2005.)

4.5 LASSI

Lassi/stirred Dahi is a common name of buttermilk, mainly popular in Pakistan and North India. It is considered a refreshing summer beverage. Lassi is slightly acidic, liquid viscous, sweet, or salty in taste, white to creamy white in color with a sweet taste and rich aroma. It can be flavored with salt or sugar and other spices depending upon the consumer preference. Lassi is prepared using pasteurized milk cultured with flavor producing culture microorganisms [74,75].

4.6 BUTTER

Butter, a fat rich dairy-based product made by churning and containing 80% fat content that is partially crystallized. Butter preparation is one of the oldest methods of preserving the fat component of milk. History reveals that its manufacturing dates back to some of the earliest historical records and reference has been made to the use of butter as a human food and medicine, for cosmetic purpose, and in sacrificial worship long before the Christian era. Butter can be manufactured from the milk of buffalo, cow, ewe, camel, mares, and goat. A cream separator is used for separating fat from milk in the form of cream. The cream can be either purchased from a fluid milk dairy or separated from whole milk by the butter manufacturer. The cream must be sweet (pH more than 6.6), free from off flavors, not oxidized, and not rancid. Pasteurization of cream is done at 80°C or more to destroy microbes and enzymes. Butter can be defined as the fatty product derived exclusively from milk of the buffalo and/or cow or its products principally in the form of an emulsion of the type water-in-oil. It can be with or without added salt and starter cultures of harmless flavor producing and/or lactic acid bacteria. Adequate heat treatment or pasteurization of milk is essential to ensure microbial safety for butter preparation. It must be free from vegetable oil, animal body fat, added flavors, off flavor, rancidity, and mineral oil [76].

4.6.1 Composition of Butter

Butter is mainly composed of milk fat, salt, moisture, curd, and salt. It also comprises some amount of acids, lactose, air, enzymes, microorganisms, vitamins, and phospholipids. The portion of principal constituents in butter is mainly influenced by the method and techniques followed by the manufacturer, and this in turn is chiefly regulated to conform to the standards of butter [77] (Table 4.4).

TABLE 4.4
Constituents of Butter

Constituents	Quantity (% w/w)
Fat	80–83
Moisture	15.5–16.0
Salt	0–3
Curd	1–1.5

4.6.2 PRODUCTION OF BUTTER

4.6.2.1 Preparation of Cream

Cultured as well as sweet cream can be used for the preparation of commercial butter. However, butter manufactured from sweet cream is most preferred because it results in sweet buttermilk having more economic value than sour butter made from the churning of sour/cultured cream (Figure 1.2). Cream should be neutralized to 0.06% lactic acid to produce butter for long storage and to 0.3% lactic acid to produce butter for early consumption. Then adjust the fat percentage of cream to 35%–40% fat. Heat the neutralized and standardized cream to 95°C for 15 seconds and cool it to 9°C (Figure 4.7).

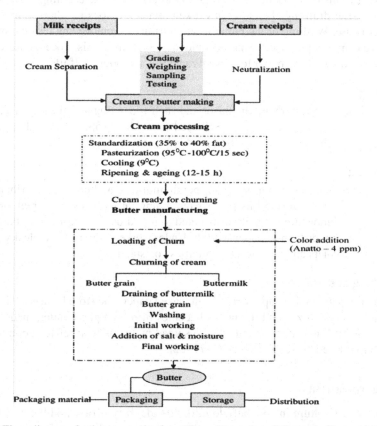

FIGURE 4.7 Flow diagram for butter production. (From Deosarkar, S.S. et al., Butter: Manufacture, In: Caballero, B., Finglas, P., Toldrá, F. (Eds.), *The Encyclopedia of Food and Health*, London, UK, 2016.)

4.6.2.2   Ripening

Ripening refers to the process of the fermentation of cream with the help of a suitable starter culture. In the case of the production of sweet cream butter, ripening can be eliminated. The key purpose of ripening the cream is to manufacture butter with greater diacetyl content. A starter culture comprising of a mixture of both flavor producing (*Leuconostoccitrovorum*, *Leuc. Dextranicum* and/or *S. diacetylactis*) and acid producing (*S. cremories* and *Streptococcus lactis*) is added. The quantity of starter culture depends on various factors and is incubated at 21°C for achieving desired acidity. Then the cream is cooled down to 5°C–100°C to achieve more acid development.

4.6.2.3   Aging

Cream is stored at a cool temperature to crystallize the butter fat globules and to ensuring proper churning and texture of the butter. In the aging tank, it is ensured that required cooling is achieved to give the fat the required crystalline structure. For aging, 12–15 hours are required. From the aging tank, the cream is pumped to the churn or continuous butter making machine via a plate heat exchanger, which brings it to the requisite temperature.

4.6.2.4   Churning

Cream is agitated, and eventually butter granules form, grow larger, and coalesce. In the end, there are two phases left: a semisolid mass of butter, and the liquid left over, which is the buttermilk.

4.6.2.5   Draining and Washing

As far as traditional churning is concerned, the machine stops when grains achieve the required size then buttermilk is drained off. With the continuous butter maker, the draining of the buttermilk is also continuous. After draining, the butter is worked to a continuous fat phase containing a finely dispersed water phase. Washing of the butter after churning to remove any residual milk solids or buttermilk was a common practice but has become rare nowadays. This process ensures that all the buttermilk is washed out of the butter to prevent rancidity and poor shelf life.

4.6.2.6   Salting

Common salt is helpful in improving the flavor and shelf life acting as a preservative. Further, the butter is worked to improve its consistency. Salt used should be 99.5%–99.8% sodium chloride, and microbial count should be less than 10/g. Salt is added at the rate of 2%–2.5%.

4.6.2.7   Working

The main purpose of working butter is to incorporate moisture and uniform distribution of added salt and moisture in butter. During this process remaining fat globules also break up and form a continuous phase, and moisture is finally distributed to retard bacterial growth in butter. It is safer to slightly over-work butter than to under-work it. Under-worked butter may be leaky in body with large visible water droplets and may develop "mottles" on standing.

4.6.2.8   Packing and Storage

The butter is finally patted into shape, wrapped in waxed paper, and stored in a cool dry place. As it cools, the butterfat crystallizes and the butter becomes firm. Whipped butter, made by whipping air or nitrogen gas into soft butter, is intended to spread more easily at refrigeration temperatures. Normally, butter is stored at −23°C to −29°C [79–82].

4.6.3   CLARIFIED BUTTER

An addition of yogurt culture in cow/buffalo milk provides a type of liquid butter called clarified butter. For preparation of clarified butter, typically a simmering of butter is done that is obtained by churning from cream (which is made by churning yogurt traditionally). After simmering, impurities

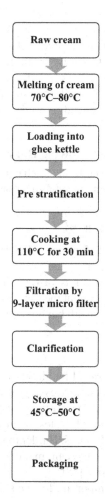

FIGURE 4.8 Clarified butter processing. (From Kessler, H.G., Food and bio process engineering, In: *Dairy Technology*, Munich, Germany, 2002.)

are skimmed from the surface, then the clear liquid fat is poured and retained while the solid residue that has settled to the bottom is discarded. Clarified butter can be flavored by adding spices. The quality of butter, the milk source used for manufacturing, and the duration of boiling time determines the color, texture, and taste of ghee. Clarified butter has been popular in the Asian Subcontinent (Pakistan, Bangladesh, and India) and across the world for centuries. Its nutritional profile reveals a rich source of good quality lipids, fat soluble vitamins, and essential fatty acids. Compositionally, it contains 62% monounsaturated fats and rich in conjugated linoleic acid (CLA) and vitamin A [83] (Figure 4.8).

4.7 ICE CREAM

4.7.1 WHAT IS ICE CREAM?

The consumption of frozen desserts is present in different types. The dairy ice creams are the combination of the different ingredients, like aerated sugar syrup which has no milk and no fat, as well as sugar, flavors, and so on.

4.7.1.1 Definition of Terms

Ice cream is defined a legal way from country to country. In Canada, ice cream contains no less than 8% milk fat, and in the US no less than 10% milk fat [85]. The industries in the United Kingdom (UK) offer different types of ice cream to consumers. To be given the authentic label of ice cream, "The product which have not less than 2.5% milk protein and prepare by the sugar, solid milk and fat emulsion, nor any other ingredient is added as well as restricted about any type of freezing, evaporation, heat treatment" [86].

4.7.1.2 A "Dairy Ice Cream" Has the Following Definition

The word ice cream is not given to any other food which cannot fulfill the requirements like no less than 5% milk fat, no fat other than milk fat, any stabilizer or flavoring agent [86].

4.7.2 How Much Is the Industry Worth?

Globally, ice cream's estimated worth is £35 billion—UK £1.48 billion and US £13 billion. Nestle and Unilever are big producers of ice cream.

However, globally the demand of ice cream is vast, the industry seeks out new innovative ideas for the consumer. They also have concerns about the improved health and about obesity. It is necessary for ice cream production to improve health but not compromise on texture and taste [87].

4.7.3 Ice Cream Manufacturing

The polyphasic system of ice cream consists of fat globules, air bubbles, and ice crystals. Its unfrozen portion is popular as a matrix. All these phases aggregate and give the structure of ice cream. The size of air bubbles and ice crystals is 20–50 μm. Fats droplets make a layer around the air bubbles, and emulsifier layer covers these air bubbles. In a frozen concentrated solution, the matrix portion comprises of polysaccharides and sugars. Hardening, freezing, aging, homogenization, pasteurization, and blending are the steps of ice cream manufacturing. In all these steps, the structure of ice cream will be continuously developed [88].

These manufacturing steps are very important for the stability and development of microstructure. Manufacturing is done in two stages: first is mix preparation and the other is freezing operation. Ingredients blending, pasteurization, homogenization, cooling, and aging are the steps of the mixing preparation. Once the ripening of mixing is done, then freezing operation will be start.

This produces millions of 12 little air bubbles; two separate phase and ice crystals are scattered into the concentrated mixture through batch/continuous process of freezing. Then the process includes packing the ice cream, hardening is done, storing it, and preparing for distribution [88,89].

4.7.3.1 Blending

First, a desired formulation has been decided, choose the ingredients and weight it. Blend the ingredients in the blending tank. The tank consists of agitator and mixers. These mixers and agitator are used for the incorporation of powders and mix with liquid solution at high speed. Two types of ingredients are the dry ingredients and wet ingredients. Dry ingredients are stabilizers, emulsifiers, flavorings, and whey powder, and wet ingredients are melted vegetable oils, cream, and water [90].

4.7.3.2 Pasteurization

After the blending process, the mix is pasteurized. The purpose of pasteurization is to decrease the microorganism to an acceptable level and safe for human use. The pasteurization process is different according to the safety laws from country to country and manufacturer to manufacturer.

For example, pasteurization of ice cream mix is at the temperature of 83°C for 20 seconds [91]. The pasteurization temperature should not increase 85°C, because high temperatures damage the milk protein [87].

4.7.3.3 Homogenization

After pasteurization, homogenization takes place. A small valve pressurizes the pasteurize mixer at 2000 psi. At this is pressure, the large fat globules are split into small droplets and produce a fine emulsion. The size of fat droplets is approximately 1 μm or less in diameter that occupy a large surface area. In ice cream mixes, usually two stages homogenization are chosen because this decreases clustering of the fat, makes thin emulsion, and helps the meltdown rate and increase air stability. The objective of the homogenization is to decrease the mass of fat globules (~2 μm) resulting in the high constancy of the fat during the ageing process [92].

4.7.3.4 Ageing

Homogenized mixes have been cooled by cooling at 4°C so bacterial growth is prevented. After this, it is transported to an ageing tank for 4–24 hours [89]. Foaming in ice cream is increased three times by the ageing process. This results in a better final product due to:

- Fat crystallizations improved
- Emulsification power is enhanced
- Protein hydration results in high viscosity [93]

4.7.3.5 Freezing

After aging, the mix is transported into a continuous freezer operating at 18°C to −22°C. It is also called as barrel freezer. Rotating blades are attached in the barrel tank, which helps the whipping mixture detach from the inner walls of the barrel. Proper aeration is done by continuously supplying air. Air bubbles make the ice cream foamy. The air content of ice cream is called over run. The product is ready for packaging, and then sends for next processing [94].

4.7.3.6 Hardening

Hardening of ice cream is done in a blast freezer at the temperature of −30°C to −40°C. Hardening should be rapid for heat transfer. Hardening is the removal of heat from the whipped ice cream [95]. Ice crystals in ice cream are prevented by the following factors:

- Temperature of the blast freezer
- Type and size of container
- Initial temperature of ice cream
- Rate of aeration in blast freezer

4.8 STORAGE AND TRANSPORTATION OF DAIRY PRODUCTS

The shelf life of the dairy products depends upon the type of processing, packaging, and storage. Unrefrigerated temperatures of the product change the freshness period, and container type is the other factors that affect the shelf life. Shelf life of cheese varies for hard/soft, cut/wax coated. The cut surface of the cheese should be wrapped in a plastic sheet. Cheese should be stored in its original packaging. Shipping of the cheese should be done in double jacket containers at temperatures below 1°C [96] (Figure 4.9).

Product	Shelf Life	
	After Opening Temp/Time	Unopened Temp/Time
Milk	35° 1 week	35° 10-14 days
Cream	35° 1 week	35° 2 weeks
Whipping Cream	35° 1 week	35° 2 weeks
Half & Half	35° 1 week	35° 2 weeks
Butter	35° 2 weeks	35° 4 weeks
Natural Cheese	35° 1-3 weeks	35° 1-4 weeks
Processed Cheese	35° 5 weeks	35° 24 weeks
Cottage Cheese	35° 7-10 days	35° 18 days
Cream Cheese	35° 10-14 days	35° 3 months
Sour Cream	35° 1 week	35° 2 weeks
Yogurt (plain)	35° 3 weeks	35° 4 weeks

FIGURE 4.9 Recommended dairy storage guidelines. (From American Dairy Association, Storing dairy products, Available at https://www.in.gov/boah/files/milkstore.pdf, 2018.)

4.9 CONCLUSION

Foods of animal origin, especially milk, have been used by human beings since prehistoric times. They contain essential nutrients for growth and health maintenance. Pakistan is one of the top milk producers worldwide, but unfortunately a small percentage of it is used for processing at industrial level. Most of it is consumed as loose milk or discarded after spoilage. Trends of milk processing into useful products must be increased as it not only increases its shelf life, but also enhances consumer acceptability and intake of milk and milk products. This can lead to better nutritional status of the population and improved economic condition of the country.

REFERENCES

1. Spreer E (2017) *Milk and Dairy Product Technology.* Abingdon, UK: Routledge.
2. FAOSTAT (2010) Food and Agriculture Organization of the United Nations. Available on http://faostat.fao.org/site/569/default.aspx#ancor. Accessed June 8, 2018.
3. Ahmad S, Anjum FM, Huma N et al. (2013) Composition and physico-chemical characteristics of buffalo milk with particular emphasis on lipids, proteins, minerals, enzymes and vitamins. *J Anim Plant Sci* 23:62–74.
4. USDA (United States Department of Agriculture) (2011) Milk for manufacturing purposes and its production and processing: Recommended requirements. Available on http://www.ams.usda.gov/AMSv1.0/getfile?dDocName=STELDEV3004791. Accessed June 8, 2018.

5. Ragab MT, Asker AA, Kamal TH (1958) The effect of age and seasonal calving on the composition of Egyptian buffalo milk. *Indian J Dairy Sci* 11:18–28.
6. Laxminarayana H, Dastur NN (1968) Buffaloe's milk and milk products – Part I. *Dairy Sci Abst* 30:177–186.
7. Sirry I, Salama FA, Salam AE et al. (1984) Studies on the physico-chemical properties of skim and standardized cow and buffalo milk. I. Effect of heating. *Deutsche Lebensmittel-Rundschau* 8:242–245.
8. Mawal RB, Barnbas T, Barnbas J (1965) Identification of cow β-lactoglobulin 'B' and buffalo β-lactoglobulin. *Nature* 205:175–176.
9. Sahai D (1996) *Buffalo Milk: Chemistry and Processing Technology.* Karnal, India: Shalini International (SI) Publications.
10. Varrichio ML, Di Francia A, Masucci F et al. (2007) Fatty acid composition of Mediterranean buffalo milk fat. *Italian J Animal Sci* 6:509–511.
11. Talpur FN, Memon NN, Bhanger MI (2007) Comparison of fatty acid and cholesterol content of Pakistani water buffalo breeds. *Pak J Anal Environ Chem* 8:15–20.
12. Angelo IA, Jain MK (1982) Physico-chemical properties of ghee prepared from the milk of cows and buffaloes fed with cottonseed. *Indian J Dairy Sci* 35:519–525.
13. Pantulu PC, Ramamurthy MK (1982) Lipid composition of skimmed milk and whey. *Asian J Dairy Res* 1:17–20.
14. Lal D, Narayanan KM (1983) Effect of lactation number on fatty acid and physico-chemical constants of milk fats. *Asian J Dairy Res* 2:191–195.
15. Kunz C, Rudloff S, Baier W et al. (2000) Oligosaccharides in human milk. Structural, functional and metabolic aspects. *Ann Rev Nutr* 20:699–722.
16. Kunz C, Rudloff S (2002) Health benefits of milk- derived carbohydrates. *Bull Int Dairy Fed* 375:72–79.
17. Urashima T, Murata S, Nakamura T (1997) Structural determination of momosialyltrisaccharides obtained from caprineclostrum. *Comp Biochem Physiol* 11:431–435.
18. Martinez-Ferez A, Rudloff S, Guadix A et al. (2006). Goat's milk as a natural source of lactose-derived oligosaccharides: Isolation by membrane technology. *Int Dairy J* 16:173–181.
19. Altman PL, Dittmer DK (1961) *Biological Handbook: Blood and Other Body Fluids.* Federation of American Societies for Experimental Biological, Washington, DC.
20. Ahmad S, Gaucher I, Rousseau F et al. (2008) Effects of acidification on physicochemical characteristics of buffalo milk: A comparison with cow's milk. *Food Chem* 106:11–17.
21. Menard O, Ahmad S, Rousseau F et al. (2010) Buffalo vs. cow milk fat globules: Size distribution, zeta-potential, compositions in total fatty acids and in polar lipids from the milk fat globule membrane. *Food Chem* 120:544–551.
22. Han X, Lee FL, Zhang L et al. (2012) Chemical composition of water buffalo milk and its low-fat symbiotic yogurt development. *Funct Food Health Dis* 2:86–106.
23. Narayanan KM, Paul TM, Anantakrishnan CP et al. (1952) Studies on vitamin A in milk. V. The vitamin A content of buffalo colostrum. *Indian J Dairy Sci* 5:45–50.
24. El-Abd MM, Ragab FH, Abd El Gawad IA et al. (1986) Study on vitamin A in milk and some milk products. *Ann Agr Sci* 24:2129–2147.
25. Singh SP, Gupta MP (1986) Influence of certain treatments on the ascorbic acid content of buffaloes' and cows' milk. *Indian Dairyman* 38:379–381.
26. Mohammad KS, Talib WA, Kashab LA (1990) Some water vitamins in different types of milk and their stabilities towards light and oxygen. *Egyp J Dairy Sci* 18:43–56.
27. Fox PF (2001) Milk proteins as food ingredients. *Int J Dairy Technol* 54:41–55.
28. Narayanan KM, Anantakrishnan CP, Sen KC (1956) Co-vitamin studies. I. Variations in tocopherol, carotene and vitamin A contents in milk and butterfat of cows and buffaloes. *Indian J Dairy Sci* 9:44–51.
29. Ibrahim EM, Mohran MA, Said MR (1983) Seasonal variation in fat, carotene and vitamin A contents of milk from buffaloes and cows herds. *J Agri Sci* 14:195–206.
30. Bourlioux P, Pochart P (1988) Nutritional and health properties of yogurt. In *Aspects of Nutritional Physiology* Basel, Switzerland: Karger Publishers, pp. 217–258.
31. Chakraborty M (1998) A study on the preparation of dahi from whole milk of cow, buffalo and their different proportionate mixture. MS Thesis, Bangladesh Agricultural University, Mymensingh, India.
32. Mustafa M (1997) A study on the preparation of fruit Dahi (Yoghurt). MSc Thesis, Bangladesh Agricultural University, Mymensingh, India.
33. FAO/WHO (1973) Code of principles concerning milk and milk products. CX 5/70, 16th Session, Rome, Italy.

34. Hasler CM, Kundrat S, Wool D (2000) Functional foods and cardiovascular disease. *Current Atherosclerosis Reports* 2:467–475.
35. Correia RTP, Borges KC (2009) Posicionamentodoconsumidorfrenteaoconsumo de leite de cabra e seusderivadosnacidade de Natal-RN. *Revista do Instituto de LaticíniosCândidoTostes* 64:36–43.
36. Dave RI, Shah NP (1998) Ingredients supplementation affects viability of probiotic bacteria in yogurt. *J Dairy Sci* (In press).
37. Zourari A, Accolas JP, Desmazeaud MJ (1992) Metabolism and biochemical characteristics of yogurt bacteria: A review. *Le lait* 72:1–34.
38. Hashim IB, Khalil AH, Afifi HS (2009) Quality characteristics and consumer acceptance of yogurt fortified with date fiber. *J Dairy Sci* 92:5403–5407.
39. Fox PF, Guinee TP, Cogan TM et al. (2000) *Fundamentals of Cheese Science.* Aspen, Gaithersburg, MD.
40. Herrington BL (2000) *Milk and Milk Processing.* New Delhi, India: Green World Publisher.
41. Abeiderrahmane N (2001) Report joint FAO Expert committee. On the code of fresh from your local drome 'dairy', htm. Food and Agriculture Organization of the United Nations
42. Thapa T (2001) Small-scale milk processing technologies: Other milk products. Discussion paper 2.2.
43. Ahmed T, Kanwal R (2004) Biochemical characteristics of lactic acid producing bacteria and preparation of camel milk cheese by using starter culture. *Pak Vet J* 24:87–91.
44. Ahmed AI, Mohammed AA, Faye B et al. (2010) Assessment of quality of camel milk and gariss, North Kordofan State, Sudan. *Res J Animal Veterinary Sci* 5:18–22.
45. Attia H, Kherouatou N (2001) Dromedary milk lactic acid fermentation: Microbiological and rheological characteristics. *J Industrial Microbiol Biotechnol* 26:263–270.
46. Farkye NY (2004) Cheese technology. *Int J Dairy Technol* 57:91–98.
47. Ramet JP (2001) The technology of making cheese from camel milk (*Camelus dromedarius*) (No. 113) Food & Agriculture Organization.
48. Mehaia MA (2006) Manufacture of fresh soft white cheese (Domiati-type) from dromedary camels milk using ultra filtration process. *J Food Technol* 4:206–212.
49. El Zubeir IE, Jabreel SO (2008) Fresh cheese from camel milk coagulated with Camifloc. *Int J Dairy Technol* 61:90–95.
50. Ibrahim A (2009) Studies on manufacture of soft cheese and fermented milk from camel's milk under the desert conditions in Egypt. PhD Thesis, Zagazig University, Zagazig Egypt.
51. Ye R, Harte F (2013) Casein maps: Effect of ethanol, pH, temperature, and CaCl 2 on the particle size of reconstituted casein micelles. *J Dairy Sci* 96:799–805.
52. Patriek FFD (2000) Fundamentals of cheese sciences. *J Sci Food Agric* 90:388.
53. Rathore B (2011) Classification of cheese. *Res J Livestock* 6:925.
54. Barbara E, Fankhausar AK, David JC (1981) *The Pocket Guide to Cheese.* 7th ed. Sydney, Australia, pp. 353–397.
55. Phillips R, Steve HB, Jenkins T (2013) *Cheese Primer.* Workman Publishing: Canada
56. Subaraman JN, Nidhi DR (2012) New era of dairy and dairy products. *J Sci Food Agric* 93:144–149.
57. Sinatara S (2008) The oldest cheese found. *J Dairy Manage* 25:189–195.
58. Charles GM (2014) The science and lore of kitchen. *Int J Food Manage* 12:43–45.
59. Meyer A (1973) *Processed Cheese Manufacture.* Silverson Mixers: London, UK.
60. Thomas MA (1973) *The Manufacture of Processed Cheese—Scientific Principles.* In *Science Bulletin.* New South Wales Department of Agriculture: Richmond, Australia.
61. Guinee TP, Caric M, Kalab M (2004) Pasteurized processed cheese and substitute/imitation cheese products. In: Fox PF (Ed.) *Cheese: Chemistry, Physics and Microbiology,* 3rd ed. Academic Press: London, UK.
62. Food and Drug Administration (2006) Food and Drug Administration. Department of Health and Human Services, Washington, DC, 21 CFR Part 133.169 to 133.180.
63. Kapoor R, Metzger LE (2008) Process cheese: Scientific and technological aspects—A review. *Compr Rev Food Sci Food Saf* 7:194–214.
64. Guinee TP (2002) The functionality of cheese as an ingredient: A review. *Aust J Dairy Sci* 57:79–91.
65. Walstra P, Geurts TJ, Noomen A et al. (2006) Milk components. *Dairy Sci Technol* 2:17–108.
66. Khaled N, Josefin L, Flavian D et al. (2015) The production of Cheddar cheese. Introduction to Dairy Technology-project work. Damanhour University, Egypt.
67. Citro V (1981) A typical local product obtained from buffalo milk. *Scienza-e-Tecnica-Lattiero-Casearia* 32:263–273.
68. Ghosh BC, Singh S, Kanawjia SK (1990) Rheological properties of mozzarella cheese: A review. *Indian J Dairy Sci* 43:70–79.

69. Kosikowski FV (1982) *Cheese and Fermented Milk Foods*. Edwards Bros: Ann Arbor, MI.
70. Jana AH (2001) Mozzarella cheese and pizza: The compatible partners. *Bev Food World* 28:14–19.
71. Merrill RK, Oberg CJ, McMahon DJ (1994) A method for manufacturing reduced fat Mozzarella cheese. *J Dairy Sci* 77:1783–1789.
72. Jana AH, Mandal PK (2011) Manufacturing and quality of Mozzarella cheese: A review. *Int J Dairy Sci* 6:199–226.
73. Mishra R, Govindasamy-Lucey S, Lucey JA (2005) Rheological properties of rannet-induced gels during the coagulation and cutting process: Impact of processing conditions. *J Texture Stud* 36:190–212.
74. Aneja RP, Vyas MN, Sharma D et al. (1989) A method for manufacturing lassi. Indian Patent no. 17374.
75. Rasane P, Kailey R, Singh SK (2017) Fermented indigenous Indian dairy products: Standards, nutrition, technological significance and opportunities for its processing. *J Pure Appl Microbiol* 11:1199–1214.
76. Frede E, Buchheim W (1994) Butter making and the churning of blended oil emulsions. *J Soc Dairy Technol* 47:17–27.
77. Bobe G, Zimmerman S, Hammond EG et al. (2007) Butter composition and texture from cows with different milk fatty acid compositions fed fish oil or roasted soybeans. *J Dairy Sci* 90:2596–2603.
78. Patton S (1952) Preparation of milk fat. 1 I. A study of some organic compounds as de-emulsifying agents. *J Dairy Sci* 35:324–328.
79. Deosarkar SS, Khedkar CD, Kalyankar SD (2016) Butter: Manufacture. In: Caballero B, Finglas P, Toldrá F (Eds.) *The Encyclopedia of Food and Health*. Academic Press: London, UK.
80. Herrmann M, Godow A, Hasse T (1995) Alternative butter production with scraped surface heat exchanger. *Deutsche Milchwirtschaft* 46:62–67.
81. Hill J (2003) The Fonterra Research Centre. *Int J Dairy Technol* 56:127–132.
82. Weissman BJ (1982) Ultrafiltration process for the preparation of cream cheese. U.S. Patent 4,341,801.
83. Ahmad N, Saleem M (2018) Studying heating effects on desi ghee obtained from buffalo milk using fluorescence spectroscopy. *PloS one* 13:0197340.
84. Kessler HG (2002) Food and bio process engineering. In: Kessler VA, (Ed.) *Dairy Technology*, Munich, Germany.
85. Goff HD, Hartel RW (2013) *Ice Cream*. Springer: New York.
86. Food Labelling Regulations (2010) Food Labelling regulations SI 1996 No. 14994, January 6, 2010, Norwich ,UK.
87. Clarke C (2008) *The Science of Ice Cream*, 3rd ed. Cambridge, UK: RSC Publishing.
88. Clarke CL, Buckley SL, Lindner N (2002) Ice structuring proteins—A new name for antifreeze proteins'. *Cryo Lett* 23:89–92.
89. Marshall RT, Goff HD, Hartel RW (2003) *Ice Cream*. Springer: New York.
90. Tharp BW, Young LS (2012) *Tharp & Young on Ice Cream: An Encyclopedic Guide to Ice Cream Science and Technology*. Destech Publications: Lancaster, PA.
91. Heuer E (2009) Formulation and stability of model food foam microstructures, PhD thesis, School of Chemical Engineering, University of Birmingham, UK.
92. Biasutti M, Venir E, Marino M (2013) Effects of high pressure homogenisation of ice cream mix on the physical and structural properties of ice cream. *International Dairy Journal* 32:40–45.
93. Goff HD (1997) Partial coalescence and structure formation in dairy emulsions. In: Damodaran S (Ed.) *Food Proteins and Lipids*. Springer: New York.
94. Huppertz T, Smiddy MA, Goff HD (2011) Effects of high pressure treatment of mix on ice cream manufacture. *International Dairy Journal* 21:718–726
95. Hui YH (2006) *Handbook of Food Science, Technology and Engineering*. Taylor & Francis Group: London, UK.
96. American Dairy Association. Storing dairy products. Available at https://www.in.gov/boah/files/milkstore.pdf. Accessed June 13, 2018.

5 Processing, Storage, and Transportation of Meat and Meat Products

Rituparna Banerjee, Arun K. Verma,
B. M. Naveena, and V. V. Kulkarni

CONTENTS

5.1 INTRODUCTION

Meat has formed a part of the human diet since ancient times. Consumption of meat runs in parallel with human development. Meat is not only considered a major source of quality protein, minerals, and vitamins, but also forms the central part of the meal and is desirable to have the appropriate quality characteristics to conform to the cultural practices followed in different parts of the world. The perishable nature of meat has led to the development of preservation techniques like drying, curing, or smoking. Later on, due to the high costs of meat or meat products and the growing demands of the increasing population, a large variety of meat products came into the market that permitted utilization of virtually every part of an animal. The increased demand that accompanies rising income has been paralleled by mounting interest in meat quality, safety, and nutritional aspects, which all give rise to appropriate legislation. The present chapter will provide a comprehensive understanding of meat composition, nutritive value, processing and preservation techniques, packaging, and guidelines for proper handling, transportation, and storage of meat and meat products.

5.2 MEAT COMPOSITION AND FUNCTION

Meat is defined by the Codex Alimentarius as "All parts of an animal that are intended for, or have been judged as safe and suitable for, human consumption." Edible animal tissues from carcasses are designated as "meat" and consist of variable amounts of muscle, adipose tissue, connective tissue, blood, blood vessels, lymphatic tissues, nerve tissue, tendons, cartilage, and bone. Meat tissues are composed of five primary chemical constituents: moisture (water), proteins, lipids (fat), carbohydrates, and inorganic matter (ash or minerals). Other components include non-protein nitrogen compounds (e.g. nucleotides, peptides, creatine, creatine phosphate, urea, etc.) and non-nitrogenous substances (e.g. vitamins, organic acids, etc.) (Table 5.1).

TABLE 5.1

Chemical Composition of Mammalian Muscle after Rigor Mortis

Composition	Wet % weight
Water	75
Protein	19
Myofibrillar	11.5
Sarcoplasmic	5.5
Stromal or connective tissue proteins	2
Lipid	2.5
Carbohydrate	1.2
Miscellaneous soluble non-protein substances	2.3
Vitamins	Minute quantity

The composition of meat tissue varies according to differences in species, physiological maturity at harvest, plane of nutrition, genetic predisposition (e.g. pale, soft, and exudative [PSE] tissue versus dark, firm, and dry [DFD] tissue), and anatomical location of cuts within a carcass. The percentages of moisture, protein, and ash decrease with increasing amounts of fat in the tissues. The percentage of carbohydrates, however, remains rather constant as the fat content of meat increases.

5.2.1 MOISTURE

In living muscle tissue, water may range from 65% to 80% of the total mass and serves as a basic component of cellular metabolism, transport medium for metabolites and waste products, thermoregulator, solvent, and as a lubricant. In postmortem muscle tissue, water is the primary component of individual cells and comprises 75%–80% of the cell mass. The myofibrils make up 75%–92% of the volume of lean muscle and play a dominant role in the water holding capacity (WHC) of the tissue. As the postmortem pH is reduced by the accumulation of lactic acid, acidification of the muscle tissue reduces the pH to 5.6–5.8. The myofibrillar protein's ability is to retain water is diminished and this may result in a corresponding increase in the percentage of protein.

5.2.2 PROTEINS

Myofibrillar, or salt-soluble proteins comprise approximately 11.5% of the total muscle proteins and can be extracted with a salt solution of ≥3 mol/L. Myosin, actin, titin, tropomyosin, troponin, nebulin, C protein, α-actinin, M protein, and desmin account for ~93% of the different contractile proteins making up the myofibril. Actomyosin (myosin and actin complex) formation during rigor mortis is one of the most important factors that influences major quality attributes; for example, the water-holding capacity of muscle tissue, intermolecular binding in a meat gel matrix (gelation), and mechanical stability of a meat emulsion.

Sarcoplasmic or water-soluble proteins account for approximately 5.5% of the total muscle proteins and are extracted with low-ionic-strength salt solutions of ~0.06 mol/L. These proteins are found in the sarcoplasm, or fluid surrounding the myofibrils, and comprise of oxidative enzymes, various heme pigments (myoglobin), mitochondrial oxidative enzymes, lysosomal enzymes, and nucleoproteins. Sarcoplasmic proteins are more effective emulsifiers in sausages or processed meat products than are stromal proteins (collagen, elastin), but not as effective as myofibrillar proteins.

Collagen is a unique triple-helical molecule and is the most abundant single protein in an animal. It comprises of 20%–25% of the total body protein with the inclusion of skin, ligaments, tendons, cartilage, and bone. During heating (60°C–70°C) slowly under moist conditions, breakage of non-covalent bonds, some covalent intermolecular and intramolecular bonds and a few peptide bonds of collagen will result in the collapse of the triple-helical polypeptide units. This conversion of a heli-cal collagen to an amorphous form (gelatin) is known as gelatinization. When it is chilled to refrig-eration temperatures (~4°C), a partial renaturation will occur, resulting in a solidified, jelly-like gel or solidified gelatin.

Elastin is a rubbery protein in a β-pleated sheet arrangement. It is present in ligaments, in arterial walls, and in the support structure for organs. The cervical ligament (*ligamentum nuchae*) in rumi-nants is primarily composed of elastin, which contains 1%–2% hydroxyproline and two unique amino acids—desmosine and isodesmosine. It is very resistant to cooking, solubilization, or enzymatic digestion because of its high content (~90%) of nonpolar amino acids and desmosine cross-links.

5.2.2.1 Muscle Proteins—Functionality

Functionality of muscle proteins can be defined as the physical and chemical performances of pro-tein during processing and storage of meat products that ultimately affect the overall quality of the products. Muscle proteins greatly contribute to the attributes of meat products (appearance, texture, juiciness, etc.) by imparting specific functionalities like water-binding, emulsification, and gelation.

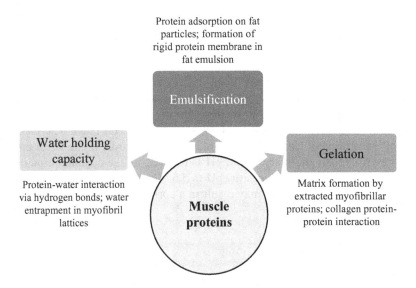

FIGURE 5.1 Functionality of muscle proteins in meat and meat products.

5.2.2.2 Water Holding Capacity (WHC)

The ability of fresh meat to retain moisture is one of the important quality characteristics of raw muscle tissue. Within the muscle cell, water is found within the myofibrils, between the myofibrils themselves, between the myofibrils and the cell membrane (sarcolemma), and between muscle cells and between muscle bundles (groups of muscle cells) [1]. Of the three groups of muscle proteins, myofibrillar proteins are responsible for much of the WHC because of their structural organiza-tion and predominance. Among the amino acids of the myofibrillar proteins, glutamic acid and lysine have charged side groups to which water is strongly attracted and bond; whereas glutamine and tyrosine contain nitrogen and oxygen atoms in side groups that have sufficient polarity, due to concentrations of electrons, to attract and bind water [2]. On the contrary, side groups of leucine, alanine, and valine are nonpolar, which, being electrically neutral, repel water.

Water is a dipolar molecule that is attracted to charged molecules (myofibrillar and stromal proteins) and is found distributed into distinct areas in muscle: bound, immobilized, and free. *Bound water* (~1%–2% of total water in fresh meat) is held tightly via myofibrillar protein charges and has reduced mobility. This water is resistant to freezing and can only be removed by severe drying processes not including conventional cooking [3]. The next fraction of water found in the muscle, *immobilized or entrapped water*, is not bound directly to the myofibrillar proteins. The water molecules may be held either by steric effects and/or by attraction to the bound water [4]. During conversion of muscle to meat, lowering of muscle pH and alteration of muscle cell structure may eventually lead to a loss of immobilized water as *drip* or *purge* [5]. *Free water* is held within muscle by weak capillary force.

Immobilized water is mostly affected in the process of conversion of muscle to meat. The goal of any meat processor is to retain this fraction of water as much as possible. Other antemortem or postmortem factors that may ultimately affect WHC are genetics, antemortem production practices, carcass chilling, and electrical stimulation. Halothane gene (*HAL*), Rendement Napole gene (*RN*), or association with porcine stress syndrome (PSS) condition may also lead to negative meat quality attributes with a lower WHC.

5.2.2.3 Emulsification

McClements [6] defines an emulsion as a system formed by two immiscible liquids (usually oil and water) in which one is dispersed (dispersed phase) as small spherical particles into the other (continuous phase). Meat emulsion is a biphasic system, in which fat globules or dispersed phase is suspended in a matrix made of proteins solubilized in a salt solution or continuous phase. In a true emulsion, the diameter of a droplet or fat globule varies between 0.1 and 100 μm [6]; whereas in a meat emulsion, it is larger than 100 μm. Therefore, meat emulsions are not considered as true emulsions, but batter or dough.

Among various muscle proteins, myofibrillar proteins have the best emulsifying properties. They are amphoteric molecules possessing both polar and nonpolar groups; on the input of mechanical energy through the shearing process, they are preferably adsorbed to the water/fat interface. The hydrophobic groups will anchor onto the fat, and the hydrophilic groups will extend into the aqueous phase. Once the fat globules are surrounded by protein, the emulsion is formed, and, on further processing (heat treatment), the denatured protein stabilizes the system. The stability of meat emulsions is attained by two mechanisms: formation of protein coatings on fat particles to reduce the interfacial tension, and immobilization of the fat particles in protein matrices through physical entrapment [7]. The effect of sarcoplasmic proteins on emulsification is relatively low [8] and of stromal proteins, it is negligible.

5.2.2.4 Gelation

Gel formation or gelation is an important characteristic of muscle protein that affects the texture and palatability of processed meat products. Gelation of muscle proteins involves formation of a three-dimensional network structure that holds water in a less mobile state [9]. During thermal gelation, myosin and other salt-soluble myofibrillar proteins exhibit complex changes in rheological characteristics depending upon specific temperatures and pH exposures [10]. Gelling properties are influenced by myofibrillar protein fraction used, type of muscle, meat species, and conditions used during processing including pH, ionic strength, pressure, heating rate, and temperature. Myofibrillar proteins produce a strong gel; conversely, sarcoplasmic proteins do not contribute to the stabilization of the product because the gel they produce is very weak. The optimum conditions for gel formation using purified myofibrillar proteins occur at about pH 6 with an ionic strength of 0.6 M and a temperature of 60°C–70°C [11]. Under similar processing conditions, proteins from white muscles generally exhibit better gelling properties than those from red muscles [12,13].

5.2.3 LIPIDS

Animal fat is composed primarily of neutral lipids (also known as triglycerides or triacylglycerols) and phospholipids that collectively range from 1.5% to 13% in muscle tissue. Neutral lipids (triacylglycerols) are glycerol esters composed of one glycerol molecule and three even-numbered long-chain fatty acids. Most fatty acids in animal fats contain an even number of carbon atoms, but a few odd-numbered carbon fatty acids are also known. In general, oleic acid (C18:1) (20%–47%) is the most abundant fatty acid in the animal body of lamb, cattle, and pigs, while palmitic (C16) (26%) is the most abundant in poultry. Saturated fatty acids are the least susceptible to lipid oxidation, followed by monounsaturated fatty acids and lastly polyunsaturated fatty acids, which are the most susceptible to free radical lipid oxidation. The most common phospholipids in muscle tissue are phosphatidylethanolamine (cephalin), phosphatidylserine, phosphatidylcholine (lecithin), and sphingomyelin. These lipids are more readily oxidized by oxygen than are triacylglycerols, resulting in the development of specific off-aromas and flavors in meat products known as warmed-over flavor (WOF).

5.2.3.1 Fat and Meat Quality

Though considered the most unpopular constituent of meat and the main culprit for labeling meat as unhealthy, fat content is an important aspect for developing sensory and nutritional values of meat. The amount and type of fat in meat influence two major components of meat quality, notably tenderness and flavor [14]. Intramuscular fat affects juiciness and flavor directly and tenderness indirectly, and accounts for 12%–14% of the variation in all palatability traits [15]. Lipids and fatty acids play an important role in generating the volatile flavor compounds and flavor characteristics of cooked meat. The basic meaty aroma of beef, mutton, pork, or chicken is the same and is derived from the water-soluble fraction of the muscle; whereas, species-specific flavors in meats originate from the involvement of lipid constituents in maillard reaction during processing. Hundreds of volatile flavor compounds derived from lipid degradation have been found in cooked meat, including aliphatic hydrocarbons, aldehydes, ketones, alcohols, carboxylic acids, and esters.

Marbling has long been recognized as a factor in eating quality of meat, especially juiciness and tenderness—a major reason may be the location of neutral lipid in fat cells within the perimysium resulting in separating muscle fiber bundles and tenderizing by opening up the muscle structure. Lipids could trap moisture in muscle and prevent its loss during processing, improving juiciness.

5.2.4 CARBOHYDRATES

Glycogen is the most abundant carbohydrate in animal tissues and is present in the liver at 2%–8%, but ranges from 0.5% to 1.5% in living skeletal muscle tissue. The initial amount of glycogen in the muscle tissues at time of slaughter affects ultimate muscle color, texture, firmness, water holding capacity, emulsifying capacity, and shelf life. At 24 hours postmortem, glycogen drops to less than 10 mmol/kg of tissue. As a consequence of the build-up of lactic acid, the pH drops from 7.1–7.3 to 5.5–5.7. Other carbohydrates that are found in animal tissues include the glycosaminoglycans and proteoglycans that are associated with the extracellular matrix of connective tissues, as well as the glycoproteins found in plasma and blood, and some hormones, glycolytic intermediates, nucleotides, nucleosides, and the glycolipids. Of all of these carbohydrates, D-glucose is the most abundant.

Animals exposed to long-term pre-slaughter stress have reduced glycogen level at slaughter, and pH decline does not proceed at a normal rate postmortem. The ultimate pH (pHu) is higher than normal (greater than 6.0) and resultant meat is darker in color, has a firm texture, high water holding capacity, and less drip loss. This meat is defined as dark, firm, and dry (DFD) meat and has a limited shelf life due to its high pH. In contrary, short-term stress results in pale, soft, and exudative meat (PSE), which is paler in color, and has a lower than normal pH that results in meat that is pale in color and does not have the ability to hold water. Additionally, muscle pH and development of lactic acid plays a central role in color development. Muscle pH plays a role in water binding, and the degree of water binding defines the meat color—a greater proportion of extracellular free water acts as a multitude of reflective surfaces and it appears pale in PSE meat. Conversely, the dark color associated with DFD meat is contributed to increased amounts of bound water as greater amount of water is held within cellular space.

5.2.5 INORGANIC MATTER

Minerals in ash are in the form of oxides, sulfates, phosphates, nitrates, chlorides, and other halides. Calcium, magnesium, sodium, and potassium are directly involved in contraction in living muscle, while magnesium and calcium contribute to muscle fiber contraction postmortem.

5.3 MEAT IN HUMAN NUTRITION

Meat is a concentrated nutrient source and considered essential to optimal human growth and development. Meat and meat products are important sources for protein, fat, essential amino acids, minerals, vitamins and other nutrients [16]. The muscle consists of 75% water, 20% protein, 3% fat, and 2% soluble non-protein substances. Out of the latter 2%, minerals and vitamins constitute 3%, non-protein nitrogen-containing substances 45%, carbohydrates 34%, and inorganic compounds 18% [17].

Protein from muscle tissue is an excellent source of essential amino acids, has a high net protein utilization (NPU 0.75–0.8), and high digestibility. Lean meat contains, on an average, 20%–24% protein, most of which is of higher biological value than plant proteins due to the presence of limiting amino acids in the latter; namely, lysine in wheat or tryptophan in maize. About 40% of the amino acids in meat protein are indispensable. Meat is also a rich source of the amino acid taurine, which is considered an essential amino acid for newborns as they do not have the ability to synthesize it.

Fat content of meat and meat products vary greatly according to animal species, age, diet, and part of the carcass used. Total fat content of meats and meat products varies around 3–25 g/100 g of food [18]. Meat fat mainly consists of triglycerides, phospholipids, and lesser amount of cholesterol. The cholesterol content of lean meat is in the range of 50–60 mg/100 g raw meat. Thus, contribution of lean meat to total maximum daily intake of cholesterol (200–300 mg) is approximately 20%–30%. Meat fat comprises mostly monounsaturated fatty acids (MUFAs) and saturated fatty acids (SFAs). MUFAs account for approximately 40% of the total fat in meat. The principal MUFA in meat is oleic acid (cis C18:1n-9). Around half of the fat (55%) in ruminant animals is present as saturated fats. Meat fats are also an important source of long-chain polyunsaturated fatty acids (PUFA), the principle ones being linoleic acid (18:2n-6) and arachidonic acid (20:4n-6). Meat contributes significantly to our intake of essential fatty acids. Beef, for example, contains useful amounts of n-3 PUFAs—α-linolenic acid (18:3n-3), eicosapentaenoic acid (EPA) (20:5n-3), and decosahexaenoic acid (DHA) (22:6n-3)—which are particularly important for heart health. The predominant SFAs are palmitic acid (16:0), stearic acid (18:0), and small amounts of myristic acid (14:0). The composition of fatty acids of meat is important in terms of its contribution to overall nutrition. Given current health recommendations that fat intake should be reduced to less than 30% of total energy intake, the PUFA:saturated ratio should be increased to above 0.4 and the ratio of n-6:n-3 PUFA should be less than 4. It is possible to achieve favorable fatty acid compositions by manipulating animal diet or by post processing modification.

Meat is generally a good source of all minerals except calcium. Red meat is a very good source of iron. Meat provides iron in readily-absorbable form. Heme iron, which accounts for about 40%–60% of the iron in meat, is several times more absorbable than non-heme iron. Absorption of iron from meat is typically 15%–25%, compared with 1%–7% from plant sources [19]. Meat also enhances iron absorption from plant foods, so the presence of meat in a meal can double the amount of iron

TABLE 5.2

Other Functional Compounds Present in Muscle Food

Conjugated linoleic acid (CLA)	Beef is a rich natural source of CLA, over 70% of which is the biologically active $c9$, $t11$ isomer shown to have anticarcinogenic and antiatherogenic effects as well as other possible health benefits; concentrations are highest in foods from ruminants (beef, lamb, dairy products); reported to be 0.46% (range 0.12%–1.20%) and 0.16% (0.06%–0.25%) of fat in meat products of ruminant and non-ruminant respectively.
Carnosine	Dipeptide composed of alanine and histidine; potent endogenous antioxidant; inhibits iron-dependent lipid oxidation in skeletal muscle.
L-Carnitine	Biosynthesized from amino acid lysine and methionine; required for mitochondrial β-oxidation of long-chain fatty acids for energy production; red meat (lamb and beef), poultry, fish, and dairy products are the richest sources.
Glutathione	A tripeptide formed in all cells (mainly liver) from three amino acids, glutamic acid, cysteine and glycine; fresh meat is a good source; presumed to be the "meat factor" that increases absorption of iron from all non-heme sources.
Bioactive peptides	Bioactive peptides displaying antihypertensive, antioxidant, antimicrobial, and antiproliferative effects have been found in the hydrolysates of meat and fish proteins.

absorbed from the other components of the meal. Beef is the richest meat source of zinc (4 mg/100 g trimmed lean beef). Of the red meats, pork contains the highest levels of selenium (13 μg per 100 g), followed by beef (7 μg per 100 g), and lamb (2 μg per 100 g). Meat is a useful source of all B vitamins, except folate and biotin. Abundant quantities of thiamine are found in pork, vitamins B_5 and B_6 in chicken, and vitamins B_6 and B_{12} in beef. Meat is a poor source of vitamin C and, except for liver, a poor source of vitamins A, D, E, and K.

Meat and meat products not only contain vital nutrients, but also additional bioactive compounds that promote human health (Table 5.2). Enriching these substances naturally in meat or meat products may be one of the avenues for the development of functional meat products.

5.3.1 MEAT BY-PRODUCTS AS HUMAN FOOD

Edible meat by-products constitute an excellent source of nutrients, like essential amino acids, minerals, and vitamins [20], and are considered part of diet in different countries. By-products such as blood, liver, lung, heart, kidney, brains, spleen, and tripe have good nutritive value [21].

Pork tail has the highest fat content and the lowest moisture content of all meat by-products. Organ meat contains 3–5 times more cholesterol than lean meat and large quantities of phospholipids. Compared to other by-products, brain has the highest amount of cholesterol (1,352–2,195 mg/100 g). Organ meat, for example brain, liver, heart, kidney, and lungs, contains a higher level of polyunsaturated fatty acids and a lower level of monounsaturated fatty acids than lean meat. The liver, tail, ears, and feet of cattle have a protein level close to that of lean meat tissue, but a large amount of collagen is found in the ears and feet [22]. The vitamin content of organ meat is usually higher than that of lean meat tissue. Kidney and liver contain about 5–10 times more riboflavin (1.697–3.630 mg/100 g) than lean meat. A single portion (100 g) of kidney and liver provide more than the daily requirement of riboflavin. Liver is the best source of niacin, vitamin B_{12}, B_6, folacin, ascorbic acid, and vitamin A. Kidney is also a good source of vitamin B_6, B_{12}, and folacin. Lamb kidneys, pork liver, lungs, and spleen are an excellent source of iron, as well as vitamins. The copper content is highest in the livers of beef, lamb, and veal. Liver also contains the highest amount of manganese (0.128–0.344 mg/100 g). However, the highest level of phosphorus (393–558 mg/100 g) and potassium (360–433 mg/100 g) in meat by-products is found in the thymus and sweet-breads [23]. Mechanically deboned meat has the highest calcium content (315–485 mg/100 g). The slaughter of large numbers of meat animals, like buffaloes, for export results in the production of buffalo offal meats at a much higher quantity than the demand for local consumption. This leads to price-cuts for these offal meats and even considerable wastage. Hence, efficient utilization of these meats adopting a cost effective way with modern technologies is needed to support an economical and viable meat production system. Verma et al. [24] evaluated the suitability of using buffalo head and heart meat in emulsion-based product preparations and to assess their quality during refrigerated storage. The researchers concluded that an acceptable product with good quality characteristics can be prepared from buffalo head meat with a combination of skeletal meat (20%) and heart meat (20%).

There has been considerable emotive and public health debate on the relative importance of meat in human diet. On one hand, muscle foods are a major source of many bioactive compounds including B vitamins, iron, zinc, and CLA [25], on the other hand meat and processed meat products are often associated with negative attributes due to high levels of saturated fatty acids, cholesterol, sodium, and high fat and caloric contents [26]. The serious health concerns resulting from the epidemic rise in cancer, coronary heart diseases, and diabetes require a holistic approach to diet and lifestyle. Lean meat, the ultimate natural functional food, if consumed in moderate quantities as part of a meal along with sufficient plant foods, can provide essential nutrient-dense supplement to the diet with beneficial effects on human health.

5.4 MEAT PROCESSING

The technology of meat processing comprises of different steps or procedures, which brings a change in biochemical, technological, and microbiological quality of processed meat products. Simple handling of meat, making it into different cut-up parts, preservation by chilling or freezing are excluded from the definition of meat processing. It involves a wide range of technological processes—particle size reduction (chopping, mincing, sectioning, chunking, flaking), tumbling, massaging, stuffing, and chemical or biochemical processes—curing or salting, smoking, drying, fermentation, and so forth.

Advantages of meat processing:

- Variety and convenience
- Utilization of low-value cuts and by-products
- Preservation and extension of shelf life
- Better marketing and distribution, better profit
- Development of new products
- Employment generation

Different types of processing methods and associated equipment are discussed below.

5.4.1 PARTICLE SIZE REDUCTION

The reduction of particle size is the first step in meat processing and is accomplished by sectioning, chunking, slicing, flaking, mincing and chopping. An improved uniformity and tenderness of the final product is achieved due to more uniform particle size and distribution of ingredients. On the contrary, due to an increase in surface area and exposure to atmospheric oxygen and contact with different machineries, reduction of the particle size may lead to higher lipid and myoglobin oxidation and reduction of shelf life. Proper care must be taken to maintain the temperature in the processing room so it does not exceed 10°C.

5.4.1.1　Mincer

Mincers are the most commonly used equipment for particle size reduction in meat processing. Intact, boneless meat cuts are comminuted by forcing them through grinder plates with holes of different sizes (3, 5, 8, and 13 mm sizes) as per the product requirement and then cutting off the particles with rotating knifes.

5.4.1.2　Slicer

Meat or meat products are cut in the form of thin slices, which is achieved by a revolving blade adjusted to get slices of different thickness.

5.4.1.3　Bowl Chopper

The mixing of ingredients and chopping can be accomplished in one step with a bowl chopper, which consists of rotating blades with a revolving bowl and forms meat batter/emulsion.

5.4.2　TUMBLING AND MASSAGING

High quality sectioned and formed, whole-muscle meat products may not be achieved without the use of a tumbler or massager. Tumbling and massaging are two different physical treatments. Tumblers use impact energy in rotating the meat pieces lifted by baffles and then falling onto the rotating drum. The speed at which the drum rotates affects the impact and needs to be optimized according to the size of the meat pieces, type of meat, or processing method used. On the other hand, massagers use frictional energy in rubbing the meat pieces against each other by rotating paddles, which may be horizontal or vertical. The vertical paddles give a better massage treatment and cause less damage to meat pieces in comparison to the horizontal ones.

Tumbling or massaging helps in enhancing the migration of curing ingredients resulting in better penetration within the meat cuts, extraction of proteins forming an exudate over the meat pieces and increased binding of products.

5.4.3　STUFFING

Meat emulsion or batter is stuffed into natural, synthetic, or semi-synthetic casings of different sizes that are permeable to water and air, and both ends are clipped. Batter should not be under or over-stuffed in the casing. Understuffing usually results in casings with wrinkles, whereas overstuffing can result in casing breakage and poor ability to peel.

5.4.3.1　Sausage Stuffer/Filler

Both hydraulic operated and manual sausage fillers may be used for filling up the meat emulsion into the casings. The unit consists of cylinder, filler tube (nozzle), and a lid. Upward movement of piston in cylinder helps in filling of emulsion in casings.

5.5　PROCESSED MEAT PRODUCTS

5.5.1　EMULSION BASED MEAT PRODUCTS

Meat emulsions are made by grinding or chopping meat and water with the addition of common salt (NaCl) into a fine meat homogenate forming the matrix in which fat is dispersed. The matrix is then capable of binding fat, water, and other non-meat ingredients. After heat processing, proteins are coagulated resulting in an immobilization of fat, water, and other ingredients. Emulsion formulation could be developed based on the ingredients and their levels and the choice of meat processor. While preparing meat emulsion, a rule of thumb is that the moisture content in the finished product shouldn't exceed four times that of the protein content. Meat products are also considered significant sources of dietary sodium and fat while lacking enough dietary fiber. Today's consumers are very much aware besides being a health conscious. They are averse to purchasing meat products rich in the components, which have negative health implications. In this connection, harmful components can be reduced, and potentially healthy ingredients can be supplemented in emulsion-based meat products through reformulation technology. Many healthy ingredients, such as natural antioxidants, besides being a beneficial to consumers can also play an important role in the quality and stability of meat products. The quality characteristics and storage stability of low fat functional chicken nuggets with 40% replaced sodium chloride and consisting high fiber ingredients like, pea hull flour, gram hull flour, apple pulp, and bottle gourd in three different combinations was investigated [27]. It was observed that sodium chloride replacement and inclusion of high fiber ingredients affected the physicochemical and textural properties of functional chicken nuggets; however, they had sensory ratings almost similar to the control. Banerjee et al. [28] determined the antioxidant potential of broccoli powder extract and observed its effects on quality and stability of goat meat nuggets. They suggested that 2% of the broccoli powder extract can be effectively used as a natural antioxidant in goat meat nuggets without affecting product acceptability.

Three important types of formulations have been developed to suit the requirements of a wide group of consumers:

- *Prime:* Lean meat content shouldn't be less than 67% of the formulation. Edible animal fat could be used as a fat source; however, no skin or other by-products are permitted.
- *Choice:* Meat should be not less than 50% and fat and by-products (in case of chicken products, skin, gizzard, and heart) could be used. Cooked meat from deboned frames also could be used.
- *Economy:* Meat content varies from 40% to 49% and edible animal fat, by-products, and other non-meat ingredients could also be used. Relatively, it costs less and facilitates incorporation of variety ingredients for health and nutrition.

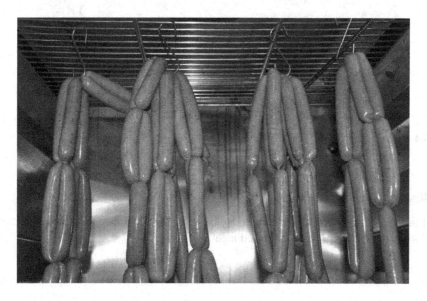

FIGURE 5.2 Meat sausage.

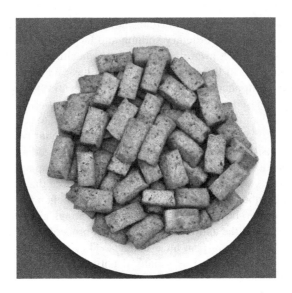

FIGURE 5.3 Meat nuggets.

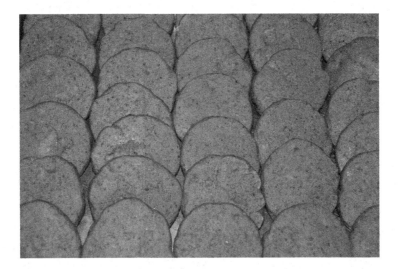

FIGURE 5.4 Meat patties.

5.5.2 RESTRUCTURED MEAT PRODUCTS

Any meat product that is partially or completely disassembled and then reformed into the same or different form can be defined as restructured meat.

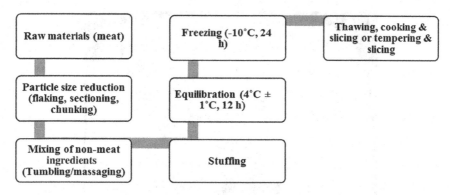

FIGURE 5.5   Restructuring process.

5.5.2.1   Advantages of Restructuring

- Restructured meat can be formed into any shape or size desired—cubes, slices, sticks, nuggets, blocks, and so forth.
- Restructuring requires little preparation time and effort. The ingredients and portion size can be easily tailored according to the consumer need.
- Tenderizing techniques can be used to provide a uniform tenderness in restructured product leading to positive consumer experience.
- Utilizing the low-value meat cuts, a new value added meat product can be developed through restructuring, which will fetch a higher profit for the manufacturer.

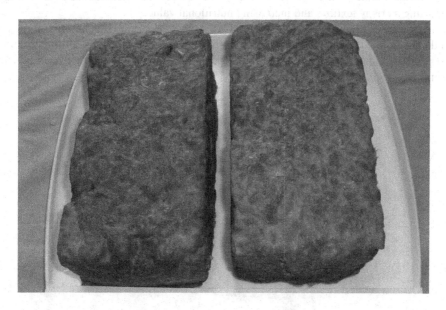

FIGURE 5.6   Restructured mutton ham.

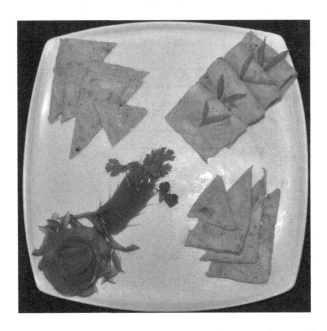

FIGURE 5.7   Restructured meat slices.

5.5.3   ENROBED MEAT PRODUCTS

Enrobing is a process in which the meat or meat products are traditionally coated with edible materials in the form of batter, which preserves the quality by preventing moisture loss, adding better taste, imparting a crispy texture, and increasing nutritional value.

Apart from water, which is used for making batter suspension, polysaccharides (Bengal gram, wheat and corn flour, starch), proteins (egg albumin, milk protein fractions, skimmed milk powder, seed proteins), and seasonings (salt, sugar, pepper, and other spices) are used as enrobing ingredients.

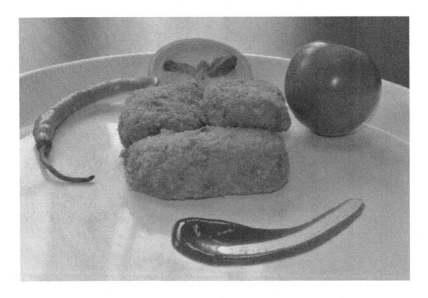

FIGURE 5.8   Enrobed meat cutlets.

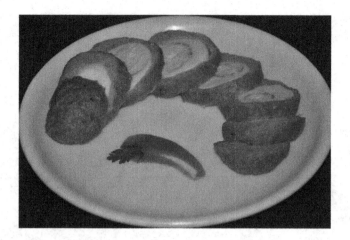

FIGURE 5.9 Enrobed eggs.

5.5.4 CURED AND SMOKED MEAT PRODUCTS

Curing is the process of adding nitrite, as well as salt or sugar, to smaller meat pieces or bigger cuts to preserve and enhance the color and flavor. Smoking helps in the application of smoke generated from burning of hardwood to meat and meat products for developing a typical color and flavor.

The principal cured and smoked meat products are made from primal cuts of pork and consist mainly of ham and bacon.

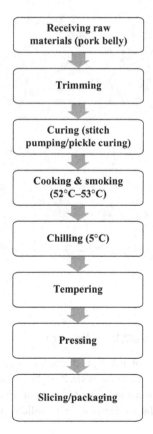

FIGURE 5.10 Processing of bacon.

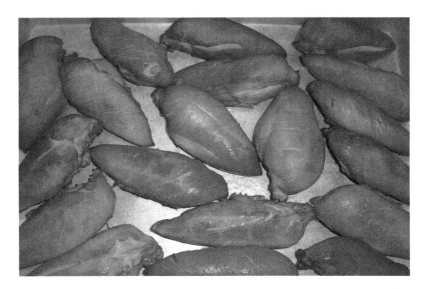

FIGURE 5.11   Smoked chicken breast.

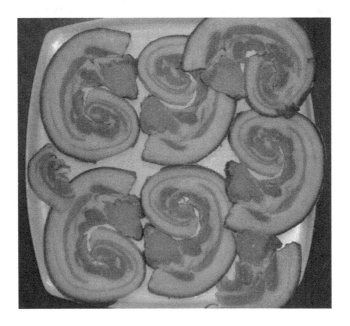

FIGURE 5.12   Ham.

5.5.5   Canned or Retort Pouched Meat Products

Canning is a process in which meat or meat products are hermetically sealed in a container and thermally processed (121°C) in order to make it shelf-stable with a considerable long shelf life and without using any further preservation methods. Meat canning essentially uses three main operations—can filling, exhaustion, and heat treatment. The solid:liquid ratio and distribution of liquid within the can is important; in order to allow a good heat transfer, 30% of the can volume must be liquid. Exhaustion is necessary to remove air from the headspace and bulk of the products inside for proper heat penetration and reduce growth of aerobic microorganisms. Heating and cooling cycles are the core of canning processes. Heating is done to inactivate the microbial and enzymatic reactions, and cooling reduces the deterioration of sensory properties of products.

Metal cans are now replaced with retort pouches—a three-layer laminate that can be processed like a can, shelf-stable, and have the convenience of frozen boil-in-bag products. Retort processing represents a unique combination of package, process, and product technology with potential, economic benefits. It is composed of an outer layer of polyester film, a middle layer of aluminum foil, and an inner layer of modified polypropylene. The outer polyester film protects the foil and provides the laminate with strength and abrasion resistance. The core layer of aluminum foil gives the laminate the necessary water, gas, odor, and light barrier properties. The polypropylene inner layer provides a strong heat seal and good product resistance required in the retort pouch. Foil laminated retortable pouches cost less and are lighter in weight than metal cans enabling easy distribution and marketing with faster processing time.

5.5.6 ROLE OF NON-MEAT INGREDIENTS IN MEAT PROCESSING

Meat processing has traditionally been associated with addition of non-meat ingredients in order to modify the sensory properties and improve shelf life. Various non-meat ingredients and their role in processing of different meat products are presented below:

Salt	Preservative effect is by the reduction of water activity (a_w) and altering osmotic pressure, which inhibits bacterial growth [29]; Salt and water form a solution for extracting myofibrillar protein, which increases emulsion stability, processing stability, water binding, and yield.
Sweetener/Sugar	Flavor enhancing effect; interacts with the amino groups of the proteins and, when cooked, forms browning products through the Maillard reaction that enhances the flavor; softens the products by counteracting the harsh hardening effects of salt.
Phosphate	Synergistic effect with salt; increase the water binding and fat emulsifying capacity of the myofibrillar proteins by increasing the pH level [30]; effective antioxidant [31] and reduces rancidity and warmed-over flavor due to metal (catalyst) chelating ability.
Nitrate/nitrite	Responsible for the development of typical cured meat color and flavor; strongly inhibitory to anaerobic bacteria, most importantly *Clostridium botulinum*, and contributes to control of other micro-organisms, such as *Listeria monocytogenes* [32].
Cure accelerators (Salt of ascorbic/erythorbic acid)	Accelerate color development; resist color fading; protect against rancidity
Water/ice	Helps in distribution of ingredients, increases binding, juiciness and yield, controls the temperature of product during processing
Binders/extenders/fillers	Reduce formulation cost, improve meat batter stability and water binding capacity, enhance nutritional value, texture, or flavor
Seasonings	Enhance flavor antimicrobial and antioxidant properties

5.6 MEAT PRESERVATION

The nutrient composition of meat makes it an ideal media for the growth of spoilage micro-organisms. It is therefore essential that adequate preservation technologies are applied to maintain its safety and quality [33].

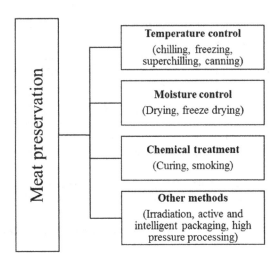

FIGURE 5.13 Approaches for preservation of meat and meat products.

5.6.1 Chilling and Freezing

The most widely used method for storage and preservation of fresh meat are chilling and freezing. Chilling is generally limited to a relatively short period, as the low temperature (2°C–5°C) is not sufficient to stop microbial growth and other deteriorative changes. At the completion of slaughter, the initial temperature of animal carcasses ranges between 30°C and 39°C. This body heat must be removed during initial chilling, and the temperature of the carcass should be reduced to 5°C or less. Beef, pork, lamb, veal, and calf carcasses are chilled in chill coolers (−4°C to 0°C). After 12–24 hours, beef carcasses are transferred to holding coolers (0°C–3°C). Pork, veal, and lamb carcasses are fabricated directly from chill coolers. Poultry and fish are generally chilled by immersion in chill coolers. It is essential to chill the meat in a way that ensures enough time for aging to take place before the meat is frozen or consumed. The relative humidity of the chiller should be maintained at around 90% to prevent excessive carcass shrinkage from moisture loss. Sufficient spacing must be provided between carcasses for thorough air circulation and ensuring rapid heat dissipation. The shelf life of meat under chilling storage depends upon the species of animal, initial microbial load, temperature and humidity condition during storage, and type of packaging used. Fresh meat in an oxygen permeable pack may have a shelf life of 5–7 days.

Freezing slows down the spoilage of meat by converting the muscle water into ice and making it unavailable for microbial growth. The freezing point of meat is approximately −1.5°C. The advantages of temperatures below the freezing point are in prolonging the useful storage life of meat and in discouraging microbial and chemical changes [34]. Under normal freezing conditions, the water content of meat forms ice crystals around nucleation sites. The sizes of these crystals depend upon the rate of freezing. If the freezing is done quickly, then the ice crystals will stay small. Ice crystals can grow within and between meat cells. The crystals have the potential to cause mechanical damage to cell membranes and the concentration of solutes into unfrozen portions of the meat during the freezing process can damage proteins, causing denaturation. These effects may lead to "drip loss" during thawing, which is unattractive to customers and causes the defrosted meat to lose weight [35]. Most nutrients are retained during freezing and subsequent storage. However, some water soluble nutrients including salts, proteins, peptides, amino acids, and water soluble vitamins are lost during thawing as drip. The fastest freezing rates are associated with the least damage because they result in small ice crystal sizes and they do not provide an opportunity for the chemicals dissolved in the moisture content of the meat to move from their original locations and *vice versa*. Several commercial methods are used to freeze meat and meat products, namely still air freezing, plate freezing, blast freezing,

TABLE 5.3
Storage Life (months) of Frozen Meat and Meat Products

Item	−12°C	−18°C	−24°C	−30°C
Beef	4	6	12	12
Lamb	3	6	12	12
Veal	3	4	8	10
Poultry	2	4	8	10
Ground beef and lamb	3	6	8	10

Source: Aberle et al. [43].

cryogenic freezing, and individual quick freeing. Cold air blast freezing is the most commonly used commercial method, wherein air velocity of about 760 meters per minute and temperature of about −30°C are the most practical and economic conditions used in the meat industry (Table 5.3).

5.6.2 SUPERCHILLING

Superchilling, also called partial freezing or deep chilling, is a process where food products are stored between the freezing point of the products and 1°C–2°C below this [36]. It allows only partial freezing of surface water, which gives insulation and maintains refrigeration capacity during storage and transportation. Storing food products at superchilling temperature was reported to have three distinct advantages: maintaining food freshness, retaining high food quality, and suppressing growth of harmful microbes [37]. Much of the superchilling work reported is focused on seafood [38]. A form of superchilling has been tried on pork [39], lamb [40], and beef [41], and there is now an increasing interest in this process for extension of chilled storage life of meat [42].

5.6.3 THERMAL PROCESSING (CANNING)

Canning is a process of preserving meat products contained in a hermetically sealed container achieved by an application of thermal sterilization procedure.

The canning process is described briefly below:

Selection, handling, and preparation of raw material	Raw materials must be clean and of good quality; inedible parts, bones, cartilages, tendon along with surplus fat should be removed; precooking can be done at 70°C for 15 minutes.
Filling the can	If meat with gravy is canned, it is important to put the gravy first followed by chunks and then the gravy again. For proper heat transfer, 30% of the can volume must be liquid. A headspace of 0.5% of the total can volume must also be considered.
Exhausting	Air from contents and headspace are removed before sealing to produce concave can ends so that any internal pressure can be checked and to minimize strain on cans during processing.
Can sealing and washing	Sealing is done by a double seaming machine. Sealed cans are washed with hot detergent solution.
Retorting	Cans are subjected to a high temperature of 121°C for 6 minutes, depending on the product, to destroy nearly all spoilage organisms.
Cooling, labeling, and storage	In commercial practice, cans are water cooled to 38°C. Cans are labeled properly providing all statutory information. Cans are kept for storage at 20°C for 1–3 months to help the contents to mature and stabilize taste or flavor.

Occasionally canned meat products may undergo spoilage, typically caused by the growth of the spore formers. Spoilage is usually characterized by swollen bulging cans due to gas production by the spore forming microorganisms. This condition develops due to under-processing, but it may also indicate a leaky can. Shelf-stable canned meat products typically have strong sulfhydryl flavor due to excessive protein denaturation during heat processing. In addition, texture of the products may get modified due to protein hardening and breakdown of connective tissue.

5.6.4   DRYING

Drying of meat under the sun or over a fire to prevent spoilage was the earliest form of food preservation. Biltong of South Africa, Pastirma of Turkey, Charque of South America, and Pemmican of North America are the classical examples of dried meat products. Reduction in the availability of water to a very low level inhibits the activity of microorganisms and enzymes. Low water activity (a_w) is probably the single reason for shelf stability of dried meat or meat products.

Dehydration can be achieved by the following methods:

Sun drying: A traditional method, whole/strips/chunks of meat are dried by direct solar radiation and natural air circulation.

Solar Drying: Solar drier lowers the air humidity by raising the temperature of the air. Drying is faster, and the quality of the final product is better when compared to sun drying.

Freeze drying: Freeze drying, or lyophilization, is a process in which water is frozen, followed by its removal from the product, initially by sublimation and then by desorption. Drying is done for 9–12 hours in vacuum chambers with pressure of 1.0–1.5 mm of mercury, and a chamber temperature as high as 43°C. The residual moisture content of freeze dried meat products is generally below 2%.

Rancidity, non-enzymatic browning, and protein denaturation are the prominent types of deterioration observed in dried meat products. They are particularly spoiled by molds and not bacteria. Hence, antioxidants and antimycotic agents are commonly employed in dried products. Packaging of dried products under modified atmospheric condition extends the storage life.

5.6.5   CURING AND SMOKING

Curing and smoking are the ancient practices for preservation of meat. Curing of meat means the addition of nitrite and/or nitrate together with salt (NaCl) to meat in different processing steps, which results in conversion of meat pigment—myoglobin to nitrosomyoglobin or cured form.

5.6.5.1   Role of Curing Ingredients

The two main ingredients that must be used to cure meat are salt and nitrite. However, other substances can be added to accelerate curing, stabilize color, modify flavor, and reduce shrinkage during processing.

- *Salt*: Flavor and preservation
- *Sugar*: Counteracts flavor of salt
- *Sodium nitrite*: Cured color development and stability, contributes to cured flavor, antimicrobial and antioxidant properties
- *Phosphates*: Improve water holding capacity and reduce oxidation
- *Ascorbate and erythorbate*: Curing aids that accelerates color development and stabilizes it
- *Spices*: Contributes to flavor

Different methods practiced for curing of meat are described briefly below:

Dry curing: Curing ingredients are mixed together and rubbed over the surface of meat cuts. The cuts are then held for few days according to their thickness for diffusion and even distribution of ingredients.

Immersion curing: It involves submerging the meat cuts into a curing solution, which results in a uniform distribution of curing ingredients throughout the meat more quickly than the dry curing method.

Artery pumping: Brine solution can be introduced into the meat cut through artery system for uniform distribution of curing ingredients.

Stitch/spray pumping: In stitch pumping, brine solution is introduced into various parts of meat cuts through a single orifice needle; whereas in spray pumping, the needle has several openings along its length and is used for uniform distribution.

Smoking of meat is the process of preserving meat by exposing it to smoke generated by smoldering wood to develop a typical appearance and flavor. A combination of heat and smoke causes a significant reduction of surface bacterial population. In addition, a physical barrier is provided by surface dehydration, protein coagulation, and absorption of resinous substance. Generally, hardwood is used for smoking, mainly oak and beech. However, for imparting specific color or flavor to some products, wood from other trees that are rich in resins may be used. The temperature of thermal degradation in the wood constituents—hemicelluloses, cellulose, and lignin—ranges from 180°C to 300°C, 260°C to 350°C, and 300°C to 500°C, respectively. The numerous components of the smoke differ in chemical and physical properties.

The gases and low-boiling compounds constitute the gaseous phase, while the higher boiling ones are dispersed in the form of fluid droplets or solid particles.

5.6.5.2 Components of Smoke

1. *Phenols*
   - Act as antioxidants (e.g. 2,6-dimethoxyphenol, 2,6-dimethoxy-4 methylphenol, 2,6-dimethoxy-4 ethylphenol)
   - Contribute to specific flavor (e.g. Guaiacol, 4methylguaiacol, 2,6-dimethoxyphenol [flavor], and syringol [aroma])
   - Antimicrobial activity that contributes to preservation (e.g. Guaiacol and its methyl and propyl derivative, creosol, pyrocatechol, methylpyrocatechol, pyrogallol, etc.)
2. *Alcohols*
   Exerts minor preservative effects (e.g. Methanol or wood alcohol)
3. *Organic acids*
   Minor preservative action play an important role in skin formation of sausage (e.g. Formic, acetic, propionic, valeric, caproic, caprylic acid)
4. *Carbonyls*
   Play a major role in browning during smoking (e.g. 2-pentanone, valeraldehyde, 2-butanone, butanal, ethanol, diacetyl, furfural, etc.)
5. *Gases*
   Most important nitrous oxide, which has been linked to the formation of nitrosamine in smoked product.
6. *Hydrocarbons*
   Polycyclic aromatic hydrocarbons (PAH) isolated from smoked meat—Benzanthracene, Dibenzanthracene, Benzapyrene, Benzepyrene, Pyrene, 4-methylpyrene, which are recognized as being carcinogens.

To avoid the problems of polycyclic aromatic hydrocarbons, nowadays liquid smoke has been used by pyrolysis of hardwood sawdust.

5.6.6 IRRADIATION

Irradiation is a process of exposing meat or meat products to a source of ionizing radiation emitted by a radioactive substance or generated by high energy accelerators, including X-rays. Irradiation is also known as "cold sterilization" as it does not significantly change the temperature or physical or sensory characteristics of the product. Radiation dose is the quantity of radiation energy absorbed by the food during processing. The units used are "Rad" or "Gray (Gy)" where 1 Gy = 100 Rads. A radiation dosage of 7 kGy has been approved by the World Health Organization (WHO) as being "unconditionally safe" for human consumption. The radiation doses approved for poultry (1.5–3.0 kGy) would destroy approximately 3–5 logs of *Salmonella*. Except for spores of *Clostridium botulinum*, all other pathogenic bacteria can be controlled within this dose range. Dosage of 0.25 kGy and 0.3 kGy is adequate to destroy *Toxoplasma gondii* and *Trichinella spiralis* in meat, respectively.

Even at low doses, irradiation of fresh meat can result in off-odor and off-flavor (rotten egg, bloody, fishy, or metallic) due to initiation or promotion of lipid oxidation or free radical formation from unsaturated fatty acids. Irradiation can also cause some color changes in meat that are greatly influenced by the packaging environment. Vacuum packaging, modified atmosphere packaging, or inclusion of antioxidants may reduce these undesirable changes.

5.6.7 HURDLE TECHNOLOGY

Hurdle technology has an immense potential to improve the microbiological stability, sensory characteristics, as well as nutritional properties of meat and meat products. It encompasses all factors used for food preservation and can be defined as a combined application of various technologies, factors, and/or agents (hurdles) to food/meat in order to maximize the preservation effect [44]. An intelligent combination of hurdles could achieve an extension of shelf life or an improvement in safety or sensory properties while maintaining meat quality. In developing countries like India, the application of hurdle technology for foods, which remain stable, safe, and tasty, if stored without refrigeration, is of paramount importance and receiving much interest. Karthikeyan et al. [45] studied the extension of shelf life of the highly perishable Indian traditional meat product, chevon (caprine) *keema*, through the application of hurdle technology. The hurdles used were water activity and pH as variable hurdles, while vacuum packaging, preservatives, and heat treatment as constant hurdles. The product with a$_w$ 0.90, pH 5.8 was found most suitable. There was a decrease in the growth rate of aerobic and anaerobic counts and complete inhibition of *S. aureus*. Sensory scores for hurdle treated *keema* declined upon storage and the product was well accepted up to the third day and fairly accepted up to the fifth day, whereas the *keema* prepared by the traditional method was acceptable only on the first day. The suitability of hot-boned pork and pork fat for processing shelf-stable pork sausages using hurdle technology was evaluated [46]. Hot-processed sausage received higher total plate counts while lactobacillus counts were high in cold-processed product throughout the storage period. Sensory evaluation revealed that hurdle-treated pork sausages from hot-boned pork were equally suitable as those from cold-boned pork up to day six at ambient temperature.

5.7 POST PROCESSING LETHALITY PROCEDURES

In the recent years, several ready-to-eat (RTE) meat products have developed to satisfy growing consumer demands for variety and convenience. These products are subjected to cooking by various methods, which provides an adequate microbiological quality. However, RTE meat products are presumed to be contaminated after cooking due to further manipulation [47]. The processing steps after cooking, such as peeling, sorting, loading, slicing, and packaging, are potential sources of recontaminations for pathogens like *Listeria monocytogenes*. The United States Department of Agriculture – Food Safety Inspection Service (USDA–FSIS) survey published in 2001 showed that 1%–10% of retail RTE meat and poultry products were contaminated with *L. monocytogenes* [48]. *L. monocytogenes* is one of the deadly foodborne pathogens that threaten the safety of ready-to-eat (RTE) meat and poultry products. This psychrotrophic organism is ubiquitous, can survive in biofilms, and resists diverse environmental conditions, such as low pH and high sodium chloride concentrations, which gives *Listeria* great persistence in the processing environments [49]. The risk of foodborne listeriosis would be higher if the contaminated products are exposed to temperature abuse. To protect the consumers from foodborne listeriosis, FSIS issued an interim final rule requiring RTE meat manufacturers to adopt one of the three alternatives to effectively control and limit the risks posed by *L. monocytogenes* [50]. These alternatives include Alternative 1—the use of a post-lethality treatment and an antimicrobial agent or process to suppress or limit the growth of this microorganism; Alternative 2—the use of a post-lethality treatment or an antimicrobial agent or process to suppress or limit the growth of this microorganism; and Alternative 3—controlling *L. monocytogenes* in the post-lethality areas through sanitary procedures only. Manufacturers choosing Alternative 2 or 3 will receive increased frequencies of inspections by FSIS. However, all manufacturers must prove that their products are free of *L. monocytogenes*.

The USDA–FSIS [51] has defined a post-lethality treatment as "a lethality treatment that is applied or is effective after post-lethality exposure. It is applied to the final product or sealed package of product in order to reduce or eliminate the level of pathogens resulting from contamination from post-lethality exposure." The preferred methods of post-lethality treatments include high pressure processing, thermal treatment/pasteurization, application of radiations, and use of pulsed light.

5.7.1 High Pressure Processing

High hydrostatic pressure (HHP) is a non-thermal technology that contributes to the increase of microbial safety and prolongs shelf life, especially in food with heat-sensitive nutritional, sensory, and functional characteristics [52]. As in package "cold pasteurization," HHP is particularly interesting as a listericidal post-processing treatment for RTE meat products [53,54]. However, the efficiency of HHP depends on the composition of food. Low a_w values and/or high solute concentration in particular have been recognized to exert a baroprotection and reduce the extent of bacterial inactivation induced by HHP [55]. HHP has been used for inactivation of pathogens in food items, with damage to the cell membrane being the primary mechanism of microbial destruction [56]. HHP can also reduce the levels of vegetative bacteria without greatly affecting the flavor of foods [57]. Studies have indicated that HPP inflicts sub-lethal injury on microorganisms, even at lower pressures than those required for their death [58]. Sub-lethally injured cells are more susceptible to antimicrobial compounds [59].

The efficiency of combining high-pressure processing (HPP) and active packaging technologies to control *L. monocytogenes* growth during the shelf life of artificially inoculated cooked ham was assessed [60]. Both antimicrobial packaging and pressurization delayed the growth of the pathogen. However, at 6°C the combination of antimicrobial packaging and HPP was necessary to achieve a reduction of inoculated levels without recovery during 60 days of storage. All HPP lots stored at 1°C led to counts <100 CFU/g at day 60. After a cold chain break, no growth of *L. monocytogenes* was observed in pressurized ham packed with antimicrobial films, showing the efficiency of combining both technologies.

Lavieri et al. [61] investigated the use of commercially available natural antimicrobials in combination with post-lethality interventions for the control of *L. monocytogenes* growth and recovery on alternatively-cured RTE ham. The post-lethality treatments of HHP (400 MPa), octanoic acid (OA), and lauric arginate (LAE) significantly reduced initial viable *L. monocytogenes* numbers compared to the control, regardless of the antimicrobial ingredient used in the formulation while post-packaging thermal treatment did not. The use of natural antimicrobial ingredients, such as vinegar and lemon juice concentrate, in combination with post-lethality interventions, such as HHP,

LAE, and OA, represents an effective multi-hurdle approach for *L. monocytogenes* control in processed meat and poultry products.

The effect of nisin application combined with HHP processing on the behavior of *L. monocytogenes* CTC1034 intentionally inoculated (at ca. 10^7 cells/g) onto the surface of RTE sliced dry-cured ham was observed [62]. The results of the study indicated that HHP, as post-processing listericidal treatment, is more effective (both immediately and long term) than the use of nisin as an antimicrobial measure. However, the both hurdles combined provided a wider margin of safety in the control of *L. monocytogenes* during the storage of RTE cured meat products.

The effectiveness of the combination of HPP at 600 MPa with the natural antimicrobials nisin and potassium lactate has been evaluated in sliced cooked ham spiked with 4-log CFU/g of *Salmonella* sp., *L. monocytogenes,* and *Staphylococcus aureus* after 3 months of storage at 1°C and 6°C [63]. In non-HPP sliced cooked ham, the addition of nisin plus lactate inhibited the growth of *L. monocytogenes* during the entire storage period while the refrigerated storage inhibited the growth of *Salmonella* sp. and *S. aureus*. The application of an HPP reduced the levels of *Salmonella* and *L. monocytogenes* to levels below 10 CFU/g. These levels continued until the end of storage at both 1°C and 6°C. HPP produced a reduction of less than 1 Log CFU/g to *S. aureus*. The combination of HPP, nisin, and refrigeration at 6°C was necessary to decrease the levels of *S. aureus* by 2.4 Log CFU/g after 3 months of storage.

Growth of *L. monocytogenes* was evaluated for up to 182 days after inoculation on RTE sliced ham and turkey breast formulated with sodium nitrite (0 or 200 ppm), sodium chloride (1.8% or 2.4%), and treated (no treatment or 600 MPa) with HHP [64]. HHP at 600 MPa for 3 minutes resulted in a 3.85–4.35 log CFU/g reduction in *L. monocytogenes*. There were no differences in growth of *L. monocytogenes* due to sodium chloride level. Sodium nitrite provided a small, but significant inhibition of *L. monocytogenes* without HHP, but addition of sodium nitrite did not significantly affect growth of *L. monocytogenes* with use of HHP.

Lavieri et al. [65] investigated the natural antimicrobials including cranberry powder, dried vinegar, and lemon juice/vinegar concentrate, and post-lethality interventions (lauric arginate, octanoic acid, thermal treatment, and high hydrostatic pressure) for the control of *L. monocytogenes* on alternatively-cured frankfurters. Lauric arginate, octanoic acid, and high hydrostatic pressure (400 MPa) reduced *L. monocytogenes* populations by 2.28, 2.03, and 1.88 $\log_{10}$ CFU/g compared to the control. *L. monocytogenes* grew in all post-lethality intervention treatments, except after a 600 MPa HHP treatment for 4 minutes.

The effect of high pressure processing (400 MPa for 10 minutes) and natural antimicrobials (enterocins and lactate–diacetate) on the behavior of *L. monocytogenes* in sliced cooked ham during refrigerated storage (1°C and 6°C) was assessed [66]. The efficiency of the treatments after a cold chain break was evaluated. The combination of low storage temperature (1°C), HPP and addition of lactate–diacetate reduced the levels of *L. monocytogenes* during storage by 2.7 log CFU/g. The combination of HPP, enterocins and refrigeration at 1°C was adjudged as most effect treatment the control of pathogen even after the cold chain break.

Porto-Fett et al. [67] evaluated the effectiveness of fermentation, drying, and HPP to inactivate *L. monocytogenes*, *Escherichia coli* O157:H7, *Salmonella* spp., and *Trichinella spiralis* in Genoa salami produced with trichinae-infected pork. The result showed that fermentation and drying and/or HPP of contaminated Genoa salami or pork are effective for inactivating *L. monocytogenes*, *E. coli* O157:H7, *Salmonella* spp., and/or *T. spiralis* larvae.

5.7.2 Pasteurization/Thermal Treatment

RTE products are most often consumed without further cooking, and therefore, the presence of pathogens presents a considerable food safety threat. This concern has prompted interest in applying post-package or post-process heat treatments to reduce surface contaminants and increasing shelf life in packaged products by microwave [68], steam [69], and hot water [70]. Roering et al. [71]

pasteurized chubs of summer sausage inoculated with *L. monocytogenes* and sealed in vacuum packages, achieving as high as 3-log reductions at 98.9°C. In-package pasteurization of RTE meat products using steam or hot water was useful in reducing the number of *L. monocytogenes* cells on the surface of RTE meat products [72,73]. In general, post-lethality in-package thermal treatment takes a relatively long time (20–40 minutes), and is highly dependent upon the thickness of products.

Flash Pasteurization (FP), uses short pulses of steam (120°C, 1.5 seconds) to decontaminate the surfaces of fine emulsion sausages, such as frankfurters or bratwurst, immediately before packaging [74]. FP inactivates 2–3 log CFU/g of *L. monocytogenes* and *L. innocua* on precooked sausage surfaces; however, the bacteria are eventually able to recover and proliferate during long-term refrigerated storage.

The use of FP to inactivate *L. innocua* on frankfurters followed by application of lauric-arginate ester (LAE) immediately prior to vacuum-packaging in a pilot plant setting was investigated [75]. Use of FP, LAE, or FP followed by application of LAE, resulted in a 2.5, 1.6, and 3.3 of log reductions of *L. innocua*, respectively. The use of FP in combination with LAE effectively inhibited the growth of *L. innocua* for 12 weeks. The use of FP in combination with LAE had little effect on frankfurter color and texture.

Selby et al. [76] determined the heat resistance of *L. monocytogenes* in two brands (A and B) of bologna differing in formulations, and evaluated the effects of post-package pasteurization on product quality. Fat content did not affect *L. monocytogenes* heat resistance in bologna at 55°C, 60°C, and 65°C; however, Brand B bologna had a numerically lower inactivation rate. Microbial heat resistance was significantly differed with changes in pasteurization temperature. Time and temperature affected cook-loss and lightness Hunter color value for both bologna brands.

Ambient steam in-package pasteurization was compared with pressurized steam pre-packaging pasteurization to reduce *L. monocytogenes* from fully cooked RTE bologna [77]. The pasteurization time using pressurized steam treatment was about 75%–90% shorter than using ambient steam treatment. Pressurized steam treatment may be integrated into a vacuum packaging unit to effectively eradicate *L. monocytogenes* from RTE meats just prior to sealing the retail packages to further reduce the treatment time, avoid post-treatment recontaminations by pathogens, and improve food safety without detrimentally affecting meat quality.

The efficacy of in-package pasteurization (65°C for 32 seconds) combined with pre-surface application of nisin and/or lysozyme to reduce and prevent the subsequent recovery and growth of *L. monocytogenes* during refrigerated storage on the surface of low-fat turkey bologna was investigated [78]. In-package pasteurization resulted in an immediate 3.5–4.2 log CFU/cm reduction in *L. monocytogenes* population for all treatments. In-package pasteurization in combination with nisin or nisin–lysozyme treatments was effective in reducing the population below detectable levels by 2–3 weeks of storage. It was claimed that a reduction in bacterial population can be achieved by a relatively short pasteurization time and antimicrobials reduced populations further during refrigerated storage.

Huang [79] developed and validated a more accurate method to analyze and calculate the inactivation of *L. monocytogenes* in frankfurter packages during post-lethality hot water immersion heating and the subsequent cooling processes. Effects of surface pasteurization on inactivation of *L. innocua* were investigated [80]. An inoculation study validated the efficacy of post-processing and the thermal lethality of *L. monocytogenes*. Pre-cooked sausage and ham, inoculated with approximately 10^7 CFU/cm^2 of *L. innocua*, were heated to a surface temperature of 70°C. Numbers of *L. innocua* were reduced by 7 log on surface-inoculated sausage.

A study was conducted to evaluate small-scale hot-water post-packaging pasteurization (PPP) as a post-lethality treatment for *L. monocytogenes* on ready-to-eat beef snack sticks and natural-casing wieners [81]. An average reduction in *L. monocytogenes* numbers of ≥2 log units was obtained using heating times of 1.0 minutes for individually packaged beef snack sticks and 4.0 minutes for packages of four sticks and seven sticks. A treatment of 7.0 minutes for packages of four natural-casing wieners achieved *L. monocytogenes* reductions of ≥1.0 log unit and average product surface temperature of 60.5°C–63.5°C. For natural-casing wieners, PPP had no detrimental effect on overall product desirability to consumers while for beef snack sticks a significant negative effect on consumer opinions of product appearance was noticed.

Muriana et al. [72] added the mixed cocktail of four strains of *L. monocytogenes* to a variety of ready-to-eat (RTE) meat products, including turkey, ham, and roast beef. All products were vacuum sealed in shrink-wrap packaging bags, massaged to ensure inoculum distribution, and processed by submersion heating in a precision-controlled steam-injected water bath. On various *L. monocytogenes* inoculated RTE deli meats, these workers achieved 2–4 log cycle reductions when processed at 90.6°C, 200 93.3°C, or 96.1°C for 2–10 minutes.

Hot water shrinkage has a promising application in controlling post-lethal surface contamination by *L. monocytogenes* in some deli meats. This intervention is likely to be cheaper than regular post-package pasteurization. It is also feasible, from a productivity standpoint, in many medium-sized companies. Delgado Suárez et al. [82] evaluated the potential of hot water shrinkage to reduce post-lethal surface contamination by *L. monocytogenes* in a turkey-based Virginia ham model. Ham slices were inoculated with 10^5 CFU/cm^2 of *L. monocytogenes* (ATCC 19114) vacuum packaged and placed in a water bath at 75°C, 80°C, 85°C, and 90°C for 0, 20, 25 and 30 seconds. Treatment at 75°C–85°C for up to 30 seconds did not affect pathogen survival, while nearly 4 log reduction was observed at 90°C for 30 seconds.

A thermal process for the surface pasteurization of ready-to-eat (RTE) meat products like turkey bologna, roast beef, corned beef, and ham for the reduction of *L. monocytogenes* was investigated [83]. The findings demonstrated that pre-package pasteurization, either alone or in combination with post-package pasteurization, is an effective tool for controlling *L. monocytogenes* surface contamination that may result from in-house handling.

Achieving a targeted lethality with minimum exposure to heat and preservation of product quality during pasteurization is a challenge. Mangalassary et al. [84] evaluated the effect of nisin and/or lysozyme in combination with in-package pasteurization of a ready-to-eat low-fat turkey bologna on the inactivation of *L. monocytogenes*. At 62.5°C, nisin-lysozyme-treated samples required 23% less time than did the control sample to achieve a 4 log reduction and 31% less time at 65°C. Lysozyme alone did not enhance antilisterial activity with heat.

The effectiveness of steam or steam in combination with an antimicrobial agent to control *L. monocytogenes* on ready-to-eat (RTE) franks was evaluated [85]. The franks were surface-inoculated to contain 6 or 3 log CFU/cm^2 of *L. monocytogenes* and treated with steam or steam in combination with an antimicrobial agent, immediately followed by vacuum-sealing. Three log CFU/cm^2 of reductions were achieved at the both inoculation levels for *L. monocytogenes* on franks. At an inoculation level of 3 logs, no outgrowth of *L. monocytogenes* was obtained on the treated franks after storing at 4.4°C or 16°C for a combined 47 days.

Huang [86] reported a study using a computer-controlled microwave heating system to pasteurize beef frankfurters surface-inoculated with *L. monocytogenes* and vacuum-packaged in plastic bags. It was observed that *L. monocytogenes* inoculated onto beef frankfurters was inactivated in a linear manner as heating progressed.

A microwave heating system equipped with a proportional–integral–differential (PID) control device was developed for in-package pasteurization of ready-to-eat meats [87]. Frankfurters, inoculated, and vacuum-sealed in plastic packages, were subjected to microwave or water immersion heating, with the package surface temperature increased to and maintained at 65°C, 75°C, or 85°C, for different periods of time, ranging from 2 to 19 minutes in total heating time. The concentration of *L. monocytogenes* decreased linearly with heating time. The observed rate of bacterial inactivation was 0.41, 0.65, and 0.94 log (CFU/package)/min at the surface temperature of 65°C, 75°C, or 85°C. When compared with water immersion heating at the same surface temperatures, the overall rate of bacterial inactivation was 30%–75% higher with microwave in-package pasteurization.

5.7.3 Pulsed Light

Different non-thermal technologies are currently being used to decontaminate food products. Among them, pulsed light (PL) can be a useful approach for the surface decontamination of foods. It consists in the application of short flashes (10^{-3} to 10^{-2} ms) of intense, broad-spectrum light (200–1100 nm). Microbial inactivation is mainly attributed to photochemical damage caused by the UV-C component [88], although photothermal damage has also been proposed [89]. The degree of inactivation achieved is highly dependent on the topography of the product, since PL has low penetration power and, also, microorganisms can hide in surface irregularities. The effect of PL is exerted at the surface level. Nevertheless, this is not a drawback for the hygienization of RTE products since post-processing contamination mainly occurs on the surface. In comparison to continuous UV systems, PL allows a greater energy input and reduces the exposure time.

Pulsed light (PL) was tested for its efficacy to reduce *L. monocytogenes* and *S. enterica* serovar *Typhimurium* on the surface of two ready-to-eat (RTE) dry cured meat products (salchichón and loin) [90]. Maximum log reductions between 1.5 and 1.8 CFU/cm^2 were obtained for both microorganisms when a fluence of 11.9 J/cm^2 was applied. Slight and particular differences in the instrumental color parameters were observed due to the treatment in both products, although no changes in the sensory analysis were detected either immediately after treatment or during 30 days storage in salchichón. Panelists perceived some changes in the sensory quality of loin immediately after treatment, but these differences disappeared along storage.

Pulsed light (PL) was tested for its utility to improve the microbial quality and safety of RTE cooked meat products [91]. The results of this study indicated that *L. monocytogenes* can be reduced by approximately 2 log CFU/cm^2 in RTE cooked ham and 1 log CFU/cm^2 in bologna using a fluence of 8.4 J/cm^2. This dose did not affect the sensory properties of ham and tripled its shelf life when compared with conventional RTE products. The efficacy of pulsed light to improve the safety of carpaccio has been investigated [92]. Beef and tuna slices were superficially inoculated with approximately 3 log CFU/cm^2 of *L. monocytogenes, E. coli, S. Typhimurium* and *V. parahaemolyticus*. Fluences of 0.7, 2.1, 4.2, 8.4 and 11.9 J/cm^2 were assayed. Treatments at 8.4 and 11.9 J/cm^2 inactivated the selected pathogens approximately by 1 log CFU/cm^2, although they modified the color parameters and had a negative effect on the sensory quality of the product. The raw attributes were not affected by fluences of 2.1 and 4.2 J/cm^2 immediately after the treatment, although changes were observed during storage. Pulsed light showed a greater impact on the sensory quality of tuna carpaccio compared to beef. None of the fluences assayed extended the shelf life of either product.

The possibility of enhancing the antilisterial capability of PL treatment by combining PL with an additional hurdle, the natural antimicrobial nisin, was explored [93]. Treatment with Nisaplin and PL resulted in a 4 to 5 log reduction for two replicate studies. The combination treatment resulted in no significant microbial growth during 28 and 48 days of refrigerated storage in the first and second replicates, respectively. These workers suggested that this combination treatment can be used as an effective antilisterial step in the production of ready-to-eat foods.

5.8 PACKAGING

Packaging is a scientific method of enclosing a food product to protect against physico-chemical changes, microbial spoilage, and to present it in the most attractive manner for consumer preference. It must contain, protect, preserve, communicate as a "silent salesman" (throughout the entire distribution process from point of manufacture to points of consumer usage), and provide convenience to satisfy the busy consumer lifestyle. Packaging materials used in food industry are broadly classified into rigid and flexible packaging materials. Rigid packaging materials include glass containers, metal (tin, aluminum, tin free steel) cans, fiber boards, cardboard boxes, and wooden boxes. Flexible packaging materials include paper, aluminum foil, plastics, laminates, co-extruded films, and retort pouches. The choice of packaging materials and a system used for a specific product depends on a variety of factors, such as the nature of the food material and associated preservation requirements and on understanding how the package and the food behave, both during and following the manufacturing process [94].

5.8.1 OVERWRAPPING

Fresh meats are placed on a semirigid tray and overwrapped with a plastic film of high-oxygen permeability, which provide ambient aerobic conditions around the product, giving it a limited shelf life. Polyethylene, Polyvinyl chloride (PVC), and Polyvinylidene chloride (PVdC) provide tight-fitting over-wraps due to the clinging properties associated with these materials. Aluminum foil or paper laminates can be used to protect cured meat against UV light.

5.8.2 VACUUM PACKAGING

The basic principle of vacuum packaging is to remove air from within the pack and maintain an oxygen-deficient environment by sealing the product in a low-O_2 permeable flexible film. The storage life of products is extended due to slower growth of anaerobic spoilage microflora and prevention of the fast-growing aerobic spoilage organisms. The packaging material used for vacuum packaging must possess high gas and moisture barrier properties and must be capable of heat sealing perfectly to deliver adequate containment [95]. For long-term storage (shelf life of approximately 5 months at 4°C) of packaged cooked meat and muscle-based, convenience-style food products, the following laminates are used in conjunction with vacuum packaging: cellophane/PVdC/LDPE, polyester/PVdC/LDPE, PA/PVdC/LDPE, metallized PA/EVA, EVA/PVdC/EVA, PA/LDPE/ionomer, PVC/PVdC/LDPE [96].

5.8.3 MODIFIED AND CONTROLLED ATMOSPHERE PACKAGING (MAP AND CAP)

In MAP, meat and meat products are packaged in vapor-barrier materials after initial alteration of gas environment, which gradually changes as a result of the interaction between the product and the package environment; whereas in CAP, after alteration of gaseous environment around the product, it is maintained at a specified composition regardless of product or any other environmental changes. Packages usually contain mixtures of two or three gases: O_2 (to enhance color stability), CO_2 (to inhibit microbiological growth), and N_2 (to maintain pack shape) [97]. Typically, fresh red meats are stored in modified atmosphere packages containing 80% O_2:20% CO_2 [98] and cooked meats are stored in 70% N_2:30% CO_2 [99] (Table 5.4).

TABLE 5.4

Gas Mixture Used in Modified Atmosphere Packaging for Meat and Meat Products

	Gas Composition		
Product	O_2	CO_2	N_2
Red meat	60–85	15–40	—
Beef/venison portion	80	20	—
Cooked meat	—	30	70
Cooked ham in slices	—	40	60
Poultry	—	75	25
Processed meats	—	—	100

Source: Ščetar et al. [101].

5.8.4 ACTIVE AND INTELLIGENT PACKAGING

Packaging in this group is characterized by its ability to extend product life by creating and maintaining in-pack conditions that differ markedly from the ambient environment; thus, creating conditions that modify or restrict microbial growth. Active packaging systems include oxygen scavengers, carbon dioxide scavengers or emitters, ethanol or ethylene emitters, temperature control and monitoring systems, and time–temperature integrated monitors. Oxygen-scavenging films have the potential to eliminate oxygen from a package providing a long shelf life. These triple-layer films have a middle layer that scavenges oxygen and plastic layers on either side for product contact and consumer handling. Antimicrobial packaging is receiving much interest nowadays; the possible ingredients for this purpose include bacteriocins, antimicrobial enzymes, silver ions, zeolite products, sorbic acids, and different combinations. Essential oils, such as thyme, oregano, and rosemary, in a packaging system have also shown promise as antimicrobials. New packaging innovations have also resulted in the development of intelligent packaging. Intelligent packaging has been defined as packaging systems, which monitor the condition of packaged foods to give information about the quality of the packaged food during transport and storage [100]. These products may feature time and temperature indicators to detect mishandling or temperature abuse of a product or to indicate when a cook-in bag product has reached a proper temperature. Other possibilities include freshness indicators in packaging that may detect levels of volatiles in a product. Other "active" possibilities are odor removers or odor emitters. The cost effectiveness of smart packaging devices is dependent on the perceived benefits derived from such systems, available consumer-attitude information seems to be in favor of such packaging concepts [102] (Table 5.5).

The increased demand for ready-to-eat meat products will serve to further advance packaging research and technologies, for use in the meat sector. The recognition of the benefits of advanced packaging by the meat industry, development of economically viable packaging systems, and increased consumer acceptance are necessary for commercial realization for use with meat and meat products in the future. In cost-sensitive markets of developing countries, like India, the pressure to reduce packaging costs is intense. While the demand for more sophisticated packaging is on the rise, with it comes additional pressures on cost for packaging suppliers. While recycling has been the mantra that both governments and manufacturers are learning to live by, reusability is an area where the packaging sector has much to offer by way of innovation. In addition, meat industry requires improved product consistency, shelf life, and acceptable appearance. Advances in packaging technology will allow meat industry to address consumer needs for food safety, palatability, cost, environmental concern, and information in global meat markets, with increased communication in the meat cold chain.

TABLE 5.5
Shelf Life of Meat and Meat Products under Different Packaging Conditions

Product	Packaging Material/Method	Shelf Life
Beef and pork	Air: PE	10–11 days, 4°C
	Vacuum PA/PE	11 days, 4°C
Beef steaks	Expanded PS Tray+ PE/PA	22–28 days, 1°C
	MAP: 70% O_2, 10% CO_2, 20% N_2	
Sausages, heat treated	Vacuum packed	6–11 weeks, 7°C
Cooked ham and frankfurters	PA/PE	4 weeks, 4°C
Pork sausage	Tray: PS, overwrap: PE	8 days, 2°C
	MAP_1: 20% CO_2, 80% N_2	16 days, 2°C
	MAP_2: 20% CO_2, 80% N_2 + O_2 absorber	>20 days, 2°C
Chicken wings	Vacuum packed and cooked (*sous vide*)	7 weeks, 2°C

Source: Ščetar et al. [101].

5.9 STANDARDS FOR HYGIENIC MEAT PRODUCTION

Meat has traditionally been viewed as a vehicle for a significant proportion of human food-borne pathogens. Although the spectrum of meat-borne diseases of public health importance has changed with changing production and processing systems, continuation of the problem has been well illustrated in recent years by human surveillance studies of specific meat-borne pathogens such as *E. coli* O157:H7, *Salmonella* spp., *Campylobacter* spp., and *Yersinia enterocolitica*. Additionally, new hazards are also becoming apparent, such as the agent of bovine spongiform encephalopathy (BSE). Furthermore consumers have expectations about suitability issues, which are not necessarily of human health significance [103].

A contemporary risk-based approach to meat hygiene requires that hygiene measures should be applied at those points in the food chain where they will be of the greatest value in reducing food-borne risks to consumers. This should be reflected in the application of specific measures based on science and risk assessment, with a greater emphasis on prevention and control of contamination during all aspects of production of meat and it's further processing. Application of Hazard Analysis Critical Control Point (HACCP) principles is an essential element. The measure of success of contemporary programs is an objective demonstration of levels of hazard control in food that are correlated with required levels of consumer protection, rather than by concentrating on detailed and prescriptive measures that give an unknown outcome [103].

5.9.1 Sources of Contamination

The microorganisms present on meat have their origins either from infection of the living animal prior to conversion of muscle into meat that is, endogenous contamination, or by contamination of the carcass postmortem, that is, exogenous contamination [104]. The main sources of contamination for meat are hides and hair, soil, contents of the stomach and gut, water, airborne pollution, utensils, and equipment. The chief source of bacteriological contamination was found to be the hide and hair of the slaughtered animals, deriving mainly from the microflora of the pasture soil, but with a higher incidence of yeasts. Then, as today, the transfer of microorganisms from the hide to the underlying tissues was found to begin during the first stage of removal of the pelt by means of knives used for skinning. Further transfer occurs via the hands, arms, legs, and clothing of the operatives [105].

Contemporary methods to control the microbial contamination of meat during production must consider the microbiological characteristics of both the exogenous and endogenous microbes, along with the process whereby the meat becomes contaminated. This can help in establishing the critical controls and reducing the hazards to the absolute minimum. This information therefore forms the basis of hygienic meat production, whether it be managed and verified at the premise level by good manufacturing (hygienic) practice and HACCP plans [106], or by the regulator through risk analysis and legislation. Various sources of the contaminations, which can pose threat to food safety in the slaughter house, are tabulated in Table 5.6.

5.9.2 General Principles of Meat Hygiene

Codex Alimentarius Commission and Recommended International Code of Hygienic Practice for Fresh Meat [103] have outlined guidelines to ensure safe production of meat as follows:

- Meat must be safe and suitable for human consumption and all interested parties including government, industry, and consumers have a role in achieving this outcome.
- The competent authority should have the legal power to set and enforce regulatory meat hygiene requirements, and have final responsibility for verifying that regulatory meat hygiene requirements are met. It should be the responsibility of the establishment operator to produce meat that is safe and suitable in accordance with regulatory meat hygiene requirements. There should be a legal obligation on relevant parties to provide any information and assistance as may be required by the competent authority.

TABLE 5.6

Sources of Contamination of Meat in Slaughter House

Source of Contamination	Description
Hide, hair, fleece	For red meat, the initial and possibly most significant potential source of exogenous contamination is from the hide/fleece of the animal [107, 108]. Most of the contaminants have fecal origin but the organisms from soil, mud, and stock supply farm may be present [109]. Dressing operation minimizing the number and extent of opening cuts through the skin can be helpful in reducing the contamination [110].
Stunning and sticking	Bacterial contamination introduced into the carcass during penetrative captive bolt stunning may become widely dispersed across the slaughter line environment and within carcass, their surfaces and edible offals [111,112]. During the act of sticking, bacteria can enter the jugular vein or anterior vena cava and travel in the bloodstream to the muscles, lungs, and bone marrow. Hygienic two-knife technique for sticking can be helpful.
Gastrointestinal tract	Accidental puncture of the stomach and intestines is a source of contamination on occasions, as is spillage from the rectum and esophagus. During decapitation enteric bacteria can be transferred via saliva and mucus, as well as direct transfer of material from the tonsils and maxillary lymph nodes. In larger species halving of the carcass into two parts by sawing through the vertebrae is done. In this case, the spinal cord can be a specified risk material due to the potential for transmission of BSE, and it must be removed from the carcass.
Physical contact with structures	The design of the slaughter line should be of enough capacity to avoid touch of animal body parts. Gross cleaning, with squeegee and shovel, and so on, must be ongoing throughout the working day to prevent the build-up of blood and debris. As part of GMP/GHP, every opportunity must be taken during breaks in production when the slaughter floor is free of carcasses and offal to rinse down the line [105].
Personnel	All persons working in the slaughter hall are an important, and extremely mobile, source of contamination, and means of cross-contamination for the meat. Movement of all personnel in the plant must be strictly controlled; movement should only be allowed from clean to dirty area. The operator of the slaughterhouse must establish a staff training program for various categories of the workers enabling them to understand and follow the procedures required to implement the GMP/GHP [105].
Equipment and utensils	The equipment used within the slaughter hall such as knives, saws, and hock cutters is a potential source of contamination must be regularly cleaned and sterilized.
The slaughter hall environment	Slaughterhouse environment should be well ventilated to avoid moisture condensation as later can help in carcass contamination and further spoilage. Poorly maintained structure may result in contamination of the meat from, for example, rust or paint flakes dropping on to the meat or into trays intended for meat. Excessive lubrication of overhead moving chains or cogs is another potential contamination hazard [105].
Vermin and pests	All measures necessary to exclude vermin and pests from the food-producing factory must be taken. Vermin and pests, which manage to gain entrance must be systematically destroyed.
Chemical contamination	Cleaning chemicals may contaminate the meat if they have not been used in accordance with the manufactures' instructions. Only chemicals suitable for use in the food industry should be used for sanitizing the slaughterhouse. All rail grease and lubricating oils should be food grade [105].

- Meat hygiene programs should have as their primary goal the protection of public health and should be based on a scientific evaluation of meat-borne risks to human health and take into account all relevant food safety hazards, as identified by research, monitoring, and other relevant activities.
- The principles of food safety risk analysis should be incorporated wherever possible and appropriate in the design and implementation of meat hygiene programs.
- Wherever possible and practical, competent authorities should formulate food safety objectives (FSOs) according to a risk-based approach so as to objectively express the level of hazard control that is required to meet public health goals.
- Meat hygiene requirements should control hazards to the greatest extent practicable throughout the entire food chain. Information available from primary production should be taken into account so as to tailor meat hygiene requirements to the spectrum and prevalence of hazards in the animal population from which the meat is sourced.
- The establishment operator should apply HACCP principles. To the greatest extent practicable, the HACCP principles should also be applied in the design and implementation of hygiene measures throughout the entire food chain.
- The competent authority should define the role of those personnel involved in meat hygiene activities where appropriate, including the specific role of the veterinary inspector.
- The range of activities involved in meat hygiene should be carried out by personnel with the appropriate training, knowledge, skills, and ability as and where defined by the competent authority.
- The competent authority should verify that the establishment operator has adequate systems in place to trace and withdraw meat from the food chain. Communication with consumers and other interested parties should be considered and undertaken where appropriate.
- As appropriate to the circumstances, the results of monitoring and surveillance of animal and human populations should be considered with subsequent review and/or modification of meat hygiene requirements whenever necessary.
- Competent authorities should recognize the equivalence of alternative hygiene measures where appropriate, and promulgate meat hygiene measures that achieve required outcomes in terms of safety and suitability and facilitate fair practices in the trading of meat.

5.10   GUIDELINES FOR TRANSPORT OF CARCASS AND MEAT PRODUCTS

The different stages in transport, from cold storage to the retail outlet, and then to the consumer refrigerator, are critical points for the overall quality and safety of the meat. A significant factor is the temperature inside the transport vehicles, and the fluctuations that occur during transit. The vehicle must be provided with a good refrigerated system, operating constantly during transportation to maintain proper chilling of the product. Another important requirement is to avoid undesirable heat infiltration, which may occur due to hot weather, sunny conditions, inadequate insulation, or air leakage. By taking precautions to avoid the above, it should be possible to achieve the recommended optimal conditions [113].

The BC Centre for Disease Control [114] gave the guidelines for the safe transportation of carcasses, poultry, and meat products. These are as follows:

- Proper transportation of carcasses and meat products will reduce the potential for contamination. The following guidelines are provided to assist those who transport meat products.
- Ensure carcasses being transported to an approved cut-and-wrap facility should be clean and not contaminated before or during transport. In some cases, it is better to leave the hide on the carcass for additional protection of the meat while en route to an approved cut-and-wrap facility. If the hide is removed, the carcass should be otherwise protected during transport.
- The operator of an approved cut-and-wrap facility should refuse any meat that appears to be diseased, unwholesome, spoiled or otherwise unfit, so it is essential to ensure protection of the carcass during transport.

- Transport vehicle should be inspected before loading. Remove items that may contaminate meat products. Vehicle, containers, and equipment used for transport should be cleaned and food contact surface be sanitized.
- Loading and unloading methods should avoid contact with any object, which can contaminate the carcass or meat products.
- Good personal hygiene should be practiced before loading and unloading.
- Provide insulated containers with securely attached lids for smaller-sized products. Provide a clean, designated protective tarp, industry-approved shipping bags/shrouds, or other suitable covers for products too large to fit in insulated containers. Tarps should be thoroughly sanitized and properly stored for future use. Securely fasten covers during transport.
- Avoid cross contamination of meat products through proper packing. Use separate containers for raw and cooked or ready-to-eat products.
- Consider the time of day and weather conditions before accepting meat products for transport. If possible, avoid transporting on days with unsuitable weather.
- Ensure carcasses and other meat products have been properly chilled to 4°C or colder at the slaughter or cut-and-wrap facility before loading. Maintain a temperature of 4°C or colder during transport.
- Hold frozen products at −18°C or colder, and ship in a way that prevents thawing and refreezing. Limit transport time when meat products are without refrigeration. Never allow meat products to be kept out of refrigeration for more than 2 hours unless other suitable means of maintaining temperatures are used.

Australian standards for the hygienic production and transportation of meat and meat products for human consumptions [115] have outlined guidelines for transportation of meat and meat products and are as follows:

- The proprietor of a meat transport business follows a system of operational hygiene process controls for the transportation of meat and meat products that is effective in ensuring the wholesomeness of the meat and meat products.
- The meat carrying compartment of a meat transport vehicle, the equipment to be used in the meat carrying compartment and the equipment to be used for the loading of meat and meat products should not be the source of contamination of meat and meat products. These should be cleaned before the commencement of operations each day and be cleaned at the end of operation each day. If the compartment and equipment are being used to transport a consignment of meat for a period greater than a day, are clean before the meat and meat products are loaded onto the vehicle and are cleaned as soon as practicable after the vehicle has been unloaded.
- Water used to clean the meat carrying compartment is potable.
- Meat transport vehicles should be maintained in a good state of repair and working order having regard to their use.
- The accumulation of material likely to cause contamination of meat and meat products during transportation is prevented.
- There should be an effective mechanism to control pest in the meat transport vehicle.
- Persons transporting meat and meat products must exercise personal hygiene practices that do not jeopardize the wholesomeness of meat and meat products.
- Wholesomeness of meat and meat product should not be compromised while transportation.
- During transport of meat and meat products exposed meat and meat products should not come into contact with any surfaces that may cause contamination; unwrapped carcass and carcass parts should be carried in closed containers and should not contaminate other meat and meat products; and there should be adequate air flow; and the introduction into

the cans of canned meat products the microorganisms that could affect the commercial sterility of the contents of the cans should be prevented; and the means of identifying the meat or meat products should not be lost.

- Meat and meat products other than shelf-stable one are transported at a temperature for a carcass, side, quarter and bone-in major separated cut, 7°C; and for any other meat or meat products, 5°C at the site of microbiological concern; or in accordance with the alternative time and temperature controls for their transport that are specified in the approved arrangement of the meat business that stores and handles them.
- Shelf-stable meat products are transported in accordance with the time and temperature controls specified for their transport in the approved arrangement of the meat business that stores and handles them.
- The transport of meat and meat products for human consumption in the same meat transport vehicle as other things does not jeopardize the wholesomeness of the meat or meat products.
- Animals, inedible material and condemned material are not transported in a meat transport vehicle.
- During transport ready-to-eat meat products are not contaminated by meat and meat products that are not ready-to-eat and cooked meat is not contaminated by raw meat.
- Meat and meat products are not loaded onto a meat transport vehicle unless the vehicle, the equipment to be used in the meat carrying compartment and the equipment to be used for the loading meet the applicable matters specified in the standard.
- If the proprietor of a meat transport business becomes aware that meat or meat products transported by the business are exposed to the conditions that may have jeopardized the wholesomeness of the meat and meat products, the proprietor notifies without delay the proprietor of the meat business that receives the meat or meat products.

5.11 SAFE MEAT STORAGE

Throughout the food industry food poisoning is a real and growing problem and meat one of its main sources. In addition to the effect of pathogens on meat, the growth of spoilage organisms leads to considerable waste and resulting financial loss. Refrigeration is the prime process controlling the growth of pathogenic and spoilage microorganisms [116]. The safety and suitability of food needs to be maintained while storage by ensuring it is stored in an appropriate environment and protected from contamination. High risk food must be stored at a temperature that minimizes the opportunity for pathogenic bacteria to grow. Food is considered to be "stored" if it is not being processed, displayed, packaged, transported, or identified for disposal [117].

It is recommended that raw materials be used on a First-In/First-Out (FIFO), first-expiry/first-out (FEFO) basis or according to a plant specified product rotation/inventory control schedule. Raw materials should be stored at temperatures that maintain proper product condition. Frozen materials should be kept frozen, unless tempering or thawing is required prior to use. The package/pallet integrity must be maintained throughout the storage period to maintain the condition of the material. Product identity in storage should allow for the in-plant tracking system [118]. Finished RTE products should be handled in a method that provides separation of raw and cooked products. They should be stored at plant-designated time/temperatures to maintain product shelf life. Frozen products should be kept frozen. A FIFO or a plant specified product rotation/inventory control schedule should also be maintained for finished products. The package/pallet integrity should be maintained throughout the storage period to maintain the condition of the finished product. Product identity in storage should allow for the in-plant tracking system to be used for recall and/or market withdrawal purposes [118]. Refrigeration and freezer storage life of raw and ready-to-eat meat products have been provided in the Table 5.7.

TABLE 5.7

Refrigeration and Freezer Storage Life of Raw and Ready-To-Eat Meat Products

Product	Refrigeration Life	Freezer Life
Fresh Meat (Beef, Veal, Lamb, and Pork)		
Steaks	3–5 days	6–12 months
Chops	3–5 days	4–6 months
Roasts	3–5 days	4–12 months
Variety meats	1–2 days	3–4 months
Fresh Poultry		
Chicken or turkey whole	1–2 days	4 months
Chicken or turkey parts	1–2 days	9 months
Giblets	1–2 days	3–4 months
Deli and Vacuum-Packed Products		
Chicken, tuna ham, macaroni salad	3–5 days	Do not freeze well
Pre-stuffed pork and lamb chops, chicken breast stuffed with dressing	1 day	Do not freeze well
Raw Hamburger, Ground, and Stew Meat		
Hamburger and stew meats	1–2 days	3–4 months
Ground turkey, veal, pork, lamb	1–2 days	3–4 months
Ham		
Ham fully cooked whole	7 days	1–2 months
Ham fully cooked half	3–5 days	1–2 months
Ham fully cooked slices	3–4 days	1–2 months
Hot Dogs and Lunch Meats (Freezer Wrap)		
Hot dogs opened pack	7 days	1–2 months
Hot dogs unopened pack	14 days	1–2 months
Lunch meats opened pack	3–5 days	1–2 months
Lunch meats unopened pack	14 days	1–2 months
Bacon and Sausage		
Bacon	7 days	1 month
Sausage, raw from pork, beef, chicken or turkey	1–2 days	1–2 months
Smoked breakfast links, patties	7 days	1–2 months
Summer sausage (labelled "Keep refrigerated") unopened	3 months	1–2 months
Summer sausage (labelled "Keep refrigerated") opened	21 days	1–2 months
Processed Chicken		
Chicken nuggets, patties	3–4 days	2 months

Source: USFDA [120].

Refrigerator or freezer storage is necessary for meat and meat products. Refrigerator and freezer temperatures do not destroy pathogenic or spoilage microorganisms, but freezer temperatures do stop their growth. McCurdy et al. [119] suggested some important points for the refrigeration and frozen storage of foods including meat products. According to them:

- Refrigerator should be maintained between 1.1°C and 4.4°C. Food placement in the refrigerator affects air circulation and efficiency. Food should not be stacked tightly, and refrigerator shelves should not be covered with foil or any material that prevents air circulation from quickly and evenly cooling the food.

- Raw meat and poultry should be securely wrapped and placed in a tray or pan to prevent leaking. Raw meat and ready-to-eat meat products should be stored separately to avoid cross contamination. Meat drawer should be designated for either raw meats or ready-to-eat meat.
- Freezer should be kept at −18°C or below (−23 to −28°C is the best) to maintain the quality of frozen foods. Use moisture-proof, freezer-weight wrap.

During storage food may become contaminated microbiologically, such as by raw foods contaminating ready-to-eat food; chemically, such as by food not being stored in food-grade containers or by chemicals being accidentally spilt onto food; and physically, from foreign objects including pests, glass, dirt, metal, and hair [117]. To prevent food from becoming contaminated during storage the following steps need to be taken:

- Food should be stored in food-grade containers and covered if there is any likelihood of contamination.
- Raw foods should be stored separately or away from ready-to-eat foods to avoid contamination from the raw food being transferred to the ready-to-eat food.
- Storage areas should be kept clean to minimize the opportunity for dirt, food scraps, and so on contaminating stored food.
- Storage areas should be kept free of pests.

5.12   CONCLUSION

In coming decades, the demand for animal derived foods, in particular meat, will continue to grow in developing countries. Though, the debate on the nutritional benefits versus the possible adverse health effects of meat consumption is still on, recent exploratory research has demonstrated the feasibility of incorporation of bioactive ingredients, natural antioxidants from spices, herbs, fruits, and other sources for reducing such health risks. New and emerging technologies, namely high pressure processing, pulsed electric field processing, power ultrasound, radiofrequency heating, and so on can also play an important role in satisfying changing consumer demands. Packaging of meat or meat products is a dynamic process and needs to be in order to meet the challenges of global marketing system. However, the broad field of meat science is much more than harvesting meat from animals and processing of products, it also includes animal welfare, antemortem stress, and its effects on meat quality, humane slaughter techniques, the basic understanding of biochemistry, and physiology for conversion of muscle to meat and meat microbiology. Meat scientists have an important role to play in this process. They are uniquely positioned to bridge the gaps between different disciplines and thereby help the meat sector to prosper. The meaningful partnership and alliance among Industry Partners, R & D Institutions, and national and international agencies for converting scientific knowledge into value added systems by improving linkages, infrastructure, regulating taxation, and food laws, as well as depicting clear plans will benefit producer, processors, and consumers, as well as to build a brand image to meat products in developing countries.

REFERENCES

1. Offer, G. and Cousins, T. 1992. The mechanism of drip production – Formation of 2 compartments of extracellular-space in muscle postmortem. *Journal of the Science of Food and Agriculture 58*: 107–116.
2. Wismer Pedersen, J. 1971. Water. In *The Science of Meat and Meat Products*, eds. J.R. Price, and B.S. Schweigirt, pp. 177–191. San Francisco, CA: W. H. Freeman.
3. Fennema, O.R. 1996. Water and ice. In *Food Chemistry*, 3rd edn., ed. O.R. Fennema, pp. 17–94. New York: Marcel Dekker.
4. Huff-Lonergan, E. and Lonergan, S.M. 2005. Mechanisms of water holding capacity in meat: The role of postmortem biochemical and structural changes. *Meat Science 71*: 194–204.

5. Offer, G. and Knight, P. 1988. The structural basis of water-holding capacity in meat. Part 2: Drip losses. In *Developments in Meat Science* (Vol. 4), ed. R.A. Lawrie, pp. 173–243. London, UK: Elsevier Science Publications.

6. McClements, D.J. 2005. *Food Emulsions: Principles, Practices, and Techniques.* London, UK: CRC Press LLC.

7. Gordon, A. and Barbut, S. 1992. Mechanism of meat batter stabilization: A review. *Critical Reviews in Food Science and Nutrition 32*: 299–332.

8. Zorba, O. 2006. The effects of the amount of emulsified oil on the emulsion stability and viscosity of myofibrillar proteins. *Food Hydrocolloids 20*: 698–702.

9. Yasui, T., Ishioroshi, M., Nakano, H. and Samejima, K. 1979. Changes in shear modulus, ultrastructure, and spin-spin relaxation times of water associated with heat-induced gelation of myosin. *Journal of Food Science 44*: 1201–1211.

10. Xiong, Y.L. 1993. A comparison of the rheological characteristics of different fractions of chicken myofibrillar proteins. *Journal of Food Biochemistry 16*: 217–227.

11. Sun, X.D. and Holley, R.A. 2011. Factors influencing gel formation by myofibrillar proteins in muscle foods. *Comprehensive Reviews in Food Science and Nutrition 10*: 33–51.

12. Xiong, Y.L. 1992. Thermally induced interactions and gelation of combined myofibrillar proteins from white and red broiler muscles. *Journal of Food Science 57*: 581–585.

13. Xiong, Y.L. 1994. Myofibrillar protein from different muscle fiber types: Implications of biochemical and functional properties in meat processing. *Critical Reviews in Food Science and Nutrition 34*: 293–320.

14. Wood, J.D., Enser, M., Fisher, A.V., Nute, G.R., Richardson, R.I. and Sheard, P.R. 1999. Manipulating meat quality and composition. *Proceedings of the Nutrition Society 58*: 363–370.

15. Jeremiah, L.E., Dugan, M.E.R., Aalhus, J.L. and Gibson, L.L. 2003. Assessment of the chemical and cooking properties of the major beef muscles and muscle groups. *Meat Science 65*: 985–992.

16. Biesalski, H.K. 2005. Meat as a component of a healthy diet—Are there any risks or benefits if meat is avoided in the diet? *Meat Science 70*: 509–524.

17. Tornberg, E. 2005. Effects of heat on meat proteins—Implications on structure and quality of meat products. *Meat Science 70*: 493–508.

18. Valsta, L.M., Tapanainen, H. and Mannisto, S. 2005. Meat fats in nutrition. *Meat Science 70*: 525–530.

19. Fairweather-Tait, S.J. 1989. Iron in foods and its availability? *Acta Paediatrica Scandinavica 361*: 12–20.

20. Aristoy, M.C. and Toldrá, F. 2011. Essential amino acids. In *Handbook of Analysis of Edible Animal By-Products*, eds. L.M.L. Nollet, and F. Toldrá, pp. 123–135. Boca Raton, FL: CRC Press.

21. Honikel, K.O. 2011. Composition and calories. In *Handbook of Analysis of Edible Animal By-Products*, eds. L.M.L. Nollet and F. Toldrá, pp. 105–121. Boca Raton, FL: CRC Press.

22. Unsal, M. and Aktas, N. 2003. Fractionation and characterization of edible sheep tail fat. *Meat Science 63*(4): 235–239.

23. Devatkal, S., Mendiratta, S.K., Kondaiah, N., Sharma, M.C. and Anjaneyulu, A.S.R. 2004. Physicochemical, functional and microbiological quality of buffalo liver. *Meat Science 68*(5): 79–86.

24. Verma, A.K., Lakshmanan, V., Das, A.K., Mendiratta, S.K. and Anjaneyulu, A.S.R. 2008. Quality characteristics and storage stability of patties from buffalo head and heart meats. *International Journal of Food Science & Technology 43*(10): 1798–1806.

25. Jimenez-Colmenero, F., Carballo, J. and Cofrades, S. 2001. Healthier meat and meat products: Their role as functional foods. *Meat Science 59*(1): 5–13.

26. Whitney, E.N. and Rolfes, S.R. 2002. *Understanding Nutrition*, 9th edn. Belmont, CA: Wadsworth.

27. Verma, A., Sharma, B. and Banerjee, R. 2009. Quality characteristics and storage stability of low fat functional chicken nuggets. *Fleischwirtschaft International 24*: 52–57.

28. Banerjee, R., Verma, A.K., Das, A.K., Rajkumar, V., Shewalkar, A. and Narkhede, H. 2012. Antioxidant effects of broccoli powder extract in goat meat nuggets. *Meat Science 91*(2): 179–184.

29. Tim, H. 2002. Sodium technological functions of salt in the manufacturing of food and drink products. *British Food Journal 104*(2): 126–152.

30. Feiner, G. 2006. *Meat Products Handbook: Practical Science and Technology.* Cambridge, UK: Woodhead Publishing.

31. Vasavada, M.N., Dwivedi, S. and Cornforth, D. 2006. Evaluation of garam masala spices and phosphates as antioxidants in cooked ground beef. *Journal of Food Science 71*: C292–C297.

32. Sebranek, J.G. and Bacus, J.N. 2007. Cured meat products without direct addition of nitrate or nitrite: What are the issues? *Meat Science 77*: 136–147.

33. Aymerich, T., Picouet, P.A. and Monfort, J.M. 2008. Decontamination technologies for meat products. *Meat Science 78*:114–129.

34. Lawrie, R.A. and Ledward, D.A. 2006. *Lawrie's Meat Science*, 7th edn. Cambridge, UK: Woodhead Publishing.

35. Sahagian, M.E. and Goff, H.D. 1996. Fundamental aspects of the freezing process. In *Freezing Effects on Food Quality*, ed. L. Jeremiah, pp. 1–50. New York: Marcel Dekker.

36. Magnussen, O.M., Haugland, A., Hemmingsen, A.K.T., Johansen, S. and Nordtvedt, T.S. 2008. Advances in superchilling of food: Process characteristics and product quality. *Trends in Food Science & Technology 19*: 418–424.

37. Kaale, L.D., Eikevik, T.M., Rustad, T. and Kolsaker, K. 2011. Superchilling of food: A review. *Journal of Food Engineering 107*: 141–146.

38. Duun, A.S. and Rustad, T. 2007. Quality changes during superchilled storage of cod (*Gadus morhua*) fillets. *Food Chemistry 105*: 1067–1075.

39. Weakley, D.F., McKeith, F.K., Bechtel, P.J., Martin, S.E. and Thomas, D.L. 1986. Effects of different chilling methods on hot processed vacuum packaged pork. *Journal of Food Science 51*: 757–760.

40. McGeehin, B., Sheridan, J.J. and Butler, F. 2002. Optimizing a rapid chilling system for lamb carcasses. *Journal of Food Engineering 52*: 75–81.

41. Jeremiah, L.E. and Gibson, L.L. 2001. The influence of packaging and storage time on the retail properties and case-life of retail-ready beef. *Food Research International 34*: 621–631.

42. Schubring, R. 2009. 'Superchilling' - an 'old' variant to prolong shelf life of fresh fish and meat requicked. *Fleischwirtschaft 89*: 104–113.

43. Aberle, E.D., Forrest, J.C., Gerrard, D.E. and Mills, E.W. 2001. *Principles of Meat Science* 4th ed. USA: Kendall/Hunt Publishing.

44. Rodríguez-Calleja, J.M., Cruz-Romero, M.C., O'Sullivan, M.G., García-López, M.L. and Kerry, J.P. 2012. High-pressure-based hurdle strategy to extend the shelf-life of fresh chicken breast fillets. *Food Control 25*(2): 516–524.

45. Karthikeyan, J., Kumar, S., Anjaneyulu, A.S.R. and Rao, K.H. 2000. Application of hurdle technology for the development of Caprine *keema* and its stability at ambient temperature. *Meat Science 54*(1): 9–15.

46. Thomas, R., Anjaneyulu, A.S.R. and Kondaiah, N. 2008. Effect of hot-boned pork on the quality of hurdle treated pork sausages during ambient temperature (37°C) storage. *Food Chemistry 107*(2): 804–812.

47. Murphy, R.Y., Duncan, L.K., Beard, B.L. and Driscoll, K.H. 2003. D and Z values of *Salmonella, Listeria innocua*, and *Listeria monocytogenes* in fully cooked poultry products. *Journal of Food Science 68*: 1443–1447.

48. Levine, P., Rose, B., Green, S., Ransom, G. and Hill, W. 2001. Pathogen testing of ready-to-eat meat and poultry products collected at federally inspected establishment in the United States, 1990 to 1999. *Journal of Food Protection 64*: 1188–1193.

49. Vázquez-Villanueva, J., Orgaz, B., Ortiz, S., López, V., Martínez-Suárez, J.V. and San Jose, C. 2010. Predominance and persistence of a single clone of *Listeria ivanovii* in a Manchego cheese factory over 6 months. *Zoonoses and Public Health 57*: 402–410.

50. Anonymous. 2003. Control of *Listeria monocytogenes* in ready-to-eat meat and poultry products; Final Rule Federal Register, June 5, Vol. 68, No. 109. Washington, DC.

51. USDA FSIS. 2012. FSIS Compliance guideline: Controlling *Listeria monocytogenes* in post-lethality exposed ready-to-eat meat and poultry products. http://www.fsis.usda.gov/shared/PDF/ Controlling_LM_RTE_guideline_0912.pdf.

52. Aymerich, M.T., Jofré, A., Garriga, M. and Hugas, M. 2005. Inhibition of *Listeria monocytogenes* and *Salmonella* by natural antimicrobials and high hydrostatic pressure in sliced cooked ham. *Journal of Food Protection 68*: 173–177.

53. CAC. 2007. Guidelines on the application of general principles of food hygiene to the control of *Listeria monocytogenes* in foods. CAC/GL 61-2007. *Codex Alimentarius Commission 1–28*.

54. HHS (Health and Human Services). 2008. Guidance for Industry: Control of *Listeria monocytogenes* in Refrigerated or Frozen Ready-to-Eat Foods. U. S. Department of Health and Human Services. Food and Drug Administration, Center of Food Safety and Applied Nutrition.

55. Patterson, M.F. 2005. Microbiology of pressure-treated foods. *Journal of Applied Microbiology 98*: 1400–1409.

56. Hugas, M., Garriga, M. and Monfort, J.M. 2002. New mild technologies in meat processing: High pressure as a model technology. *Meat Science 62*(3): 359–371.

57. Cheftel, J.C. and Culioli, J. 1997. Effects of high pressure on meat: A review. *Meat Science 46*(3): 211–236.

58. Patterson, M.F., Quinn, M., Simpson, R. and Gilmore, A. 1995. Sensitivity of vegetative pathogens to high hydrostatic pressure treatment in phosphate buffered saline and foods. *Journal of Food Protection 58*: 524–529.

59. Kalchayanand, N., Sikes, T., Dunne, C.P. and Ray, B. 1994. Hydrostatic pressure and electroporation have increased bactericidal efficiency in combination with bacteriocins. *Applied and Environmental Microbiology* 60: 4174–4177.

60. Marcos, B., Aymerich, T., Monfort, J.M. and Garriga, M. 2008a. High-pressure processing and antimicrobial biodegradable packaging to control *Listeria monocytogenes* during storage of cooked ham. *Food Microbiology* 25(1): 177–182.

61. Lavieri, N., Sebranek, J., Cordray, J., Dickson, J., Horsch, A., Jung, S., Manu, D., Mendonça, A. and Stecher, B.B. 2015. Control of *Listeria monocytogenes* on alternatively cured ready-to-eat ham using natural antimicrobial ingredients in combination with post-lethality interventions. *Journal of Food Processing and Technology* 6(10): 1–7.

62. Hereu, A., Bover-Cid, S., Garriga, M. and Aymerich, T. 2012. High hydrostatic pressure and biopreservation of dry-cured ham to meet the food safety objectives for *Listeria monocytogenes*. *International Journal of Food Microbiology* 154(3): 107–112.

63. Jofré, A., Garriga, M. and Aymerich, T. 2008. Inhibition of *Salmonella* sp., *Listeria monocytogenes* and *Staphylococcus aureus* in cooked ham by combining antimicrobials, high hydrostatic pressure and refrigeration. *Meat Science* 78: 53–59.

64. Myers, K., Montoya, D., Cannon, J., Dickson, J. and Sebranek, J. 2013. The effect of high hydrostatic pressure, sodium nitrite and salt concentration on the growth of *Listeria monocytogenes* on RTE ham and turkey. *Meat Science* 93(2): 263–268.

65. Lavieri, N.A., Sebranek, J.G., Brehm-Stecher, B.F., Cordray, J.C., Dickson, J.S., Horsch, A.M., Jung, S., Larson, E.M., Manu, D.K. and Mendonca, A.F. 2014. Investigating the control of *Listeria monocytogenes* on alternatively-cured frankfurters using natural antimicrobial ingredients or post-lethality interventions. *Meat Science* 97(4): 568–574.

66. Marcos, B., Jofré, A., Aymerich, T., Monfort, J.M. and Garriga, M. 2008. Combined effect of natural antimicrobials and high pressure processing to prevent *Listeria monocytogenes* growth after a cold chain break during storage of cooked ham. *Food Control* 19(1): 76–81.

67. Porto-Fett, A.C., Call, J.E., Shoyer, B.E., Hill, D.E., Pshebniski, C., Cocoma, G.J. and Luchansky, J.B. 2010. Evaluation of fermentation, drying, and/or high pressure processing on viability of *Listeria monocytogenes*, *Escherichia coli* O157: H7, *Salmonella* spp., and *Trichinella spiralis* in raw pork and Genoa salami. *International Journal of Food Microbiology* 140(1): 61–75.

68. Schalch, B., Eisgruber, H. and Stolle, A. 1995. Microwave reheating of vacuum-packaged cooked sausage cold cuts for shelf-life improvement. *Fleischerei* 45: 3–4.

69. Cygnarowicz-Provost, M., Whiting, R.C. and Craig, J.C. 1994. Steam surface pasteurization of beef frankfurters. *Journal of Food Science* 59: 1–5.

70. Cooksey, D.K., Klein, B.P., McKeith, E.K. and Blaschek, H.P. 1993. Reduction of *Listeria monocytogenes* in precooked vacuum-packaged beef using post-packaging pasteurization. *Journal of Food Protection* 56: 1034–1038.

71. Roering, A.M., Wierzba, R.K., Ihnot, A.M. and Luchansky, J.B. 1998. Pasteurization of vacuum-sealed packages of summer sausage inoculated with *Listeria monocytogenes*. *Journal of Food Safety* 18: 49–56.

72. Muriana, P., Quimby, W., Davidson, C. and Grooms, J. 2002. Post-package pasteurization of ready-to-eat deli meats by submersion heating for reduction of *Listeria monocytogenes*. *Journal of Food Protection* 65(6): 963–969.

73. McCormick, K.E., Han, I.Y., Acton, J.C., Sheldon, B.W. and Dawson, P.L. 2005. In-package pasteurization combined with biocide-impregnated films to inhibit *Listeria monocytogenes* and *Salmonella* Typhimurium in turkey bologna. *Journal of Food Science* 70: M52–M56.

74. Kozempel, M., Goldberg, N., Scullen, O.J., Radewonuk, E.R. and Craig, J.C. 2000. Rapid hot dog surface pasteurization using cycles of vacuum and steam to kill *Listeria innocua*. *Journal of Food Protection* 63: 457–461.

75. Sommers, C., Mackay, W., Geveke, D., Lemmenes, B. and Pulsfus, S. 2012. Inactivation of *Listeria innocua* on frankfurters by flash pasteurization and lauric arginate ester. *Journal of Food Processing & Technology* 3(147): 1–4.

76. Selby, T., Berzins, A., Gerrard, D., Corvalan, C., Grant, A. and Linton, R. 2006. Microbial heat resistance of *Listeria monocytogenes* and the impact on ready-to-eat meat quality after post-package pasteurization. *Meat Science* 74(3): 425–434.

77. Murphy, R.Y., Hanson, R.E., Duncan, L.K., Feze, N. and Lyon, B.G. 2005. Considerations for postlethality treatments to reduce *Listeria monocytogenes* from fully cooked bologna using ambient and pressurized steam. *Food Microbiology* 22: 359–365.

78. Mangalassary, S., Han, I., Rieck, J., Acton, J. and Dawson, P. 2008. Effect of combining nisin and/or lysozyme with in-package pasteurization for control of *Listeria monocytogenes* in ready-to-eat turkey bologna during refrigerated storage. *Food Microbiology* 25(7): 866–870.

79. Huang, L. 2007. Numerical analysis of survival of *Listeria monocytogenes* during In-package pasteurization of frankfurters by hot water immersion. *Journal of Food Science* 72(5): E285–E292.

80. Ahn, J., Lee, H.Y., Knipe, L. and Balasubramaniam, V. 2014. Effect of a post-packaging pasteurization process on inactivation of a *Listeria innocua* surrogate in meat products. *Food Science and Biotechnology* 23(5): 1477–1481.

81. Ingham, S.C., DeVita, M.D., Wadhera, R.K., Fanslau, M.A. and Buege, D.R. 2005. Evaluation of small-scale hot-water postpackaging pasteurization treatments for destruction of *Listeria monocytogenes* on ready-to-eat beef snack sticks and natural-casing wieners. *Journal of Food Protection* 68(10): 2059–2067.

82. Delgado Suárez, E.J., Chairéz Espinosa, A., Rodas Suárez, O., Quiñones Ramírez, E.I. and Rubio Lozano, M.S. 2015. Hot water shrinkage as a post-lethal intervention against *Listeria Monocytogenes*: Preliminary assessment in a Turkey-based Virginia ham model. *Journal of Food Safety* 35(2): 145–153.

83. Gande, N. and Muriana, P. 2003. Pre-package surface pasteurization of ready-to-eat meats with a radiant heat oven for reduction of *Listeria monocytogenes*. *Journal of Food Protection* 66(9): 1623–1630.

84. Mangalassary, S., Han, I., Rieck, J., Acton, J., Jiang, X., Sheldon, B. and Dawson, P. 2007. Effect of combining nisin and/or lysozyme with in-package pasteurization on thermal inactivation of *Listeria monocytogenes* in ready-to-eat turkey bologna. *Journal of Food Protection* 70(11): 2503–2511.

85. Murphy, R.Y., Hanson, R., Johnson, N., Scott, L., Feze, N. and Chappa, K. 2005. Combining antimicrobial and steam treatments in a vacuum-packaging system to control *Listeria monocytogenes* on ready-to-eat franks. *Journal of Food Science* 70(2): M138–M140.

86. Huang, L. 2005. Computer-controlled heating to in-package pasteurize beef frankfurters for elimination of *Listeria monocytogenes*. *Journal of Food Process Engineering* 28: 453–477.

87. Huang, L. and Sites, J. 2007. Automatic control of a microwave heating process for in-package pasteurization of beef frankfurters. *Journal of Food Engineering* 80(1): 226–233.

88. Gómez-López, V.M., Ragaert, P., Debevere, J. and Devlieghere, F. 2007. Pulsed light for food decontamination: A review. *Trends in Food Science & Technology* 18: 464–473.

89. Takeshita, K., Shibato, J., Sameshima, T., Fukunaga, S., Isobe, S., Arihara, K. and Itoh, M. 2003. Damage of yeast cells induced by pulsed light irradiation. *International Journal of Food Microbiology* 85: 151–158.

90. Ganan, M., Hierro, E., Hospital, X.F., Barroso, E. and Fernández, M. 2013. Use of pulsed light to increase the safety of ready-to-eat cured meat products. *Food Control* 32(2): 512–517.

91. Hierro, E., Barroso, E., De la Hoz, L., Ordóñez, J.A., Manzano, S. and Fernández, M. 2011. Efficacy of pulsed light for shelf-life extension and inactivation of *Listeria monocytogenes* on ready-to-eat cooked meat products. *Innovative Food Science & Emerging Technologies* 12(3): 275–281.

92. Hierro, E., Ganan, M., Barroso, E. and Fernández, M. 2012. Pulsed light treatment for the inactivation of selected pathogens and the shelf-life extension of beef and tuna carpaccio. *International Journal of Food Microbiology* 158(1): 42–48.

93. Uesugi, A.R. and Moraru, C.I. 2009. Reduction of *Listeria* on ready-to-eat sausages after exposure to a combination of pulsed light and nisin. *Journal of Food Protection* 72(2): 347–353.

94. Tung, M.A., Britt, I.J. and Yada, S. 2001. Packaging considerations. In *Food Shelf-life Stability: Chemical, Biochemical and Microbiological Changes*, eds. N.A.M. Eskin and D.S. Robinson, pp. 129–145. Boca Raton, FL: CRC Press LLC.

95. Robertson, G.L. 2006. *Food Packaging – Principles and Practice*, 2nd edn. Boca Raton, FL: CRC Press.

96. ICPE (Indian Centre for Plastics in the Environment). 2005. Packaging of meat and poultry products. Available from: www.icpeenvis.nic.in/icpefoodnpackaging/pdfs/19_meat.pdf.

97. Jakobsen, M. and Bertelsen, G. 2002. The use of CO_2 in packaging of fresh red meats and its effect on chemical quality changes in the meat: A review. *Journal of Muscle Foods* 13: 143–168.

98. Georgala, D.L. and Davidson, C.L. 1970. Food package. British Patent 1199998.

99. Smiddy, M., Fitzgerald, M., Kerry, J.P., Papkovsky, D.B., O'Sullivan, C.K. and Guilbault, G.G. 2002. Use of oxygen sensors to non-destructively measure the oxygen content in modified atmosphere and vacuum packed beef: Impact of oxygen content on lipid oxidation. *Meat Science* 61: 285–290.

100. Ahvenainen, R. 2003. Active and intelligent packaging: An introduction. In: *Novel Food Packaging Techniques*, ed. R. Ahvenainen, Cambridge, UK: Woodhead Publishing.

101. Ščetar, M., Kurek, M. and Galić, K. 2010. Trends in meat and meat products packaging—a review. *Croatian Journal of Food Science and Technology* 2(1): 32–48.

102. Lähteenmäki, L. and Arvola, A. 2003. Testing consumer responses to new packaging concepts. In *Novel Food Packaging Techniques*, ed. R. Ahvenainen, pp. 550–562. Cambridge, UK: Woodhead Publishing.

103. CAC. 2005. Code of hygienic practice for meat (CAC/RCP 58-2005). Codex Alimentarius Commission, Rome, Italy.

104. Lawrie. R.A. 1998. *Lawrie's Meat Science*, 6th edn. Cambridge, UK: Woodhead Publishing.

105. Collins, D.S. and Huey, R.J. 2014. *Gracey's Meat Hygiene*. Hoboken, NJ: John Wiley & Sons.

106. Pennington, T.H. 2000. Introduction. In *HACCP in the Meat Industry*, ed. M. Brown, pp. 3–9. Boca Raton, FL: CRC Press.

107. Sheridan, J.J. 1998. Sources of contamination during slaughter and measures for control. *Journal of Food Safety 18*: 321–339.

108. Koohmaraie, M., Arthur, T.M., Bosilevac, J.M., Guerini, M.N., Shackelford, S.D. and Wheeler, T.L. 2005. Post-harvest interventions to reduce/eliminate pathogens in beef. *Meat Science 71*: 79–91.

109. Broda, D.M., Boerema, J.A. and Brightwell, G. 2009. Sources of psychrophilic and psychrotolerant clostridia causing spoilage of vacuum-packed chilled meats, as determined by PCR amplification procedure. *Journal of Applied Microbiology 107*: 178–186.

110. Bell, R.G. and Hathaway, S.C. 1996. The hygienic efficiency of conventional and inverted lamb dressing systems. *Journal of Applied Microbiology 81*: 225–234.

111. Daly, D. J., Prendergast, D. M., Sheridan, J. J., Blair, I. S. and Mcdowell, D. A. 2002. Use of a marker organism to model the spread of central nervous system tissue in cattle and the abattoir environment during commercial stunning and carcass dressing. *Applied and Environmental Microbiology 68(2)*: 791–798.

112. Buncic, S., McKinstry, J., Reid, C. and Anil, M. 2002. Spread of microbial contamination associated with penetrative captive bolt stunning of food animals. *Food Control 13*: 425–430.

113. Koutsoumanis, K. and Taoukis, P. 2005. Meat safety, refrigerated storage and transport: Modeling and management. In *Improving the Safety of Fresh Meat*, ed. J. Sofos, pp. 503–561. Cambridge, UK: Woodhead Publishing.

114. BCCDC. 2012. Guidelines for the Safe Transportation of Carcasses, Poultry and Meat Products. http://www.bccdc.ca/resource-gallery.

115. Browne, G. 2007. Australian standard for the hygienic production and transportation of meat and meat products for human consumption.

116. James, S. 1996. The chill chain "from carcass to consumer". *Meat Science 43*: 203–216.

117. Auhtority, A.N.Z.F. 2001. Safe food Australia: A guide to the Food Safety Standards: Australia New Zealand Food Authority.

118. Harris, K. and Blackwell, J. 1999. Guidelines for developing good manufacturing practices (GMPs), standard operating procedures (SOPs) and environmental sampling/testing recommendations (ESTRs). Ready-to-eat (RTE) products. Desarrollado por los Representantes de las Industrias Productoras de Alimentos Listos para el Consumo. EE.UU.

119. McCurdy, S.M., Peutz, J.D. and Wittman, G. 2009. *Storing Food for Safety and Quality*. University of Idaho Cooperative Extension System.

120. USFDA. 2016. Food Facts. How to cut food waste and maintain food safety. https://www.fda.gov/downloads/food/resourcesforyou/consumers/ucm529509.pdf.

6 Biotechnological Approaches for Improving Quality and Safety of Animal Origin Foods

Bushra Ishfaq, Mariam Aizad, and Rizwan Arshad

CONTENTS

6.1 INTRODUCTION

Biotechnology is a technical approach that uses living organisms or substances from these organisms to create or modify a product or to develop microorganisms for specific purposes to improve animals and plants. Advances in the field of biotechnology derived to a wide area of science, namely medicine, agriculture, environmental science, food science, and animal sciences etc. Among allied sciences and agricultural science, animal health, and production have possibly promoted mostly by biotechnology. The use of biotechnology will lead to a discrete shift in the economic returns from livestock. Livestock production currently accounts for about 43% of the gross value of agricultural production. In developed countries livestock accounts for more than half of agricultural production, while in developing countries the share is about one-third. However, this latter share is growing fast because of rapid growths in livestock production resulting from population growth, urbanization, change in lifestyles, dietary habits, and increasing disposable incomes. The biotechnology among livestock production is growing rapidly than any other sectors and, by 2020, livestock component is expected to become the most significant agricultural sector in terms of value-added products [1]. Although it is hoped that biotechnology will improve the lifespan of every individual in the world and allow more sustainable living, vital decisions may be dictated by profitable considerations and the socioeconomic goals that society considers to be the most important.

Biotechnology is basically the use of biological principles for manipulating living organisms or their derivatives to either improve or multiply a product. Among numerous techniques of biotechnology, such as cloning of genes, gene transfer, genetic manipulation of animal and plant embryo transfer, genetic manipulation of rumen microbes, chemical, and biological treatment of low quality animal feeds for enhanced nutritive value, genetically engineered immune-diagnostic, and immune-prophylactic agents, as well as veterinary vaccines, are finding their ways into research and development programs of developing countries. The main obstruction to the successful application of biotechnology in livestock sector relates to the cost of adoption and acceptability [2]. In this chapter, biotechnological interventions in the areas of animal genetics and breeding along with conservation of animal genetic resources, nutrition, health and survival, and quality improvement of livestock products were mentioned.

Globally, there has been a continuous increase in the demand for livestock and livestock-related product. However, today the world production merely meets the demand to a significant extent. No wonder this has made scientists try to improve livestock and livestock-associated derivatives. With genetic manipulation and related technologies gaining importance, research interests to improve livestock using genetic engineering has become a buzzword; day by day more focus is being put in this regard [3]. Therefore, the objective of this review paper was to investigate the use of biotechnology in animal production and productivities.

6.2   ROLE OF BIOTECHNOLOGY IN LIVESTOCK PRODUCTIVITY

Biotechnology is regarded as a means to the rapid growth in agricultural production through tackling the production limits of small-scale or resource-poor farmers, who contribute more than 70% of the food produced in developing countries [4]. Agricultural biotechnology as the solution to the problem of global food insecurity has also been reviewed by Soetan [5]. It has the potential to address some of the problems of developing countries like food insecurity, unfavorable environmental and climatic conditions, and others.

Agricultural biotechnology has provided animal agriculture with safer, more efficacious vaccines against pseudo rabies, enteric collibacilosis, and foot-and-mouth disease (FMD) [6]. Disease detection in crops and animals are more efficiently and rapidly done using DNA probes. Biotechnology as a key tool to break through in medical and veterinary research has been reviewed by Soetan and Abatan [7].

Livestock recycle nutrients on the farm, produce valuable output from land that is not suitable for sustained crop production, and provide energy and capital for successful farm operations [8]. Livestock can also help maintain soil fertility in soils lacking adequate organic content or nutrients [9]. Adding animal manure to the soil increases the nutrient retention capacity (or cation-exchange capacity), improves the soil's physical condition by increasing its water-holding capacity, and improves soil structure. Animal manure also helps maintain or create a better climate for microflora and microfauna in soils.

Grazing animals improve soil cover by dispersing seeds, controlling shrub growth, breaking up soil crusts, and removing biomass that otherwise might be fuel for bushfires [8]. These activities stimulate grass tilling and improve seed germination and, thus, improve land quality and vegetation growth. Livestock production also enables farmers to allocate plant nutrients across time and space by way of grazing to produce manure, land that cannot sustain crop production, and makes other land more productive [8].

Biotechnology has enhanced increased animal production through artificial insemination (AI), and has also improved animal health and disease control through the production of DNA recombinant vaccines [7]. Microorganisms have broadened the environments they live in by evolving enzymes that allow them to metabolize numerous man-made chemicals (i.e., xenobiotics) [10].

6.3   BIOTECHNOLOGY APPROACHES APPLIED TO LIVESTOCK SYSTEMS

6.3.1   ANIMAL NUTRITION AND FEED UTILIZATION

In developing countries poor nutrition is a big hurdle for domestic animal production. Both quality and quantity of feed resources are poor, and a large proportion of animal feed is fibrous with varying levels of digestibility and nutritive values. Gene-based technologies are mostly used to improve animal nutrition, either through modifying the feeds to make them more digestible or through modifying the digestive and metabolic systems of the animals to enable them to utilize the available feeds [11]. The digestive tract of livestock is manipulated by modifying the microbial flora and type, which includes mainly the rumen in ruminants and intestinal tract in monogastrics. These include development of transgenic bacteria with enhanced cellulolytic activity, capability to cleave lignohemicellulose complexes, reduced methane production capability decreased proteolytic and/or deaminase activities, increased capability for nitrogen "fixation," and better ability for microbial production of specific amino acids. The first successful transmission of foreign genes was reported in rumen bacteria, namely *Bacteriodes ruminicola* [12]. Transgenic rumen microbes also play an essential role in the detoxification of plant poisons [13] as well as inactivation of antinutritional factors. The use of recombinant bovine somatotropin (rBST) in dairy cows increases both milk yield and production efficiency and decreases animal fat [14]. The scarcity and the increasing cost of feed ingredients among developing countries indicated that there is a need to improve feed utilization. Aids to animal nutrition, such as enzymes, probiotics, single cell proteins, and antibiotics in feed, are extensively applied in intensive production systems universally to improve the nutrient components of feeds and the productivity of livestock. The genetic modification (GM) of crop seeds is used for the production of livestock feeds containing energy rich protein sources for animals. The first GM crops produced in commercial scale for livestock feed were herbicide tolerant soybean and canola, and corn and pest-protected cotton in 1996 in the United States (US) [15]. Feeds derived from GM plants, like grain, silage, and hay, have contributed to increases in growth rates and milk yield [16]. The GM crops containing better amino acids can be used to reduce nitrogen excretion in pigs and poultry. An increased level of amino acids in grains means that the essential amino acid requirements of pigs and poultry can be met by diets that are lower in protein.

6.3.2   ANIMAL HEALTH AND SURVIVAL

The biotechnology for animal health has been developed in numerous regions that include transgenesis, disease prevention, diagnosis, treatment, and control [1,17]. Effective management and control of a disease involve accurate diagnosis. In low-income regions, the Polymerase chain reaction (PCR), monoclonal antibodies, and recombinant antigens are the molecular diagnostic techniques that are either previously used or being tested. Application of monoclonal antibodies has concluded that the breakdown of vaccines (e.g., of rabies) to provide protection due to the diversity in the antigenic composition of the causative virus around all regions of the world [18]. The development of basic DNA detection techniques is the improved diagnostic tools of which the most significant tool is PCR methodology by Mullis [19]. Advanced biotechnology-based diagnostic experiments make it possible to identify the disease-causing agent(s) at a species/sub-species/type level and to evaluate the impact of disease control programs. Advancements used in biotechnology has enabled the application of enzyme-linked immunosorbent assay (ELISA) that uses recombinant antigens developed via gene cloning and sequencing for detection of antibodies and provides information on responses to single epitopes or antibody recognition sites. In addition, highly specific and sensitive diagnostic techniques used to detect the disease-causing agents are nucleic acid hybridization (NAD) and restriction endonuclease mapping (REM). A good example to explain the specificity of NAD is its application in diagnosing infections caused by peste des petite ruminants (PPR) virus from rinderpest [20]. The diagnostic techniques applied in small ruminants and cattle include; nucleic acid probes (NAP) for heartwater (*Cowdri ruminantium*), *Chlamydia psitacci*, Paratuberculosis and Bluetongue [21] restriction endonuclease reaction (RENR) for diagnosis of *Corynebacterium pseudotuberculosis* [22]; PCR for categorizing subtypes of Bluetongue from different geographical regions [23]; monoclonal antibodies (MAB) for distinguishing false positive anti-*Brucella* titres caused by *Yersinia enterocolitica* and true positive anti-*Brucella* titres in latent infected animals [24]; and MAB to diagnose the Toxoplamosis, Pasteurellosis, *Mycoplasma* sp., PPR, and Boder disease [20].

Conventional methods of controlling major livestock diseases include chemotherapy, vector control, vaccination, slaughtering of infected livestock, and controlled livestock movements, as well as grazing management. To control vector, a continuous application of pesticides is required. These practices are often unaffordable to farmers in developing country. Moreover, resistance by parasites is often encountered with the use of these drugs or pesticides, and reinfection following administration of drugs against parasitic diseases frequently occurs. Moreover, in many cases, drugs are not readily available locally. In a few cases where they are available, they are ineffective, either because they have been partly preserved or they are not genuine. Immunization is the most cost-effective methods of preventing specific diseases. An effective vaccine can generate long-lasting immunity and sometimes life-time immunity.

Additional methods of disease prevention and control, such as vector control and quarantine, are widely applied. Vaccination is a sustainable means of providing health safety in comparison to vector control and quarantine due to cost implication. The vaccines that are extensively utilized are either attenuated or inactivated and have proved very efficient in generating resistance. However, a few limitations are observed with live attenuated vaccines, such as their stability, possibility of recombination with wild strains, and the complexity in discriminating vaccinated animals from their infected counterparts. As a result, sub-unit vaccines developed by recombinant technology producing pure protective antigens for formulation with adjuvant [25], pathogen attenuation by gene deletion [26], and vectored vaccines have been constructed to avoid the limitations of conventional attenuated vaccines. Highly effective vaccines against animal diseases, such as rinderpest and pig cholera, have been in use for more than 20 years and have assisted to significantly reduce the incidence of these diseases world-wide. A recombinant hormone bovine somatotropin (BST) is a genetically engineered synthetic analog of the natural growth hormone [27]. The regular administration of BST to lactating dairy cows increases milk yield by 15%–30% and increases efficiency of milk production. Porcine somatotropin (PST) as well as recombinant growth hormone stimulatory peptides (e.g., growth hormone releasing factor, GRF) along with BST have been shown to increase growth rates by 8%–38% in cattle, sheep, and pigs. Other growth-promoting agents, like anabolic steroids and beta agonists, have been shown even larger effects but public concerns over the possible residual effects in meats have led to being banned in most developing countries.

6.3.3 Animal Genetics and Breeding

Genetic improvement of livestock depends on the gain of genetic variations and appropriate methods for exploiting these variations. Genetic diversity provides a defense against alterations in the environment and also gives a solution in selection and breeding for adaptability and production on a range of environments. Maintaining genetic diversity should always be the objective of animal breeding and genetics. This provides a cushion against environmental fluctuations and, hence, an avenue for utilizing selection and mating systems to produce animals for diverse production environments. The biotechnology applied to animal breeding and genetics is mostly directed towards increasing breeding efficiency of livestock particularly within organized breeding schemes and conservation of animal genetic resources.

6.3.4 Genetic Engineering

The first successful gene transfer method in animals (mouse) was based on the microinjection of foreign DNA into zygotic pronuclear. However, microinjection has several major short comings including low efficiency, random integration, and variable expression patterns that mainly reflect the site of integration. Research has focused on the development of alternate methodologies for improving the efficiency and reducing the cost of generating transgenic livestock.

These include sperm-mediated DNA transfer [28–37], intracytoplasmic injection (ICSI) of sperm heads carrying foreign DNA injection or infection of oocytes [38–42] and/or embryos by different types of viral vectors [43,44], RNA interference technology (RNAi) [45], and the use of somatic cell nuclear transfer (SCNT) [46]. To date, SCNT, which has been successful in 13 species, holds the greatest promise for significant improvements in the generation of transgenic livestock. Furthermore, there are some common ways of manipulating the animal genome.

6.3.5 Conservation of Genetic Resources

Developing countries are endowed with the majority of the global domestic animal diversity landraces, strains, or breeds. Few livestock breeds in these countries are in immediate danger of loss due to indiscriminate crossbreeding with exotic breeds. The significance of indigenous livestock breeds lies in their adaptation to local biotic and abiotic stresses and to conventional husbandry practices. Conservation of indigenous animal genetic resources should be one of the major priority livestock development activities for developing countries. The terms conservation, preservation, *ex situ*, and *in situ* are used here according to the definition given by the Food and Agriculture Organization (FAO) [47]. There are several approaches, differing in efficiency, technical feasibility and costs, to conserve animal genetic resources. Developing and utilizing a genetic resource is considered the most rational conservation strategy. *Ex-situ* approaches include: maintenance of small populations in domestic animal zoos; cryopreservation of semen (and ova); cryopreservation of embryos; and various combinations of these. Cryopreservation of gametes, embryos, or DNA segments can be a relatively effective and safe approach for breeds whose populations are too small to be conserved by any other means. Technology used for cryopreservation of semen and embryo is suitably developed to be applied in developing countries. Cryopreservation of oocytes followed by successful fertilization and live births has been achieved in the mouse. Cryopreserved bovine oocytes have been successfully matured and fertilized in vitro and zygotes developed to blastocyst stage [48].

6.4 BIOTECHNOLOGY TOOLS APPLIED TO IMPROVE LIVESTOCK PRODUCTS

Biotechnological interventions of recent years have appeared as an important tool to improve various livestock products including milk and meat products. The biotechnological techniques can be applied to improve the quality traits of animal originated products, production of hormones, functional and exclusive livestock products, enzymes, biopreservation of livestock products, quality control, and meat authentication as outlined below:

6.4.1   IMPROVEMENT IN THE QUALITY OF LIVESTOCK PRODUCTS

Major genes ensure meat quality offers excellent opportunities for increasing level of meat quality and reducing variability. Identification, isolation, and modification of useful genes are some of the important aspects of biotechnology research and development. The genes that affect the tenderness of meat before slaughter are *CLPG* in sheep, *myostatin* in beef, and *RN* in pork [49]. Manipulation of the lipoprotein receptor and leptin genes causes improvement in the quality of carcass, thereby the cholesterol and fat content of meat can be controlled.

6.4.2   PRODUCTION OF HORMONES

The pituitary-derived somatotropin (ST) is used as an agent to improve growth and carcass composition. Insertion of the *pST* gene inside the genome of pigs causes 35% loss of fat and 8% increase in protein content. Recombinant DNA technology has provided a mechanism for large scale production of somatotropin by inserting the ST gene in laboratory strain *E. coli*. Bovine and ovine ST improves growth rate by 20% and lean to fat ratio by 40% in ruminants.

6.4.3   FUNCTIONAL AND DESIGNER LIVESTOCK PRODUCTS

In order to improve the product, attempts can be made to develop strains of starter cultures capable of enhanced antichlolestermic attributes, enhanced anticarcinogenic attributes, and enhanced antagonistic influence on enteropathogenic microorganism. Consequently, it is important to take attention towards the construction of new and improved strains by using modern techniques of molecular biology, namely plasmid transfer, transduction, protoplast fusion, and cloning [50]. Genetically engineered microbial strains can play a vital role in formation of process resulted high quality fermented livestock products.

6.4.4   BIOPRESERVATION

Biopreservation can be defined as the utilization of non-pathogenic microbes and their metabolites for the extension of shelf life of the product and to improve the microbiological safety [51]. The main aim of biopreservation is the use of microflora and their metabolites to extend the shelf life of the product and increase safety of the food. Fermentation is one of the most common examples of biopreservation, which is the process of adding the microbes to the food or being natural. It refers to the production of acid, breakdown of complex compounds, production of many useful vitamins, such as riboflavin, vitamin C, vitamin B12, and many other compounds. It also increases the antifungal properties and improvement of flavor as well as aroma. Fish can be processed by the enhancement of acid in fish muscle or by adding antimicrobials [52]. The identification and development of many protective cultures of bacteria shows some antibacterial properties against the spoilage organisms and pathogens. The antimicrobial activities of microbiota can be shown by many compounds, such as bacteriocins, organic acids, acetaldehydes and diacetyl, CO_2, enzymes, and H_2O_2.

There is reduction in the standards of food processing as well as the microbiological due to the use of modern technologies, but the spoilage of food products and food-related diseases are not eliminated in industrialized countries. The damage of the original texture, nutritional value, and flavor of the food is called food spoilage, which makes the food unfit for the consumption and is harmful for the people. The import of raw seafood from the developing countries and using it in precooked form results in the outbreaks of the illness due to food borne problems [53]. The most common cause of food borne illness is food being spoiled by the pathogens. About 250–350 million people are affected annually by food borne illnesses, and about 500 deaths occur due to this problem. The main cause of illness is that 22%–30% illness is due to eggs, meats, poultry, dairy products, and sea food in USA [54]. Such outbreaks are caused by many pathogens, such as *Listeria monocytogenes, Campylobacter jejuni, Clostridium botulinum, Salmonella, Staphylococcus aureus,* and *Escherichia coli O157:H7* [53]. Physical treatments and chemical preservatives are used by the industries in order to achieve the improvement in the standards of food safety. There are many drawbacks of preservation techniques, which include the change in the nutritional and organoleptic quality of the food, toxicity of chemicals, and the demands of the consumers for the minimal processed food having no additives. This target can be achieved by using traditional methods of food preservation along the use of Lactic acid bacteria (LAB) and their metabolites [53]. The use of LAB as biopreservatives is due to their non-pathogenic and safe properties [55]. Chemical additives are being changed with natural products due to the demand for safe food and to prevent damage to the environment. The selection, production, as well as improvement of the beneficial microbes are being done by the biotechnologists and the technical application in food.

6.4.5 BACTERIOCIN

Bacteriocin are complex proteins or peptides that are biologically active and have antibacterial properties against closely related species. These are not antibiotics, which are produced by bacteria and are concerned with therapeutic antibiotics that cause allergic reactions and other medicinal problems in human beings [56]. These are different from therapeutic antibiotics that are proteinaceous and are digested by proteases in the human gut. The protein increases their action and intensity [57]. The first bacteriocin, which was discovered by Andre Gratia and his group in 1925, was Colicine [58]. As these peptides kill the pathogenic bacteria that can compete for niche, so their production is an advantage for the producers of feed and food. As bacteriocins have a narrow host range and are effective against similar bacteria, so their role is very important in food resources [59].

6.4.6 LAB BACTERIOCINS

In recent years a great number of bacteriocins were characterized in lactic acid bacteria (LAB). Most of these bacteriocins are of small size, heat resistant, and have no modification through translation. Studies have shown that there are 2–3 bacteriocins produced in LAB but commercial producers only produce one of them. In food industry bacteriocin-producing bacteria can be used as a protective culture that's why LAB is most attractive and commonly used strain in food industry as preservative. These strains are considered safe due to their characteristics like:

1. They are a simple protein in nature and can be inhibited by gastric enzymes (proteolytic).
2. They are tested on laboratory animals and are proven to be non-toxic and non-immunogenic.
3. Thermal resistance is one of the key characters that they can survive pasteurization and even sterilization.
4. They are good bactericidal and can kill broad range of gram-positive and some of the gram-negative bacteria.

Plasmid of bacteria contains the genetic determinants, which are used for the manipulation of their varieties through change in the peptide analogues to introduce desired characters [53]. For the selection of bacteriocin-producing strains features that should be considered are as following:

1. Strain should be having a status as generally regarded as safe (GRAS).
2. Desired bacteriocin should be highly effective against pathogens to be inhibited.

3. Should be thermally stable.
4. Must improve the safety aspect of the product.
5. There should be no side effects on the quality and safety of product.

6.4.7 PRODUCTION OF ENZYMES

Today's enzyme industry as we probably know it is the after effect of quick advancement seen principally over the previous four eras on account of the development of present-day biotechnology. Since ancient times, enzymes have been used in the production of different food products including sourdough, wine, cheese, vinegar, and beer, and for manufacturing of linen, indigo, and leather. These procedures depended on either enzymes are delivered by precipitously developing microorganisms or through the enzymes present in rumen, calves, and papaya. Such enzymes were not used in well characterized and pure form.

During the most recent century, fermentation process development was targeted at enzymes production by using particular production strains, after this it became possible to manufacture the enzymes on large scale as in purified and well-characterized forms. This advancement permitted the production of enzymes into industrial and products, for instance, inside the starch industries and detergent textiles.

The utilization of recombinant gene technology has additionally enhanced assembling forms and empowered the commercialization of enzymes that could already not be created. Moreover, the most recent advancements inside present-day biotechnology, presenting protein engineering and coordinated advancement, have additionally upset the improvement of industrial enzymes. These advances have made it conceivable to give tailor-made enzymes showing new exercises and adjusted to new process conditions, empowering a further extension of their modern utilize. The outcome is a profoundly differentiated industry that is as yet becoming both as far as complexity and size.

The industrial enzymes mostly show hydrolytic actions when they are used for the degradation of naturally occurring substances. Due to the extensive uses in dairy and detergent industry, proteases are considered as dominant enzyme types. The second largest group of enzymes is cellulases, carbohydrates, and amylases that are used in detergent, starch, baking, and textile industry [60].

As delineated in Table 6.1, the industrial enzymes are mostly consumed in technical industries for example detergent, textile, starch, and fuel alcohol industries. Generally speaking, the assessed estimation of the overall utilization of recent enzymes has risen from $1 billion in 1995 to $1.5 billion in 2000. This development, be that as it may, has stagnated in a portion of the major technical industries above all else the detergent industry [61]. The speediest development over the previous decade has been found in the animal feed and baking industries, yet development is additionally being produced from applications set up in an abundance of different ventures crossing from organic synthesis to paper, personal care, and pulp. This survey will, fragment by portion, talk about the most essential late improvements in the specialized utilization of enzymes and will consider the latest innovative advances that have encouraged these advancements.

6.4.7.1 New Technologies for Enzyme Discovery

Naturally occurring microorganisms have throughout the years been an extraordinary way of enzymes variety. The accessibility of sequence data and advancements in bioinformatics has expanded hugely the proficiency of gene isolation from nature known as gene of interest. Reasonable protein engineering and the likelihood of acquainting little changes with proteins, based on their structure and the related biophysical and biochemical properties, acquainted another important instrument with protein advancement in the 1980s. Guided advancement is the most recent expansion to the tool kit [62].

Variant libraries are generated that are, therefore, presented to a screening or selection method, due to more or less introduction of mutations. The improved and isolated variants from one round

TABLE 6.1
Enzymes Used in Various Industrial Segments and Their Applications

Industry	Enzyme Class	Application
Detergent (laundry and dish wash)	Protease	Protein stain removal
	Amylase	Starch stain removal
	Lipase	Lipid stain removal
	Cellulase	Cleaning, color clarification, anti-redeposition (cotton)
	Mannanase	Mannanan stain removal (reappearing stains)
Starch and fuel	Amylase	Starch liquefaction and saccharification
	Amyloglucosidase	Saccharification
	Pullulanase	Saccharification
	Glucose isomerase	Glucose to fructose conversion
	Cyclodextrin-glycosyltransferase	Cyclodextrin production
	Xylanase	Viscosity reduction (fuel and starch)
	Protease	Protease (yeast nutrition—fuel)
Food (including dairy)	Protease	Milk clotting, infant formulas (low allergenic), flavor
	Lipase	Cheese flavor
	Lactase	Lactose removal (milk)
	Pectin methyl esterase	Firming fruit-based products
	Pectinase	Fruit-based products
	Transglutaminase	Modify visco-elastic properties
Baking	Amylase	Bread softness and volume, flour adjustment
	Xylanase	Dough conditioning
	Lipase	Dough stability and conditioning (*in situ* emulsifier)
	Phospholipase	Dough stability and conditioning (*in situ* emulsifier)
	Glucose oxidase	Dough strengthening
	Lipoxygenase	Dough strengthening, bread whitening
	Protease	Biscuits, cookies
	Transglutaminase	Laminated dough strengths
Animal feed	Phytase	Phytate digestibility—phosphorus release
	Xylanase	Digestibility
	β-Glucanase	Digestibility

of screening are then utilized as beginning material in the accompanying rounds of recombination and additionally new assorted variety age (Figure 6.1).

As of late, different endeavors at understanding the imperative parameters in coordinated advancement have risen and effective cases of consolidating sane building with coordinated development have been accounted for [63,64]. Generally, new, energizing innovation is anticipated to out-compete current advances, yet we expect that time will exhibit how the consolidated utilization of normal outline, coordinated advancement, and nature's assorted variety will be far better than any solitary standing innovation.

6.4.7.2 Enzymes for Starch Conversion

The enzymatic transformation of starch to high-fructose corn syrup is an entrenched procedure and gives a wonderful case of a bioprocess in which the back to back utilization of a few enzymes is important. The enzymes used in the starch industry business are likewise subjected to steady upgrades.

The initial phase in the process is the transformation of starch to oligo maltodextrins by the activity of α-amylase. The associative infusion of steam puts outrageous requests on the thermostability of the compound. Utilizing conventional α-amylases, the pH must be acclimated to a high level and

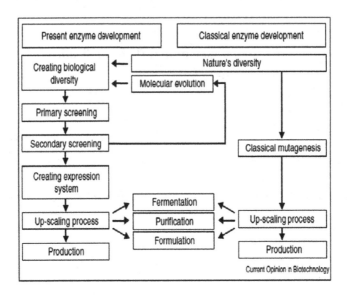

FIGURE 6.1 The steps involved in classical versus state of the art development of enzymes.

calcium must be added to settle the enzyme. New α-amylases with upgraded properties, for example, acid tolerance, improved thermostability, corrosive resilience, and capacity to work without the expansion of calcium, have, as of late, been created [65] that offer clear advantages to the business. Efforts of engineering have likewise been embraced to create enhanced forms of the enzymes, such as glucose isomerase and glucoamylase, utilized later simultaneously [66].

6.4.7.3 Enzymes for the Feed Industry

Enzymes have been used in feed industry for the last decade. It's a well-established practice in the industry to use enzymes as additives, for example xylanase and glucanase, in feed for monogastric animals that are unable to fully degrade the plant carbohydrates like ruminants. In recent years, natural phosphorus bounds in the phytic acid of cereal-based feeds for monogastrics has been the main focus because 85%–90% of plant phosphorus is bound to phytic acid that can only be available by the addition of phytase enzyme, which breaks the bond between phosphorus and phytic acid. The main source of inorganic phosphorus in feed was spongiform encephalopathy, which was banned in different countries. Another concern is the release of phosphorus in the environment. Western countries followed the standards to minimize the release of phosphorus to environment. Phytase enzyme was resulted in significant reduction of phosphorus release from monogastric, which attracted the feed industry towards this enzyme. Now phytase is the largest produced enzyme in the feed industry. Uptake of nutrients other than phosphorus is also reported by the use of phytase [67]. Now, the recent advances in the feed industry aim to improve the performance and applications of phytases [68]. Advancement in enzyme identification resulted in new species of fungal enzymes that have been reported to be 4–50 folds more activity than the previous phytases [69]. New techniques for developing better strains resulted in better catalytic activity of phytases, for example the specific activity of *Aspergillus fumigatus* phytase was increased to four fold by the study of three-dimensional structures [70]. Another use for enzymes in the feed industry is to make phytase thermally stable for the application of pelleted feed products. This is attained by the introduction of consensus phytase that makes it stable for pelleting under the temperature of about 80°C [71]. The focus of feed industry is not only phosphorus availability but also the utilization of enzyme for enhancements of nutritional value of different feed products for example the digestibility of soy bean meal to get the more available protein.

6.4.7.4   Enzymes for the Food Industry

Application of enzymes is broad in food industry that ranges from texturizing to flavoring as illustrated in Table 6.1. Almost in all processed food enzymes are involved from raw material to the final product in many ways. For the optimization and better results, many advances have been made in enzymes to avoid possible side effects. To improve the textural and viscoelastic properties of different products like sausage, yogurt and noodles, transglutaminase have been studied [72]. The problem is the availability of enzymes at a commercial level, and, for instance, the availability of transglutaminase at industrial level; the only economical source is from *Streptoverticillium* sp. and this limits the availability in market. For this obstacle, researchers are working on recombinant technology for the production of enzyme by *Escherchia coli* [73]. In baking industry the main focus is on lipolytic enzymes [74]. Recent studies suggested the use of lipases as emulsifiers to replace synthetic emulsifiers as they convert the lipids of wheat to emulsifying agents *in situ*. Staling in bread industry is also in consideration to understand the proper mechanism of bread staling and its prevention by the enzymatic activity when xylanases and amylases are used [75]. Researchers have confirmed that the capacity of water binding and retaining of starch and hemicellulose of bread is being the critical substrates of amylase and xylanase that controls the properties of elasticity and softness. Three-dimensional structure of amylase, which has been determined recently, revealed the deep sight of mechanism for amylase action [76]. Elasticity of bread is the character of degradation of amylopectin to certain level and amylase is being used to prevent the crystallization of degraded amylopectin after gelatinization, which imparts the proper amylopectin network in bread. Beside the above mentioned enzymes, new enzymes are being introduced day by day in food industry (which should be illustrated in literature) like the use of laccase in juice industry for the purpose of purification. It is also used in beer industry for flavoring. These are the recent publication about enzymes in beverage industry. Understanding the mode of function of new and different enzymes can help in advancement in food industry.

6.4.8   Quality Control

Ensuring a satisfactory level of food quality and safety is absolutely necessary to provide enough protection for consumers and to facilitate trade. The use of modern biotechnology has proved to be rapid, sensitive, and an accurate detection and analysis method of bacterial contaminants and pathogens or their toxins. Genetic engineering, PCR, microarray, amplified polymorphic DNA (RAPD), or amplified fragment length polymorphism (AFLP) marker systems can be used. Microarrays are biosensors consisting of a large amount of parallel hybrid receptors (DNA, proteins and oligonucleotides). They can be used for the detection of pathogens, pesticides, and toxins and offer significant potential for monitoring the quality and safety of raw materials.

6.4.9   Meat Authentication

There is always been a demand to check the origin of meat precisely and quickly. Now another demand is to check the origin in processed meat products because of religious, economic, and some health issues. The past decade was important for food industry due to the development of nucleic acid base analytical techniques. Meat authentication had been done through by the application of PCR, but a limited number of studies were on buffalo meat. In recent years, different techniques were coupled with PCR to differentiate between cattle and water buffalo meat. Random amplified polymorphic DNA, forensically informative nucleotide sequencing, nucleotide sequencing, restriction fragment length polymorphism, and hybridization were techniques used to couple PCR for meat authentication [77].

There were complications in the PCR technique, which was simplified by the development of florescence-based formats that ease the DNA detection protocols and overcome the limitation of PCR.

Heteroduplex and single strand conformation polymorphism had limitations that require the confirmatory testing through sequencing for the positive results to identify the variation in sequencing. In contrast to these, single nucleotide primer extension (SNaPshot) assay gives a simple and specific assay through sequencing data and do not require confirmatory testing [78].

SNaPshot was recently used to verify the meat from game animals and domestic species [79]. This method uses the mitochondrial cytochrome *b* (cyt *b*) gene region to build an assay for the authentication and differentiation of different buffalo species.

6.4.10   AUTHENTICATION OF HALAL MEAT

If seen in history, consumption of meat by the Muslim was free from the concept of adulteration as it was sold fresh and available in the market in a specific area. By the advancement in our life style and preferences around the globe, the need of preservation emerged to avoid the deterioration of processed products of meat [80]. With the increase of technological advances, cases of fraud and gaining of profit through adulteration was introduced. To overcome these frauds and adulterations, new techniques were introduced for the safety and authenticity of meat. Identification of meat genome through DNA-based identification was one of the great steps towards safety parameters. Consumer confidence was rebuilt by the authentication of meat and its derivative products. Currently, the global issue concerns the substitution of expensive meat with the cheaper ones. Consumers, who are vegetarian, also have concerns about the adulteration of food with meat particles. Authentication of species and animals is the concern of Muslims so they know whether the meat is from a halal source or haram [81]. The level of porcine and equine contents is not tolerable because of their religious doctrine. That is why the limit of detection should be as low as possible to avoid the identification errors. For this purpose, the development of more sensitive techniques are needed.

6.5   CONSTRAINTS ON APPLYING THE BIOTECHNOLOGY

In developing countries the application of modern biotechnological techniques and breeding approaches to the livestock breeds used in small holder production systems is constrained by several factors. The key controls on applying biotechnologies have been concluded and include:

1. The lack of an accurate and ample database on livestock and animal owners so that programs can be accomplished.
2. The biodiversity existing within species and breeds in agro-ecological systems, the fact that models of biotechnological intervention vary particularly between developed and developing economies.
3. The fact that many animal species and breeds having distinct characteristics, such as developmental, production, disease resistance, and nutrient utilization.
4. The lack of skilled scientists, technicians, and fieldworkers to improve and apply the technologies, both in the government and in the private sectors. In order to translate technologies into products there is the lack of an interface between industry, universities, and institutions.
5. The high cost of technological inputs, such as materials and biological equipment, are the major constrains in the failure to access technologies from the developed world at a reasonable rate in order to make a rightful, positive, and sustainable contribution to livestock production and the economic welfare of farmers.
6. The failure to address issues of biosafety and to conduct risk analysis of new biological, gene products, transgenic and modified food items, and above all the negligible investment in animal biotechnology.

6.6 CONCLUSION

The biotechnology has resulted in discrete benefits in relations to animal improvement and economic returns to the farmers as well as to feed the increasing population of the world. Developments in different biotechnology laboratories have considerably altered animal production globally, and the developing world attained benefits in a few areas of conservation, animal improvement, healthcare (including diagnosis and control of disease), upgrading feed resources, and quality improvements to livestock products making them safe for public health. To adopt biotechnology among livestock sector, there is a dire need to provide training along with publicizing material regarding these technologies to farmers, for which proper development conditions available in a number of countries in the region. Although it is true that there is a certain bit of risk involved within the technology, this is an utmost reality that to feed an ever-growing population of the world accepting this technology is an absolute compulsory; there is no going back from here. A comprehensive investigation of both the advantages and the disadvantages will contribute in leading the future of environmental and agricultural biotechnology, since the entire objective is to accomplish a safe environment and improved agricultural productivity. These uncertainties and concerns about the application of biotechnology to achieving a safe environment and agriculture are addressed and lead to significant impact on the future of biotechnology. Although animal production is being improved significantly by advances made in thousands of biotechnology laboratories around the world, benefits are reaching the developing world in only a few areas of conservation, animal improvement, healthcare (including diagnosis and control of disease), and the augmentation of feed resources. It resulted in distinct benefits in terms of animal improvement and economic returns to the farmers. Over the past decade, the International Livestock Research Institute (ILRI) has concentrated on biotechnological applications, especially in Africa and several developing countries. Now it has multi-institutional programs to develop and apply biotechnology. The evolving realm will have to respond to the many gene-based technologies now being developed with a sense of commitment, trained manpower, infrastructure, and funding.

6.7 RECOMMENDATIONS

- In all circumstances, biotechnologies developments required the involvement of stakeholders in a systematic scheme to progress research and advancements as well as transfer to target groups.
- Government and national agricultural research systems are liable for a majority of the processes essential to successfully development and disseminate relevant biotechnologies.
- To deliver biotechnologies for use by target groups, there is need for cooperation between government and benefiters.
- The more emphasis must be given to promote a massive campaign to popularize biotechnology among livestock farmers and commence and institute obligatory steps to assist them accordingly.

REFERENCES

1. Abraham H, Pal SK (2014) Animal biotechnology options in improving livestock production in the horn of Africa. *Int J Interdiscip Multidiscip Res 1*:1–8.
2. Kahi AK, Rewe TO (2008) Biotechnology in livestock production: Overview of possibilities for Africa. *Afr J Biotechnol 7*:4984–4991.
3. Onteru S, Ampaire A, Rothschild M (2010) Biotechnology developments in the livestock sector in developing countries. *Biotechnol Genet Eng Rev 27*:217–228.
4. Rege JEO (1996) Biotechnology options for improving livestock production in developing countries, with special reference to Sub-Saharan Africa. In: Lebbie SHB, Kagwini E (Eds.), *Small Ruminant Research and Development in Africa. Proceedings of the Third Biennial Conference of the African Small Ruminant Research Network*, UICC, Kampala, Uganda, December 5–9, 1994. ILRI, Nairobi, Kenya, p. 322. http://www.fao.org/wairdocs/ilri/x5373b/x5473b05.htm.

5. Soetan KO (2008) Agricultural biotechnology: The solution to the problem of global food insecurity. *Proceedings of the 1st International Society BioTechnology Conference (ISBT)*, December 28–30, Gangtok, India.

6. Stenholm CW, Waggoner DB (1992) Public policy and animal biotechnology in the 1990s: Challenges and opportunities. In: MacDonald JF (Ed.), *Animal Biotechnology – Opportunities and Challenges*, NABC National Agricultural Biotechnology Council, Ithaca, NY, Report 4, pp. 25–35.

7. Soetan KO, Abatan MO (2008) Biotechnology: A key tool to breakthrough in medical and veterinary research—A review. *Biotechnol Mol Biol Rev 3*:88–94.

8. Delgado C, Rosegrant M, Steinfeld H, Ehui S, Courbois C (1999) Livestock to 2020: The next food revolution. Food, agriculture, and the environment. Discussion Paper 28 IFPRI/FAO/ILRI, IFPRI, Washington, DC.

9. Ehui S, Li-Pun H, Mares V, Shapiro B (1998) The role of livestock in food security and environmental protection. *Outlook Agric 27*:81–87.

10. Okpokwasili GC (2007) Biotechnology and clean environment. *Proceedings of the 20th Annual Conference of the Biotechnology Society of Nigeria (BSN)*, November 14–17, Ebonyi State University, Abakaliki, Nigeria.

11. Madan ML (2005) Animal biotechnology: Applications and economic implications in developing countries. *Rev Sci Tech 24*:127–139.

12. Thomson AM, Flint HJ (1989) Electroporation induced transformation of bacteroides ruminicola and bacteroides uniformis by plasmid DNA. *FEMS Microbiol Lett 61*:101–104.

13. Singh B, Bhat TK, Singh B (2001) Exploiting gastrointestinal microbe for livestock and industrial development. *Asian-Australasian J Anim Sci 14*:567–586.

14. Fereja GB (2016) Use of biotechnology in livestock production and productivites: A review. *Int J Res-Granthaalayah 4*:100–109.

15. Alexander TW, Reuter T, Aulrich K, Sharma R, Okine EK, Dixon WT, McAllister TA (2007) A review of the detection and fate of novel plant molecules derived from biotechnology in livestock production. *Anim Feed Sci Technol 133*:31–62.

16. Novoselova TA, Meuwissen MPM, Huirne RBM (2007) Adoption of GM technology in livestock production chains: An integrating framework. *Trends Food Sci Technol 18*:175–188.

17. McKeever DJ, Rege JEO (1999) Vaccines and diagnostic tools for animal health: The influence of biotechnology. *Livest Prod Sci 59*:257–264.

18. Wiktor TJ, Koprowski H (1980) Antigen variants of rabies virus. *J Exp Med 152*:99–112.

19. Joshi M, Deshpande JD (2010) Polymerase chain reaction: Methods, principles and application. *Int J Biomed Res 1*:81–97; Suhre K, Gieger C (2012) Genetic variation in metabolic phenotypes: Study designs and applications. *Nat Rev Genet 13*:759–769.

20. Lefevre PC, Diallo A (1990) Diagnosis of viral and bacterial diseases. *Rev Sci Tech OIE 9*:951–965.

21. Blancou J (1990) Utilization and control of biotechnical procedures in veterinary science. *Rev Sci Tech OIE 9*:641–659.

22. Knowles DP, Gorham JR (1990) Diagnosis of viral and bacterial diseases. *Rev Sci Tech OIE 9*:733–757.

23. Dahiya S, Prasad G, Minakshi, Kovi RC (2005) PCR for categorizing subtypes of Bluetongue from different geographical regions. *Indian J Biotechnol 4*:373–377.

24. Schwarz NG, Loderstaedt U, Hahn A, Hinz R, Zautner AE, Eibach D, Fischer M, Hagen RM, Frickmann H (2015) Microbiological laboratory diagnostics of neglected zoonotic diseases (NZDs). *Acta Tropica 165*:40–65.

25. Mohan T, Verma P, Rao DN (2013) Novel adjuvants and delivery vehicles for vaccines development: A road ahead. *Indian J Med Res 138*:779–795.

26. Pascual DW, Suo Z, Cao L, Avci R, Yang X (2013) Attenuating gene expression (AGE) for vaccine development. *Virulence 4*:384–390.

27. Bauman DE, Eppard PJ, De Geeter MD, Lanza LM (1985) Response of high-producing dairy cows to long-term treatment with pituitary somatotropin and recombinant somatotropin. *J Dairy Sci 68*:1352–1362.

28. Baccetti B, Spadafora C (2000) Sperm-mediated gene transfer: Advances in sperm cell research and applications. Proceedings of the workshop. Siena, Italy May 23-6, 1999. Conclusions. *Mol Reprod Dev 56*:329–330.

29. Chan AW, Luetjens CM, Schatten GP (2000) Sperm-mediated gene transfer. *Curr Top Dev Biol 50*:89–102.

30. Khoo HW (2000) Sperm-mediated gene transfer studies on zebrafish in Singapore. *Mol Reprod Dev 56*:278–280.

31. Lauria A, Gandolfi F (1993) Recent advances in sperm cell mediated gene transfer. *Mol Reprod Dev 36*:255–257.
32. Lavitrano M, Forni M, Bacci ML, Di Stefano C, Varzi V, Wang H, Seren E (2003) Sperm mediated gene transfer in pig: Selection of donor boars and optimization of DNA uptake. *Mol Reprod Dev 64*:284–291.
33. Lavitrano M, Forni M, Varzi V, Pucci L, Bacci ML, Di Stefano C, Fioretti D et al. (1997) Sperm-mediated gene transfer: Production of pigs transgenic for a human regulator of complement activation. *Transplant Proc 29*:3508–3509.
34. Maione B, Lavitrano M, Spadafora C, Kiessling AA (1998) Sperm-mediated gene transfer in mice. *Mol Reprod Dev 50*:406–409.
35. Nakanishi A, Iritani A (1993) Gene transfer in the chicken by sperm-mediated methods. *Mol Reprod Dev 36*:258–261.
36. Shamila Y, Mathavan S (1998) Sperm-mediated gene transfer in the silkworm Bombyx mori. *Arch Insect Biochem Physiol 37*:168–177.
37. Smith K, Spadafora C (2005) Sperm-mediated gene transfer: Applications and implications. *Bioessays 27*:551–562.
38. Cai QF, Wan F, Huang R, Zhang HW (2011) Factors predicting the cumulative outcome of IVF/ICSI treatment: A multivariable analysis of 2450 patients. *Hum Reprod 26*:2532–2540.
39. Li MW, Baridon B, Trainor A, Djan E, Koehne A, Griffey SM, Biggers JD, Toner M, Lloyd KC (2012) Mutant mice derived by ICSI of evaporatively dried spermatozoa exhibit expected phenotype. *Reproduction 143*:449–453.
40. Lu Z, Zhang X, Leung C, Esfandiari N, Casper RF, Sun Y (2011) Robotic ICSI (intracytoplasmic sperm injection). *IEEE Trans Biomed Eng 58*:2102–2108.
41. Umeyama K, Saito H, Kurome M, Matsunari H, Watanabe M, Nakauchi H, Nagashima H (2012) Characterization of the ICSI-mediated gene transfer method in the production of transgenic pigs. *Mol Reprod Dev 79*:218–228.
42. Yu Y, Zhao C, Lv Z, Chen W, Tong M, Guo X, Wang L, Liu J, Zhou Z, Zhu H, Zhou Q, Sha J (2011) Microinjection manipulation resulted in the increased apoptosis of spermatocytes in testes from intracytoplasmic sperm injection (ICSI) derived mice. *PLoS-One*. doi:10.1371/journal.pone.0022172. Accessed on March 26, 2018.
43. Ishii Y, Reese DE, Mikawa T (2004) Somatic transgenesis using retroviral vectors in the chicken embryo. *Dev Dyn 229*:630–642.
44. Kimura O, Yamaguchi Y, Gunning KB, Teeter LD, Husain F, Kuo MT (1994) Retroviral delivery of DNA into the livers of transgenic mice bearing premalignant and malignant hepatocellular carcinomas. *Hum Gene Ther 5*:845–852.
45. Wise TG, Schafer DS, Lowenthal JW, Doran TJ (2008) The use of RNAi and transgenics to develop viral disease resistant livestock. *Dev Biol (Basel) 132*:377–382.
46. Mir B, Zaunbrecher G, Archer GS, Friend TH, Piedrahita JA (2005) Progeny of somatic cell nuclear transfer (SCNT) pig clones are phenotypically similar to non-cloned pigs. *Cloning Stem Cells 7*:119–125.
47. FAO (Food and Agriculture Organization of the United Nations) (1992) The management of global animal genetic resources: Proceedings of an FAO expert consultation. FAO Animal Production and Health paper 104. FAO, Rome, Italy, 309 pp.
48. Lim JM, Reggio BC, Godke RA, Hansel W (1999) Development of in-vitro-derived bovine embryos cultured in 5% CO2 in air or in 5% O2, 5% CO2 and 90% N2. *Hum Reprod 14*:458–464.
49. Meadus WJ (1998) Molecular techniques used in the search for genetic determinants to improve meat quality. *Can J Anim Sci 78*:483–492.
50. Gupta S, Savaliya CV (2012) Application of biotechnology to improve livestock products. *Vet World 5*:634–638.
51. De Martinis, Elaine CP, Bernadette DGM, Franco BDGM (2001) Inhibition of Listeria monocytogenes in a pork product by a Lactobacillus sake strain. *Int J Food Microbiol 42*:119–126.
52. Stiles ME (1996) Biopreservation by lactic acid bacteria. *Antonie van Leuwenhoek 70*:331.
53. Nath S, Chowdhury S, Sarkar S, Dora KC (2013) Lactic acid bacteria – A potential biopreservative in sea food industry. *Int J Adv Res 1*:471–475.
54. Mead PS, Slutsker L, Dietz V, McCaig LF, Bresee JS, Shapiro C, Griffin PM, Tauxe RV (1999) Food-related illness and death in the United States. *Emerg Infect Dis 5*:607–625.
55. Caplice E, Fitzgerald GF (1999) Food fermentations: Role of microorganisms in food production and preservation. *Int J Food Microbiol 50*:131–149.
56. Deraz SF, Karlsson EN, Hedström M, Andersson MM, Mattiasson B (2005) Purification and characterisation of acidocin D20079, a bacteriocin produced by Lactobacillus acidophilus DSM 20079. *J Biotechnol 117*:343–354.

57. Saavedra JM, Abi-Hanna A, Moore N, Yolken RH (2004) Long-term consumption of infant formulas containing live probiotic bacteria: Tolerance and safety. *Am J Clin Nutr 79*:261–267.
58. Jacob F, Lwoff A, Siminovitch A, Wollman E (1953) Definition de quelques termes relatifs a la Iysogenie. *Am Inst Pasteur 84*:222–224.
59. Deegan LH, Cotter PD, Hill CC, Ross P (2006) Bacteriocins: Biological tools for bio-preservation and shelf-life extension. *Int Dairy J 16*:1058–1071.
60. Godfrey T, West SI (1996) Introduction to industrial enzymology. In *Industrial Enzymology*, 2nd ed. Macmillan Press, London, UK.
61. McCoy M (2000) Novozymes emerges. *Chem Eng 19*:23–25.
62. Tobin MB, Gustafsson C, Huisman GW (2000) Evolution: The 'rational' basis for 'irrational' design. *Curr Opin Struct Biol 10*:421–427.
63. Voigt CA, Kauffman S, Wang ZG (2000) Rational evolutionary design: The theory of in vitro protein evolution. *Adv Protein Chem 55*:79–160.
64. Altamirano MM, Blackburn JM, Aguayo C, Fersht AR (2000) Directed evolution of a new catalytic activity using the α/β-barrel scaffold. *Nature 403*:617–622.
65. Bisgaard-Frantzen H, Svendsen A, Norman B, Pedersen S, Kjærulff S, Outtrup H, Borchert TV (1999) Development of industrially important α-amylases. *J Appl Glycosci 46*:199–206.
66. Sauer J, Sigurdskjold BW, Christensen U, Frandsen TP, Mirgorodskaya E, Harrison M, Roepstorff P, Svensson B (2000) Glucoamylase: Structure/function relationships and protein engineering. *Biochem Biophys Acta 1543*:275–293.
67. Kies AK, Hemert KHF, Sauer WC (2001) Effect of phytase on protein and amino acid digestibility and energy utilization. *Worlds Poult Sci J 57*:109–126.
68. Lei XG, Stahl CH (2001) Biotechnological development of effective phytases for mineral nutrition and environmental protection. *Appl Microbiol Biotechnol 57*:474–481.
69. Lassen SF, Breinholt J, Østergaard PR, Brugger R, Bischoff A, Wyss M, Fuglsang CC (2001) Expression, gene cloning and characterization of five novel phytases from four Basidiomycete fungi: Peniophora lycii, Agrocybe pediades, a Ceriporia sp. and Trametes pubescens. *Appl Environ Microbiol 67*:4701–4707.
70. Tomschy A, Tessier M, Wyss M, Brugger R, Broger C, Schnoebelen L, van Loon APGM, Pasamontes L (2000) Optimization of the catalytic properties of Aspergillus fumigatus phytase based on the three-dimensional structure. *Protein Sci 9*:1304–1311.
71. Lehmann M, Kostrewa D, Wyss M, Brugger R, D'Arcy A, Pasamontes L, van Loon APGM (2000) From DNA sequence to improved functionality: Using protein sequence comparisons to rapidly design a thermostable consensus phytase. *Protein Eng 13*:49–57.
72. Kuraishi C, Yamazaki K, Susa Y (2001) Transglutaminase: Its utilization in the food industry. *Foods Rev Int 17*:221–246.
73. Yokoyama K, Nakamura N, Seguro K, Kubota K (2000) Overproduction of microbial transglutaminase in Escherichia coli, in vitro refolding and characterization of the refolded form. *Biosci Biotechnol Biochem 64*:1263–1270.
74. Collar C, Martinez JC, Andreu P, Armero E (2000) Effect of enzyme associations on bread dough performance. A response surface study. *Food Sci Technol Int 6*:217–226.
75. Andreu P, Collar C, Martínez-Anaya MA (1999) Thermal properties of doughs formulated with enzymes and starters. *Eur Food Res Technol 209*:286–293.
76. Dauter Z, Dauter M, Brzozowski AM, Christensen S, Borchert TV, Beier L, Wilson KS, Davies GJ (1999) X-ray structure of Novamyl, the five-domain 'maltogenic' α-amylase from Bacillus 350 protein technologies and commercial enzymes stearothermophilus: Maltose and acarbose complexes at 1.7 Å resolution. *Biochemistry 38*:8385–8392.
77. Wang Q, Zhang X, Zhang HY, Zhang J, Chen GQ, Zhao DH, Ma HP, Liao WJ (2010) Identification of 12 animal species meat by T-RFLP on the 12S rRNA gene. *Meat Sci 85*:265–269.
78. Murphy K, Geiger T, Hafez M, Eshleman J, Griffin A, Berg KD (2003) A single nucleotide primer extension assay to detect the APC I1307K gene variant. *J Mol Diagn 5*:222–226.
79. D'Andrea M, Merigioli A, Scarano MT, Pilla F (2009) Cattle breed traceability in meat and cheese using DNA polymorphisms detected by the Snapshot method. *Italian J Food Sci 21*:365–373.
80. Nakyinsige K, Che Man YB, Sazili AQ (2012) Halal authenticity issues in meat and meat products. *Meat Sci 91*:207–214.
81. Doosti A, Ghasemi Dehkordi P, Rahimi E (2014) Molecular assay to fraud identification of meat products. *J Food Sci Technol 51*:148–152.

7 Fish Processing, Storage, and Transportation

*Muhammad Ammar Khan, Huijuan Yang,
and Asghar Ali Kamboh*

CONTENTS

7.1 INTRODUCTION

Fisheries are an important source of income, nutrition, and food worldwide. The food obtained from any sea life is regarded as seafood. These include sea mammals (whales and dolphins), fin fish and shellfish (mollusks, crustaceans, and echinoderms), edible sea plants (seaweeds and microalgae), and fish eggs. According to the Food and Agriculture Organization (FAO), worldwide production of fish was almost 202 MMT in 2016 [1]. Almost 54% of it was captured [2], whereas the remaining was reared as aquaculture. Marine fishes are harvested in large amount due to their unique flavor. Marine fish account for almost 85%, whereas the remaining are captured from freshwaters including rivers, lakes, and ponds. Asia produced more than two-thirds of the world production (Figure 7.1). China alone accounts for more than one third of the global total and half of the Asian productions, respectively. Almost 85%–88% of the fish are consumed by humans, whereas the remaining

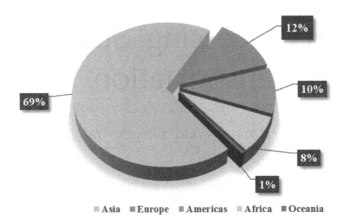

Asia Europe Americas Africa Oceania

FIGURE 7.1   Worldwide production of fish.

10%–12% is used as feed for broiler chicken farming. Most popular species of fishes used for farming and processing include herring, cod, tuna, mackerel, flounder, and salmon.

Seafood harvest is used as food, oil, as fish food, fertilizer, feed for domestic pets, medicine, and non-food purposes. By-products of fish are also of great economic value. By-products of marine and freshwater fishes include pearls, pigments, as well as uses in soap and glass productions. Flesh obtained from animals is called meat. It includes skeletal muscle, fat, and offal. The meat packing industry often restricts the term meat to include the flesh of mammalian species (pigs, cattle, etc.), and exclude flesh of fish and poultry from it. However, being composed of muscles of similar nature, the flesh obtained from fish is also called fish meat. People who consume fish meat and other seafoods, but not the flesh of mammals and birds, are called Pescatarians; whereas vegetarians do not consume flesh of any animal, including fish and poultry. The per capita consumption of fish of Iceland, Japan, and Portugal is the greatest in the world. Other foods derived from fish include, roe (fish egg), surimi (fabricated fish food from fish gel), and fish gelatin (prepared from skin, bones, scales, etc.).

Fish include all forms of aquatic animals, including finfish (fin fish), mollusks, crustaceans, and it refers to any animal that lives in fresh or saltwater. Fish are the most diverse group of vertebrates. Almost forty thousand species of vertebrates have been reported so far in the world, and about thirty thousand of them are those of fish [3]. They are classified as Pisces, Mollusca, or Crustacea, and distinguish from marine mammals, such as whales and dolphins, and birds. In fisheries, the term fish refers to any aquatic animal, including mollusks and crustaceans, which are harvested from water bodies, including oceans, ponds, fish farms, and others. Finfish are paraphyletic (descended from common ancestors, i.e. monophyletic, but some of their descendants form separate groups) aquatic vertebrates that are ectothermic (cold blooded) and craniate (possess skull), lack limbs with digits, have fins for relocation, gills for breathing throughout their life, and an elongated body with scaly skin having slimy glandular secretions. Although each criterion has exceptions. Fishing is a general term that means catching the fish to fulfill dietary needs or for the purpose of sports and recreation, while the related term fishery includes all the organized efforts to catch the fishes. Fish farming is a type of aquaculture meant for the production of fish using commercial methods. Fishing means harvesting or hunting of seafood. More than eight thousand fresh-water species of fish, as well as more than eleven thousand marine species of fish have been reported so far. In addition, shellfish are also very diverse; however, only a few common species of shellfish are captured by humans for consumption. Fish of different species may tolerate temperatures ranging from subzero to 38°C. Based upon trophic level, fish are carnivorous, herbivorous, omnivorous, or scavengers, and are found on surfaces, as well as bottoms of lakes, rivers, and oceans. Several fish, born in freshwater, spend their adult lives in the ocean, and return to freshwaters to spawn, and vice versa. Based upon fat content, fish may be classed as either whitefish or oily. Whitefish are those having very low fat and include haddock and cod. Fish vary based on mode of reproduction, as well. Few undergo internal fertilization and give birth to young ones, whereas others lay eggs, which are fertilized after deposition in water. Eggs of fish are also consumed by humans. Eggs of marine fish buoy in water [4], whereas those of freshwater ones remain under water and adhere to other objects.

7.2 CLASSIFICATION

Classification of fish is important to assess their economic value. Fish are usually classified based upon anatomy, habitat, and fat content. Knowing fish anatomy is essential, because processing of fish muscles and organs may require diverse methods. Fish have a backbone, possess gills, and contain limbs in the shape of fins. Fish have heads with a brain and sensory organs, trunks with a body cavity having internal organs, and a tail. A few fish also have functional lungs. Mostly fish skin contains scales and slimy glandular secretions. Finfish and shellfish are two major types of fish based upon anatomy. There are two types of fish, namely vertebrates and invertebrates (Figure 7.2). Vertebrate fish are called finfish, whereas the invertebrates include crustaceans and mollusks. Finfish are the types of fish having bony (salmon) or cartilaginous (shark) skeletons. Finfish are further divided into two main categories: lean (white, <5% fat) and oil-rich (fatty, >5% fat) fish. Lean fish have oils stored only in their liver. Lean fish are further sub-divided into three classes, including round, flat, and cartilaginous fish. Cod is an example of a round lean fish. Lemon and black sole are examples of flat lean fish. Rock salmon and shark are examples of cartilaginous fish. Fatty fish have oils distributed throughout their flesh. Eel, herring, mackerel, salmon, sardines, and trout are examples of fatty fish.

Based upon habitat, finfish can be classified into marine or freshwater fish. Freshwater fish may further be classified into freshwater aquarium or pond fish. Marine means "of or pertaining to the ocean or sea," whereas saltwater is more precisely classified based upon the salt content of the water body and is measured by specific gravity (relative density). For example, the specific gravity of marine or saltwater ranges between 1.022 and 1.035. Saltwater fishes pass some or all their lives in salt water (salinity >0.05%), either in oceans or lakes. They are of five different types. Coastal fishes, also called offshore or neritic fishes, include the ones that live between the shoreline and the edge of the continental shelf of the sea. On the other hand, deep-sea fishes inhabit the area below the photosynthetic zone of the ocean, because enough light cannot penetrate below a certain depth, thus photosynthesis cannot occur. Moreover, pelagic fishes, such as mackerel, herring, and tuna, live near

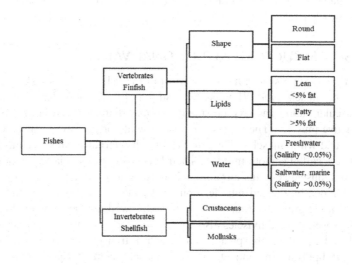

FIGURE 7.2 Common classifications of fishes.

TABLE 7.1
Classification of Saltwater Fishes

Coastal fish (offshore fish/neritic fish)	Live between the shoreline and the edge of the continental shelf of the sea
Deep sea fish	Inhabit below the photic zone of the ocean
Pelagic fish	Inhabit near the surface or in mid waters of the sea and lakes
Demersal fish	Inhabit on or near the bottom of the sea or lakes
Coral reef fish	Remain attached to coral reef

the surface in mid-waters of the sea or lakes. On the other hand, demersal fishes stay on or near the bottom of the sea or lakes. Furthermore, coral reef fishes remain attached to coral reefs (Table 7.1).

Freshwater fish are those that spend some or all their lives in freshwater, such as rivers and lakes, with a salinity of less than 0.05%. Freshwater fish species are usually classified by the water temperature in which they survive. The water temperature affects the amount of oxygen available as cold water contains more oxygen than warm water. There are three main freshwater fish types: cold-water, warm-water, and cool-water [5]. These fish prefer particular temperature ranges for survival but can tolerate certain temperature extremes. Cold-water fish species survive in the coldest temperatures, preferring a water temperature of 10°C–16°C degrees. Common cold-water fishes include brook-, rainbow-, and brown-trout. Cool-water fish species prefer water temperatures between the cold-water and warm-water species, around 16°C–27°C. Common cool-water species include northern pike and yellow perch. Warm-water fish species can survive in a wide range of conditions, preferring a water temperature around 27°C. Warm-water fish can survive cold winter temperatures in northern climates but thrive in warmer water. Common warm-water fish include largemouth bass, bluegill, catfish, and crappies. Several fishes born in freshwater spend their adult lives in the ocean and return to freshwaters to spawn, and vice versa.

Shellfish are classified into two categories: mollusks and crustaceans [6]. Mollusks have an unsegmented soft body, partially or wholly enclosed in a shell. They are further divided into three major groups: uni-valve mollusks, bi-valve mollusks, and cephalopods. Uni-valve mollusks possess one shell, and bi-valve mollusks have two shells. Cephalopods contain an internal shell and don't have an external one. Crustaceans are characterized by hard segmented shells and flexible joints. They have a segmented body covered with crust, namely the exoskeleton. Prawns, shrimp, crabs, and lobsters are crustaceans.

7.3   FISH MUSCLE STRUCTURE: NUTRITIONAL VALUE

Three types of muscles are present in most fish. Most of the fish muscles are skeletal. Fish contain three types of skeletal muscles: red [7], white [8], and pink [9]. The muscles containing high myoglobin content, vascularization and oxygen supply, a small diameter, and large blood volume are called red or oxidative muscles. The reverse are called white or glycolytic muscles. Pink muscles are in between red and white muscles. The muscles of fish internal organs, such as those of stomach and intestines, are called smooth muscles. Their heart contains special types of muscles called cardiac muscles. Red muscle contains more mitochondria than white muscles, but lesser sarcoplasmic reticulum. Additionally, the red muscles contain two to five times more amounts of lipid in the cells, more vitamins, greater amounts of glycogen, as well as nucleic acids than those of the white muscles. Moreover, the red muscles also contain greater amounts of enzymes responsible for tricarboxylic acid cycle, pentose phosphate shunt, electron transport chain, synthesis of glycogen, and those involved in lipolysis. In contrast, the white muscles contain higher activity of Adenosine Triphosphatase (ATPase), greater amount of glycolytic acids and more water content. The fish fillet is formed of large lateral muscles that spread on both sides of the fish body. The segments of fish muscles are called *myotomes* [10], due to the presence of thin connective tissue membranes called *mycommata* [11]. Each myotome is composed of muscle fibers (generally <20 mm in length and up to 1 mm diameter), which run parallel to the longer axis of the fish. The fiber bundles are surrounded by a membrane known as *sarcolemma*. These thin fibrils merge into mycommata, and their junction is called the myotome–mycommata junction. A muscle fiber is similar to a cell that contains elongated, thread-like structures of myofibrils (1000–2000 in each bundle), each having a diameter up to 5 μm. The myofibrils are segmented into sarcomeres, which are composed of thin (actin) and thick (myosin) filaments. These segmented myofibrils form alternate arrangements of anisotropic (A) and isotropic (I) bands, which are separated from each other by Z-lines [12]. The crustacean muscles also contain prominent A and I bands. The fibers are of two types, tonic (Type I), which have long (10 μm) sarcomeres, and phasic (Type II) fibers, which have shorter (2–3 μm) sarcomeres. The skeletal muscle fibers can further be divided into two types; slow-twitch and fast-twitch, which are mainly composed up of type I and type II fibers, respectively [13]. The muscles based upon type I fibers enable the fish to swim for long distances, while the muscles based upon type II are used in powerful activities that usually require short-term bursts, such as jumping and sprinting. White muscles are usually composed up of fast-twitch fibers, whereas red muscles are composed up of slow-twitch fibers.

Seafood is an important source of nutrients for humans. They contain all the important nutrients including water, proteins, lipids, vitamins, and minerals, but lack carbohydrates (Figure 7.3).

Water is the most important constituent of living cells. Fish muscles contain 60%–75% of water. The water present in the muscles is the most important indicator of fresh fish meat quality. It is usually present in three compartments in the muscles. However, a fourth type of water may also exist in the secondary meat products subjected to further processing treatments [14]. The first compartment of water is that of chemically bound water [15]. This compartment usually comprises almost 5% of total muscle water. Based upon the amount of water, it is the smallest compartment of water in any type of meat. This water is held by strong covalent forces, and as a part of water of hydration in various chemicals of cells. Although a continuous exchange of this water takes place with water of the subsequent compartment, yet no significant loss of chemically bound water takes place under usual processing conditions. The second compartment constitutes the bulk water compartment of fish muscles [16]. Based upon the amount of water, it is the largest compartment of water in any type of meat. It contains almost 80%–85% of muscle water. It is held in intramuscular spaces of myofibrils of fishes, so it is called myofibrillar water, or simply myowater [17]. It is held by weak forces in the muscles, such as with hydrogen bonding. Moreover, the interactions of intramuscular fats (marbling) with myofibrillar proteins strongly influence the amount of myowater. This water is lost when the external forces overcome the internal forces of hydrogen bonding, or the proteins and fats holding this water are denatured. Moreover, the water of this compartment also remains in constant exchange with physically bound water, as well as with the water of third compartment.

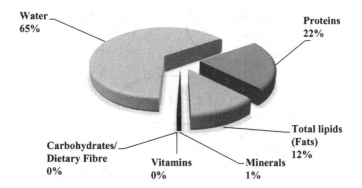

FIGURE 7.3 Nutritional profile of fish fillet.

The third compartment comprises of free water, also called capillary water [18]. It is held between the myofibrillar muscles and is the second largest compartment of water in the muscle. The amount of water in this compartment may range almost 10%–15%. It is held by weak capillary forces and is the most easily prone to loss. In the fresh or minimally processed meat, these three compartments account for almost all the water of muscle. However, most recently a fourth type of water has been reported by a few authors [14]. The denaturation of myofibrillar proteins under cooking and high-pressure processing conditions results in release of myowater, as well as free water. Moreover, the denatured proteins arrange themselves into new orientations and develop into a three-dimensional (3D) matrix, which irreversibly holds the released water. This represents the fourth compartment of water in further processed meat products.

Fish is a source of high quality protein, having all the essential and nonessential amino acids [19]. Moreover, it contains a number of important vitamins and minerals. Furthermore, fatty fish contain lipids, especially essential fatty acids. The flesh of fishes contains almost 17%–23% proteins [20], which are composed of a good array of amino acids. The loss of water during cooking and other processing techniques, however, may increase the proteins to as much as 35%. Fish flesh is abundant in two essential amino acids, namely methionine (Met, $C_5H_{11}NO_2S$) and lysine (Lys, $C_6H_{14}N_2O_2$). Biological value (BV) is a term generally used to describe the proportion of proteins absorbed from a certain food, which gets incorporated into the total proteins of body, and is measured in terms of nitrogen used by tissue synthesis divided by nitrogen absorbed from the food [21]. It indicates the readiness of the digested proteins to be used in the protein synthesis in the cells. BV of fish proteins is 76. Fish proteins are rich sources of all types of essential and non-essential amino acids (especially, methionine and lysine). Since, they do not contain collagenous fibers and tendons, hence their digestibility is quite high in the body. Moreover, fish-protein treatment can reduce plasma cholesterol level, and particularly gives higher content of high-density lipoprotein (HDL) [22]. There are three main types of proteins in fish muscle, namely water-soluble proteins, salt-soluble proteins and connective tissue proteins. The water-soluble proteins are mainly sarcoplasmic proteins, which account for almost 20%–35% of the total muscle proteins and include myoglobin and many enzymes. The sarcoplasmic proteins have low water holding capacity (~20%), low molecular weight (Kilo Dalton, kDa). Myoglobin is the most predominant sarcoplasmic protein [23], which is composed of a protein chain and non-protein heme molecule. It is responsible for color of meat. The most predominant amino acid present in myoglobin is histidine (His, $C_6H_9N_3O_2$). The heme molecule of the myoglobin contains central iron, which makes bonds with a variety of ligands, which determine the resulting meat color (Figure 7.4).

Color is an important indicator of fish meat quality. Color of meat will be purple if Fe^{+2} has no ligand (myoglobin), cherry red if Fe^{+2} has O_2 ligand (oxymyoglobin), cherry red if Fe^{+2} has CO

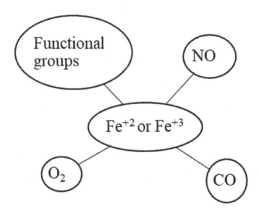

FIGURE 7.4 Ligands responsible for meat color.

ligand (carboxy-myoglobin), and brown if Fe^{+3} has no ligand (metmyoglobin) [24]. The myoglobin contents vary in animal muscles depending upon species and age of the animal. For example, chicken breast has 0.05, chicken leg has 2, pork/veal muscle has 3, young beef has 8–10, and old beef has >15 mg/g myoglobin. The enzymes present in sarcoplasmic proteins mainly include calpains and cathepsins [25]. Several other enzymes are also present in sarcoplasmic proteins. The main functions of enzymes include postmortem glycolysis and protein hydrolysis. Salt soluble protein constitutes almost 60%–75% of fish flesh. They mainly comprise of myofibrillar protein. The most predominant protein, myosin, constitutes almost 55% of the myofibrillar proteins of fish. The remaining 40%–45% proteins include actin (43 kDa), troponin, and tropomyosin. Almost 1%–5% of myofibrillar proteins comprise of desmin, synemin, actinin, and nebulin. These proteins have high WHC (~70%–80%). The ionic strength of these proteins is higher than 0.3%. They also possess high fat binding properties. Stromal proteins constitute almost 10%–15% of total muscle proteins. They are mainly connective tissue proteins involved in connecting various tissues with each other. Collagen (70 kDa) is the most abundant (almost 3% of total protein in fish muscle, almost 20%–25% of total body proteins including skin, bones, tendons, etc.) proteins among the structural and connective tissue proteins. It is widely used in gelatin preparation (produced after hydrolysis of collagen) and cosmetic surgical treatments.

Lipids in fishes vary based upon species and habitat. Fish are classified into lean (<5% fat) and fatty (>5% fat) fish based upon the amount of fats present in them. Most fish contain up to 12% lipids. However, fish fats are characterized by lower cholesterol (77–86 mg) than terrestrial animals [26]. However, shrimp and crab possess high cholesterol contents. Lipids are structural components of cell membrane. They are essential for normal growth and metabolism of animals and humans. Lipids are composed of fatty acids linked with ester bonds with glycerol molecules. Fatty acids can be saturated (SFA) or unsaturated (Figure 7.5).

It is a recommendation of the United Kingdom (UK) Food Standards Agency to consume a minimum of two portions of seafood per week, while the half should be oil-rich fishes, such as mackerel, fresh tuna, salmon, sardines, trout, and herring. Almost 21% of fish lipids are SFA. Unsaturated fatty acids can be monounsaturated (MUFA) or polyunsaturated (PUFA). In fish, almost 41% fats are PUFA, while 37% are MUFA. Omega-3 (ω-3 or n-3) fats are PUFA, which contain a double bond between the third carbon atom (omega minus 3) of the chain from the methyl end. The ω-3 fatty acids reduce cholesterol and triglycerides in the blood and possess anti-oxidant properties. The fatty fishes, such as salmon, trout, sardines, tuna, and mackerel, are considered the healthiest, because fat harbors a lot of fat-soluble nutrients. There are three important ω-3 fatty acids, namely α-linolenic acid (ALA), eicosapentaenoic acid (EPA), and

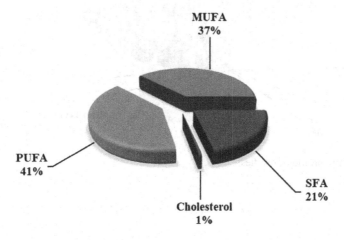

FIGURE 7.5 Lipid profile of fish flesh.

docosahexaenoic acid (DHA). These are also considered as essential fatty acids. The primary sources of ω-3 fatty acids are marine algae and phytoplanktons, which are bioaccumulated in carnivorous fishes by consuming herbivorous fishes. Lipids are essential for humans, because they are important constituents of cells, and account for almost 10%–12% of human brain. DHA is important component of human brain [27], skin and retina [28]. It can be synthesized from α-Linoleic acid (C: 18, ALA). Moreover, fish muscles are also good source of ω-6 fatty acids. Particularly, α-Linoleic acid is an example of ω-6 fatty acids. Daily minimum requirement of ω-3 and ω-6 fatty acids is almost 3 and 12 g, respectively. An increase in ω-6 to ω-3 fatty acid rations can cause obesity and risks of cardiovascular diseases [29].

Vitamins play important function in regulating normal metabolism in humans. Fish flesh is vital source of water-soluble, as well as fat-soluble vitamins (Figure 7.6). Niacin is the most predominantly found vitamin in fish flesh, followed by vitamin C. An additional function of fish fats is to contain many fat-soluble nutrients, including vitamins, such as vitamin A, D, E, and K. Whitefish are those characterized by less than 1%, whereas oily fish contain up to 25% of body weight. Fat-soluble vitamins are housed on these fats, thus consuming fish contribute to healthier functioning of human body.

Vitamin A (retinol) is important for normal growth and tissue differentiation. Moreover, it has important role for proper eye functioning and its deficiency can result into eye function impairment and eyesight loss. Vitamin D (cholecalciferol) is responsible for Ca absorption and retention in bones. Vitamin E (α-Tocopherol) is an important antioxidant. Vitamin K (K1: phylloquinone, phytomenadione, K2: menaquinone) has an important role in blood clotting.

Fish flesh is an important source of wide array of minerals (Figure 7.7). Mineral are essential for optimum body and functioning. Fish contains significant amounts of potassium and phosphorus. Other minerals present in high amounts are sodium, Magnesium and Calcium. Zinc, iron, iodine and selenium are also found in fish flesh, however, in trace amounts. Shellfish, such as oysters, are good sources of zinc [30], whereas several types of fishes and seafoods are good sources of iodine [31].

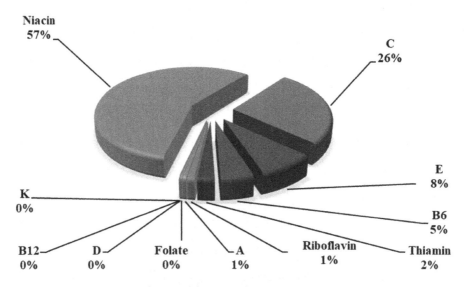

FIGURE 7.6 Vitamin profile of fish flesh.

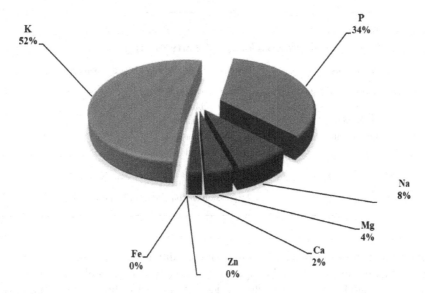

FIGURE 7.7 Mineral constituents of fish flesh.

7.4 SEAFOOD CONSUMPTION: BENEFITS AND DRAWBACKS

Fish flesh contains a wide array of nutrients, which are usually deficient in nutritional sources of terrestrial origin. Consuming fish has been associated with reduced risk of heart attacks and strokes [32], brain development and skin diseases. The control of these diseases has been associated with the nutrients found in fish flesh, especially are the ω-3 fatty acids, vitamins and mineral. Particularly, ω-3 fatty acids are important constituents of brain, thus aid proper brain functioning [33]. Moreover, depression and bipolar disorder are other important diseases, which are related to brain functioning, which have been reported to be controlled by consuming ω-3 fats obtained from fish [34]. Type 1 diabetes, which is an autoimmune disease that is characterized by an attack of the immune system on insulin-producing cells in the pancreas is also reported to be reduced by consumption of ω-3 fats in children and adults [35]. Additionally, ω-3 fats are also components of retina [36]. Macular degeneration, which is a disease associated with vision impairment and blindness, is also reported to be reduced by dietary consumption of ω-3 fats [37]. EPA obtained by consuming fatty fishes reduces productions of leukotriene B4 and cytokine tumor necrosis factor, hence helps in reduction and prevention of asthma [38]. Sleep disorders have also been found to be negatively correlated with consumption of fish and ω-3 fatty acids [39]. Similarly, another report correlated poor sleep with low consumption of fish. Better sleeping efficiency was associated with fish consumption in another study (Table 7.2).

Osteomalacia and rickets in humans have been associated with a deficiency of vitamin D. Moreover, vitamin D has been associated with utilization of calcium and phosphorus in humans. It is expected that over 40% of people worldwide are deficient in vitamin D, which is widely available from fish and fish products including fish oil. Furthermore, higher biological value of fish is essentially an important property [40], because N obtained from fish proteins is retained in our body for optimum growth and maintenance. Moreover, the essential amino acids absorbed from fish and its

TABLE 7.2

Benefits and Drawbacks of ω-3 Fatty Acids

Drawbacks	Benefits of ω-3 Fatty Acids (<3 g per day)
Increased oxidation	Type I diabetes control
Hemorrhagic stroke of brain	Control of blindness—component of retina
Disturb homeostasis	Anti-inflammatory
Immune intolerance	Prevention of asthma
	Allergy control
	Sleep disorder control
	Component of brain
	Depression and bipolar disorder prevention

products are available for vital functions in the body. Additionally, the digestibility coefficient of fish proteins (the ability of proteins to be digested by humans) is quite high. Similarly, net protein utilization (NPU) is another useful indicator, which is a product of both the biological value and digestibility coefficient. It is the direct measure of nitrogen retained in the body from the nitrogen absorbed from the food [21]. Fish contains all essential and non-essential amino acids that are why the biological value of fish proteins is quite high. Moreover, fish proteins contain several important antibodies.

All living organisms naturally harbor parasites, and fish do as well. Thorough cooking often eliminates the hazard. However, traditional recipes may involve partial cooking or eating fish raw, which poses the risk of serious illness to healthy, as well as immunocompromised, persons. Parasite infections, such as those of roundworms, flukes, and tapeworms, are more prevalent in salmon and mackerel, which live in freshwaters [41]. In Japan, consumers eat raw salmon. Freezing overnight, salting, vinegar application, and proper cooking may kill these parasites [42]. Vitiligo, also called leukoderma, is a condition where milky-white patches develop on the skin. Patches of hair can turn white. Melanocytes are color producing cells. Vitiligo develops in humans if melanocytes die. This problem may worsen by consumption of milk-related foods and citrus fruits after fish eating. Seafood may contain heavy or toxic metals and some other contaminants. Fish and shell fish accumulate toxic metals, such as arsenic, lead, mercury, and cadmium, in their tissues [43]. They concentrate mercury in their bodies by the process of bioaccumulation. Mercury is often stored in the tissues of fish as methylmercury, which is highly toxic [43]. Carnivorous fish consume the fish containing mercury. Since carnivorous fish consume many fish containing mercury, their methylmercury concentration is much higher than those of the consumed ones. This process is termed as biomagnification. Minamata disease, first reported in May 1956 in Minamata, a town in Japan, is an example of mercury poisoning in humans [44]. Fish consumption high in mercury are associated with problems related to brain development, nervous system, and failure of vital organs, including kidney and lungs. Other contaminants may include dioxins and polychlorinated biphenyls, which may cause cancer and interference with the endocrine system, thus causing problems in reproductive development and optimal growth in humans. These contaminants may also be found in fish products, including fish oil supplements and fish feed for chicken, thus may affect a variety of foods. Consumption of ω-3 fatty acids from seafood is very beneficial; however, its over consumption may disturb homeostasis. Firstly, ω-3 fatty acids may undergo oxidation, which could be toxic and induce intolerance in humans. Secondly, over eating ω-3 fatty acids (up to 3 g per day) can increase the risk of developing hemorrhagic stroke of brain ruptures. Anaphylaxis, the most severe seafood allergy, results as an overreaction of human immune system to fish products including gelatin, hydrolyzed fish collagen, and atelocollagen [45]. Some fish contain poisons as defense mechanisms against predators. Fugu fish contain tetrodotoxin [46]. Sea bass, grouper, and red snapper can cause Ciguatera poisoning resulting from ciguatoxins [47]. Shellfish poisoning including four syndromes; namely, amnesic shellfish

TABLE 7.3

Toxicity and Diseases Caused by Fish Eating

Vitiligo	Patches of hair can turn white
Minamata disease	Mercury poisoning
Anaphylaxis	Seafood allergy
Shellfish poisoning	Scombrotoxic fish Poisoning
	Brevetoxins
	Okadaic acid
	Saxitoxins
	Ciguatoxin
	Domoic acid

poisoning, diarrheal shellfish poisoning, neurotoxic shellfish poisoning and paralytic shellfish poisoning. These syndromes can result in humans by consumption of mussels, clams, oysters and scallops. Shellfish consume algae that possess biotoxins including brevetoxins [48], okadaic acid [49], saxitoxins [50], ciguatoxin [47], and domoic acid [51]. Consuming fish may result into food poisoning or allergy. Food poisoning is a type of illness that is a response of the human gut to harmful bacteria. It is generally a single-time illness. If such illness takes place frequently after eating fish and other seafood, then it is an allergy. Eating these fish can cause Scombrotoxic fish poisoning or histamine fish poisoning in humans [52]. Scombroid fishes, such as tuna and mackerel, as well as non-scombroids fishes like mahi-mahi and amberjack, may undergo bacterial spoilage if they are not refrigerated or frozen after harvest and can cause scombroid poisoning. Histidine is an amino acid, and, after bacterial spoilage of fish, it can be converted to histamine. Consumption of spoiled fish containing high levels of histamines can result histamine fish poisoning in human disease. Since, anchovy fishes largely feed on marine algae (sources of domoic acid), hence concentration of domoic acid keeps increasing in their bodies. Domoic acid and ciguatoxin may cause death to humans (Table 7.3).

7.5 PRIMARY PRODUCTION

A fish hatchery is the facility that releases juvenile fish into the wild population or to increase the population of a species' or for recreational purposes. Commercial fish farming dates back to at least 40,000 years and was first reported in Egypt. There are two types of aquaculture, namely pisciculture and mariculture. The former refers to the raising of fish for commercial purposes in tanks and enclosures for the production of food, whereas the latter involves the growing of fish in marine water, either in an enclosed section of an ocean, tanks, or ponds filled with seawater. Fish has been used as a staple food in many cultures worldwide. The main purposes for rearing fish include meeting domestic and international dietary, calorie, and nutritional demands; reducing poverty by increasing household income, enhancing yield, food security, quality and safety; and production of new fish species by selective breeding. The commercial farming of fish may have many additive benefits as compared to wild populations, such as controlled water quality, protection against predators, ensuring uniform species population, ensuring feed quality and quantity for rapid growth, and production of desired fish populations to supplement the wild fish types in natural habits. Construction of fish ponds is not only beneficial in terms of fish production, but also ensuring arrival of birds, enhancing greenery in the nearby land, possibility of developing it into recreational locality for boating and fishing, and enhance environmental upgradation. There could be some disadvantages as well, such as the nutritional profile cannot be as diverse as those of natural fish populations, plus there is greater risk of diseases. However, these problems may be overcome by ensuring good quality diet in the fish ponds, using antibiotics, proper housekeeping practices, and clean water. Moreover, the quality and safety of the fish flesh obtained from the commercial fish ponds depends upon the quality of diet and medical care. Fish ponds can be created on any area of land; however, one-acre ponds can be the best manageable. The average depth of the fish ponds could be 6–8 feet, because shallow ponds may not allow the fish free movement, while deeper ponds may cause trouble for catchers, losses of feed, and problems in housekeeping. The best time and species for fish production should be consulted with the local fishery department. Prior to filling the pond, it must be ensured that all the vegetation is properly removed from the pond. An over or under population of fish may result in poor sanitary conditions, onset of diseases, and lower yield. An average of three fish per square meter is a good choice, though the size of fish may determine the actual population of fish. Worldwide, the most important fish species used in farming are carp, tilapia, salmon, and catfish. The breeds with the highest demand and price in the local market should be preferred, because storage and transportation to other areas may incur additional charges and lower profitability. A good quality diet is necessary for ensuring high quality and nutritious fish flesh. The required nutrients should be supplied to fish through natural food, as well as purpose designed supplementary feeds, having an array of essential vitamins, micro-minerals, essential fatty acids, and other essential nutrient elements.

Fish are often kept alive until delivered to the consumer and eaten to ensure freshness. Floating cages, as well as holding basins are used to keep the fish in their natural environment until required for consumption. The quality of fish, however, may deteriorate by these practices, in cases of poor water quality, inappropriate keeping practices, nutritional deficiencies, and onset of infectious and parasitic diseases.

7.6 TRANSPORTATION

Significant monetary losses have been associated with the detrimental changes occurring in fishes during transportation. Fishes generally have very small shelf life, once harvested and removed from water. So, they are immediately transported to cold stores and warehouses, in order to ensure minimal losses during processing. They may be transported live or frozen, though transportation of live fish requires a lot of care. They are transported by ships, land or air transport. Transportation incurs expenses, because the traveling vehicles have to be specialized and fishes need to be kept at cool temperatures prior to and during transportation. Additionally, the economic losses associated with transportation may further increase, because the quality of fish muscles deteriorates under stressed transport conditions. In order to prevent the additional damages, conditioning and starving practices of fishes are performed prior to their transportation in order to acclimatize them to new conditions. Restrains are applied in the pond and quite corner of the canal by cloths, and fish are kept there for a period of time before transferring them to the transport carrier (Table 7.4).

TABLE 7.4
Requirements Prior to Transportation of Fishes

Restrains prior to transportation	Acclimatize fish to confined transport environment
Starving for 24 hours	Digestive tract of fish remains clear
Higher diffused oxygen level	Reduce fish metabolism
Low temperature	Reduce oxygen requirement. Reduce ATP metabolism
Use of buffers	Prevent pH decrease due to accumulation of fish excreta
High fish densities	Restrict fish activity
Low transportation time	Minimize transportation losses on fish quality
Insulated tanks	Prevent temperature shock

Fishes acclimatize to these conditions and do not overreact during the transportation in the closed containers. Moreover, the fishes need to be starved for 24 hours, so that the digestive tract of the fish may remain clear [54]. During the conditioning stage, the fish get acclimatized to confined conditions, stay less excited and require less energy for metabolism. During this process, fish also recover from the stress and minor injuries faced during the capture. Additional expenses could be in terms of fulfilling the demands of fish for higher oxygen and lower temperatures. The higher diffused oxygen level and lower temperatures in the transportation tanks are beneficial to ensure restrained metabolism of fishes. Lower temperature not only reduces the oxygen requirements, but also ensures lower depletion of muscle ATP during transportation. Buffers should be used in the tanks to prevent a drop of pH due to increased concentration of metabolic wastes, such as carbon dioxide and ammonia as results of respiration and metabolic activities of the fishes [55]. Higher fish densities are suitable to lower activity, but it may result in increased oxygen consumption, as well as higher muscular and metabolic activities. Lastly, transportation times inversely affect the quality of fishes. Insulated tanks reduce the shocks during travel, as well as loss of temperature and oxygen. Moreover, efficient loading and handling practices, as well as system of mechanical refrigeration in transportation tanks and continuous monitoring of temperature and dissolved oxygen are important to ensure optimum fish quality. The leakage of seafood packages in aircrafts requires hefty investment to repair the damages, so fish might be packed in dry ice or gel, rather than in ice.

7.7 PRIMARY PROCESSING

Separation of economically valuable parts from low value ones and by-products is important for ensuring profitability to the fish rearing business. The preliminary processing of raw fish and preparation of raw fish products is called primary processing. Fish processing by humans was first evidenced during the early Holocene period (11,700 years ago) [56]. However, over the years, processing technology has significantly modernized. Modern fish processing plants conduct many unit operations to preserve the nutrition of the fish, portion, and convert them into valuable products. The major unit operations are described in the following text (Figure 7.8).

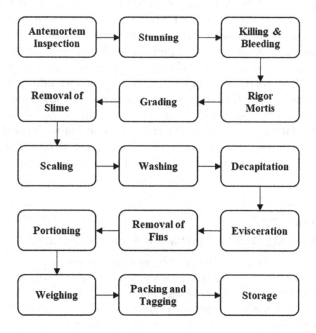

FIGURE 7.8 Primary processing of fish.

Antemortem inspection refers to diagnostic tests performed to avoid any fish containing pathogenic organisms entering the human food chain. Aquarists are able to diagnose most infectious and parasitic diseases using a simple light microscope. The most common antemortem tests for fish include gill and fin biopsy, skin scrape, as well as blood and fecal analysis. The investigations of clips of primary and secondary lamellae are useful tools for assessing the quality of the gills. The individual gill filaments of the primary lamellae can be observed with the naked eye. However, the epithelial and endothelial cells comprising secondary lamellae can only be observed using microscope. The reduction in surface area of the secondary lamellae is indicative of damage to the gills. The lesions on fish skins or fins indicate infection, so fins could be used to identify whether the infection is bacterial, fungal, or parasitic. Similarly, fecal examination of fish might also be useful for determination of parasitic infections. Complete blood samples are, however, taken for detailed analysis to confirm the type and extent of pathogenic bacterial attack, and analyze the risk of entering zoonotic diseases into human food chain. The report of the antemortem inspection is prepared by trained personnel, which is viewed and verified by a competent veterinary practitioner. Fishes not suitable for processing are separated, and information regarding any threat related to zoonotic disease dispersion are provided to related institutions. Only the healthy fishes pass into the processing site.

Recently, humane handling and killing of animals have been highly demanded by most civilized cultures. Seafood is also not an exception. Stunning is used to render the seafood unconscious prior to killing or getting killed during stunning. It also significantly influences final product quality, because the fishes do not go into a stress condition. Traditional stunning practices include percussive stunning (hitting the fish's head with a wooden piece), which is considered the best for stunning large fish, such as salmon and trout; pithing, (also known as ikejime, or ikijime, sticking a sharp spike through the brain of the fish), also useful for large species such as tuna and salmon; shooting of large fish; as well as electrical stunning, which could be used for larger number of fishes. The HS1 is a modern electrical stunning machine [57], which subjects the trout to an electric field of 250 V/m r. m. s. with a sinusoidal waveform of 1,000 Hz for 60 seconds. Under these conditions, fish are stunned first, followed by unconsciousness until death. This machine is widely used in the UK for processing of trout (Table 7.5).

Air asphyxiation is the oldest fish killing method, which can take the fish 55–250 minutes to die. At higher temperatures, fish lose consciousness more quickly. Moreover, putting fish in baths of ice water up to 1 hour can kill them of anoxia by slowing down the metabolic rate and oxygen needs. It is useful for killing zebrafish [58]. CO_2 narcosis (drowsiness) produces acidic pH in water, which injures the brains. Salmon and trout get immobilized in 2–4 minutes but remain conscious until subsequent stunning or killing [59]. Salt baths are used for killing some fish, such as eels, whose slime on the skin is lost by salting. They keep on moving to avoid salt until they become motionless [60]. Similarly, ammonia baths are also used for killing fish. Exsanguination (cutting the highly vascular body regions) without stunning is the most widely adopted practice, during which fish remain conscious for 15 minutes or more [61]. Some fish, such as eels, remain conscious up to 30 minutes after decapitation (removing head, throat cutting) and evisceration. Stripping is the method in which live fish are cut to remove the blood and organs. Killing fish without stunning is very painful, so has been abandoned by most societies, and stunning practices

TABLE 7.5

Stunning Methods for Humane Slaughter of Fishes

Percussive stunning	Hitting the fish's head with a wooden piece
Pithing	Sticking a sharp spike through the brain of the fish
Shooting	Used for large fish
Electrical stunning	Used for many types of fishes
HSI	Modern machine, used for stunning trout

TABLE 7.6

Killing and Methods for Fishes

Air asphyxiation	55 to 250 minutes to die, quicker at higher temperatures
Baths of ice water	Kill fish in up to 1 hour by slowing metabolic rate
CO_2 necrosis	Immobilizes fish in 2 to 4 minutes by decreasing pH of water
Salting or ammonia baths	Slime on skin is lost to salt, and fish become motionless
Exsanguination	Cutting highly vascular regions of fish body
Decapitation	Removal of head, cutting throat
Stripping	Live fish are cut to remove blood and organs

are used for humane slaughtering of fishes. The bleeding of fishes normally yields uniform white fillets. The bleeding of the live fresh fish yields the best results. Cutting the fish prior to *rigor mortis* results in muscle contractions that force the blood out of the fish tissues. The bled fish should be immediately chilled. Rough handling of caught fishes, while they are still alive, can result into discoloration of the fillet, bruises, rupture of blood vessels, and hematoma (blood oozing into the muscle tissues) (Table 7.6).

Rigor mortis is an important stage of death happening in fish, as well as all the animals. The onset of *rigor mortis* and its resolution critically affects the meat quality. Respiration in all living animals and fish yields 36 adenosine triphosphate (ATP) molecules by glycolysis, citric acid cycle, and electron transport chain. The ATP molecule breaks down into adenosine diphosphate (ADP) for muscle contraction and relaxation. Uptake and release of Ca^{+2} take place during relaxation and contraction of muscles, respectively. Ca^{+2} is released from sarcoplasmic reticulum in the muscle cells because of stimulus (electrical signal). Ca^{+2} ions enter the muscle cells and bind to the regulatory proteins, troponin and tropomyosin, changing the shape of actin. ATP provides energy to slide the actin over myosin within the myofibril to cause contraction (muscle shortening). Myosin ATPase enzyme catalyzes the hydrolysis of ATP into ADP, which results in the release of energy and increases the Ca^{+2} concentration from 0.1 to 10 M during the contraction. ATP is needed to release the myosin and actin from each other (muscle relaxation), as well as return the Ca^{+2} ions out of the cell. During the relaxation, the concentration of Ca^{+2} ions returns to 0.1 M, and the ATP molecule re-associates with the myosin heads on the thick filaments. The removal of Ca^{+2} ions brings the actin back to its shape, which then releases the myosin. Muscles can be classified as white or red based upon the biological function. For short-term and rapid contractions, fast-twitch white muscles are used, which get energy by glycolysis for the re-synthesis of ATP. For sustained and low amplitude contractions, slow-twitch red or dark muscles are used, which regenerates ATP by aerobic mitochondrial metabolism. The red and white muscles are made up of red and white muscle fiber. Both red, as well as white muscles are present in fish. The muscle fibers near the skin surface are usually red, whereas those inside are white. During postmortem, sarcoplasmic reticulum or mitochondria lose the ability to sequestrate calcium, resulting in depletion of ATP into adenosine diphosphate (ADP) and H^+ ions (i.e. drop in pH). The fish muscles immediately after death are soft and elastic. Afterward, (aerobic as well as anaerobic) glycolysis ceases postmortem due to inhibition of enzymes (e.g. phosphofructokinase) or depletion of glycogen. During postmortem, the muscle tissues switch from aerobic to anaerobic glycolysis, during which glycogen yields lactate, resulting in the formation of 2–3 ATP molecules. Soon after the depletion of muscle glycogen (which is less than 1% in fish and animal muscles), the anaerobic respiration also stops. Since ATP required for the release of actin and myosin filaments, as well as for pumping out of Ca^{+2} ions, is not available postmortem, hence, muscle stiffening takes place. This process is called *rigor mortis*. Moreover, the sarcoplasmic reticulum and mitochondria of pre-rigor fish lose the ability to sequester Ca^{+2}. This accelerates

ATP hydrolysis and re-synthesis and ultimately completes the depletion of ATP and decrease in pH. Enzymes are also involved in the onset of *rigor mortis*.

Carcass temperature, processing conditions, as well as species characteristics significantly affect the rate and extent of chemical, biological, and microbial reactions leading to *rigor mortis*. Under ice bath conditions (hypothermia), the onset of *rigor mortis* in fish takes place within a few hours. Rigor sets in when the ATPs of fish are completely consumed that result in binding the proteins in the muscle into a network, thus causing the stiffening and hardening of the fish muscles. Few more enzymes break down (proteolysis) the fish protein network after a couple of days in ice and result in re-softening. The formation of ice crystals under ice bath conditions causes physical damages to the cells and membrane bound organelles, which results in leakage of cell constituents. The leachates contain several enzymes that find substrates and, thus, the extent of several chemical reactions increases. Moreover, salts are also used to enhance the efficiency of ice bathing. Penetration of salts into cells and their reaction with leachates also increase the rate of chemical reactions taking place in the muscle.

In the case of starving, the energy reserves of fish are significantly depleted and onset of rigor is very fast. Similarly, in cases of stressing or injury, fish undergo *rigor mortis* quite rapidly. Stunning conditions also influence the onset of rigor; hypothermia gives relatively faster onset of rigor than that attained after percussion. Under normal conditions, the higher concentration of ADP in muscle cells leads to re-synthesis of ATP by aerobic glycolysis, but this is limited in the dead fish, because of anoxia (absence of oxygen) and glycogen. The rate and extent of pH decline also influences the quality of fish muscles, because the postmortem biochemical events of cells are significantly affected by pH. During the conversion of ATP into ADP and P, there is also formation of H+ ions, hence the inability of muscles to resynthesize ATP after fish death results in significant decrease in fish muscle pH.

Fish processing should be delayed until resolution of rigor. Rigor is resolved under the action of proteases after some time depending upon species, muscle type, antemortem history (stress, health, nutritive status, fasting, etc.), and slaughter method. Pre-rigor filleting results in significant drop in the yield. Since rapid contractions are the job of fast-twitch white muscles, so rigor tension is mainly attributed to them. During *rigor mortis*, the dark muscles of fish may shrink up to 52%, whereas white muscles may shrink up to 15%. This difference in extent of shrinking among muscles of various types results in splitting of layers of muscle bundles. This condition is usually referred to as gaping. Gaping problems can also take place in muscles because of rough handling. The removal of the skeletal system removes the constraints required for fish muscles to hold its shape, thus results in post-rigor shrinking and gaping. Another consequence of pre-rigor filleting is extensive drip loss. Cooking quality of fish is also influenced by the time of rigor. For instance, pre-rigor cooking of fish flesh results in soft and pasty texture, during rigor cooking of fish flesh yields tough but not dry texture, and post-rigor cooking of fish flesh yields firm, succulent, and elastic texture (Table 7.7).

Sorting and grading are very important in fish processing. These can be done manually, as well as by mechanical graders. Grading and sorting of the fish is performed based upon species, sizes, freshness, and physical condition. Fish thickness is highly correlated with fish length, so mechanical sorters use these characteristics for sorting fishes.

TABLE 7.7
Problems in Fish Meat Related to Improper *Rigor Mortis*

Pre-rigor Filleting	Excessive Drip Loss, Yield Drop
During rigor filleting	Gaping
Pre-rigor cooking	Soft and pasty texture
During rigor cooking	Tough, but not dry texture

Slime on the fish skin is a protection mechanism against harmful conditions, which is very prominent when the fish is dying. It may account for 2%–3% of body weight in some freshwater species. Its excretion stops prior to *rigor mortis*. It is a perfect medium for microbial growth, so needs washing. Moreover, slime may result in yellowish-brown spots on the fish skin. Washing of slime is done in salted water manually as well as mechanically. Moreover, it can be removed by soaking in 2% baking soda solution, followed by washing in a cylindrical rotating washer.

The removal of scales from fish skin is a difficult process. Manual scaling is extremely labor intensive. Blanching of fish for 3–6 seconds in boiling water can be useful prior to scaling. Mechanized scalers are commonly used in fish processing plants. Mechanical scaling units, however, can leave 10%–20% scales, which can be removed by secondary scaling using electrical handheld scalers. It should be noted that scaling practices do not cause any mechanical damage to the fish.

Washing of the fish slime and other residues is very important for ensuring smooth processing and avoiding any contamination. Soaking as well as spraying can be used as effective washing techniques.

Decapitation refers to the removal of the head from the fish. The heads of fish account for almost 10%–20% of the total weight, but it is mostly considered an inedible part and is wasted. However, a significant amount of fish flesh can be recovered from it, so careful de-heading is required. Usually, small freshwater fishes are de-headed manually. Manual de-heading is very slow process, so mechanical de-heading devices are also used these days. The amount of meat lost depends upon the de-heading procedure, type of head cut, and skill of the operator of the mechanical de-heading device. Usually, mechanical de-heading devices can process 20–40 fishes per minute of the uniform size and species.

Evisceration of fish is usually performed manually. Gutting includes cutting of fish belly, removal of internal organs, as well as cleaning the body cavity. Cutting the gall bladder should be avoided to prevent contamination. The surfaces should be rinsed and disinfected prior to and after gutting to avoid contamination. Mechanical evisceration of larger, uniform sized fishes is also done, however, 10%–20% residues of viscera may not be removed, which are manually removed later.

Removal of fins is usually done after the gutting process. Sometimes, fish are sent for frozen storage after gutting. In such cases, fins are not removed from the fishes. But, during steak or fillet production, removal of fins is performed. Knives, scissors, or special rotating disc knives can be used for fins removal. Automated fin removal devices are also available, but they can only be used for large uniform sized fishes.

Portioning means cutting and slicing of fish into small pats. Most of the raw finfish is sold as whole fish without any further processing. However, several secondary fish products are also produced worldwide. If the fish is sold after evisceration (removal of internal organs), it is called a drawn fish. If the fish is scaled as well as eviscerated, then it is known as a dressed fish. If the head, tail, and fins of dressed fish are removed then it is termed a pan-dressed fish. Two major types of portioning are usually practiced including steaking and filleting. Steaking refers to slicing of de-headed whole fish by cutting the fish perpendicular to the fish backbone. Fish cut into cross-section slices of the backbone are called fish steaks. Filleting is another important technique in which the flesh of each side of the fish is deboned (separated from the backbone). The cutting of fish flesh lengthwise along the backbone is called filleted fish. Butterfly fillets refer to two fish fillets held together. Steaking has a higher technological efficiency than that of filleting, though both are equally popular among fish consumers. Steaking can be done by knives as well as by a band saw. Mechanical slicing of the larger uniform sized fishes is preferred in the fish industry. A mechanized slicer can produce steaks of 20–40 fishes per minute. Block (boned) fillet is a type of fillet in which some bones are retained; however, ribs are further cut during further processing. Small pieces of filleted fish are called fish sticks. Moreover, only de-heading to cut whole fish into two halves is also a preferred practice for some fishes. Meat-bone separator machines can recover the leftover flesh on the fish backbone. Furthermore, the fillets could be skin on, as well as skinless. Skinning operations can also be performed manually and with mechanical devices. Skin on fish fillets are more preferred for roasting, whereas skinless fillets are preferred for caning purposes. Moreover, fish cakes, fish fingers, surimi, and fish roe are also important fish products.

The objectives of packing the seafoods include preservation of nutritional and quality attributes, increasing its shelf life, as well as enhance the selling value of the seafoods. Packaging material of a wide variety can be used. In addition, ordinary packaging, vacuum packaging, controlled and modified atmospheric packaging, etc. can be used to enhance the shelf life and preserve the nutritional components of seafoods. These days a growing trend has been observed toward active packaging. Active packaging materials scavenge metals from the foods, absorb oxygen present in the package, perform antibacterial role, and exhibit antioxidant properties, thus increase the monetary profits associated with the seafoods. The packaged products are tagged with suitable information usually in the forms of codes (numbers, alphabets, barcodes, QR codes, etc.) for future identification of the products, traceability and possible recall.

7.8   SECONDARY PROCESSING: VALUE ADDITION

Raw fish is cheaper than the products manufactured from them. So, additional profitability has been associated with further processing of fishes. Secondary or further processing refers to all the processing methods intended to develop secondary products from the raw fish, including ready-to-cook and ready-to-eat fish products. Value addition refers to the additional activities intended to change the nature of a product for increasing its sale value and customer acceptance. Frozen fish cannot be processed without thawing. Defrosting is performed under controlled conditions (4°C for overnight) to thaw frozen fish. Thawing is extremely detrimental to fish yield, quality, and safety. Almost 4%–10% myowater (the water held by myofibrillar bundles) of fish is lost during thawing. The water-soluble nutrients, such as vitamins, minerals, and proteins, also leach down along with myowater and are an invitation for microorganisms. So, the thawing practices should be performed in properly disinfected environment. The loss of water reduces the yield, as well as deteriorates the quality and the nutritional value of fish meat.

Mechanically deboned fish meat is obtained by removing the residues of fish flesh from bones, head, and tail, and is considered of the low economic value. This fish flesh can be processed into fish paste, called surimi, which gives very soft texture upon cooking. Surimi can also be made from smaller and low-value fish. Ready-to-eat seafood, such as fish sausages, can be prepared from surimi. Moreover, low-grade fish can be processed to extract fish oil, which is of high economic value because of higher omega-3 fatty acid contents. The fish waste left after the oil extraction is called fish meal, which is further processed and dried to be supplied as poultry feed.

7.9   STORAGE AND DISTRIBUTION

Preservation techniques increase the economic value of products by preventing nutrition deterioration and contribute to public health by minimizing microbial contamination. Freshly caught fishes have limited shelf life and should be preserved as soon as possible. However, some fish stores may keep live fish in glass containers filled with water. The undesirable textural and flavor changes taking place in fish flesh are owed to the onset of *rigor mortis*, tissue degradation due to oxidative changes in protein and lipids, as well as enzymatic activity and microbial spoilage. Fishes may undergo preliminary storage prior to final storage, because they are often moved from the source of catching to the shore, and then transported to fish processing sites. The objective of appropriate preservation practices is to protect the fish from deterioration of nutrition, quality, and safety. The most important and common storage techniques include refrigeration, freezing, and drying. Moreover, smoking, salting, canning, and pickling are also traditional primary processing techniques, which are used for preservation and value addition of fish.

7.9.1 REFRIGERATION

The common principle of refrigeration is described in Figure 7.9. Initially, a hot gas is compressed under high pressure in a compression chamber, due to which the temperature of the gas further rises, and the gas becomes heat-supersaturated getting ready to radiate the absorbed heat. In the next step, the hot compressed gas is passed through a series of condensing coils, which are directly exposed to the air. Since the temperature of the air is significantly lower than that of the compressed heat-supersaturated gas, the hot gas radiates heat into the atmosphere, and the temperature of the gas is significantly dropped. This gas then enters the refrigeration chamber, in which it is passed through an expansion valve. In the expansion valve, the pressure of the gas is released, due to which its temperature is further dropped. Moreover, a vacuum is created among the gas molecules, due to which its ability to absorb the temperature increases. This is the entirely opposite process to that occurring in the compressor. Here, cold gas also becomes unsaturated. This cold unsaturated gas then passes into the evaporator of the refrigeration box, where due to being heat-unsaturated, it absorbs heat from the foods, thus the temperature of the foods is dropped. The temperature of the gas rises, and finally the hot gas is directed toward the compressor, where it is again heat-supersaturated, and the cycle carries on.

Refrigeration involves chilling, pre-cooling, and cooling, with a final temperature of just above freezing (0°C–4°C). The temperature of the cooling room is maintained at −2°C to ensure temperature differential. Fish may be chilled at <15°C prior to refrigeration to avoid too much temperature differential at the time of refrigeration. Most modern processing plants carry on a portion of their activities at chilling temperatures to avoid any rise of biochemical and enzymatic activities. Usually, food is allowed at this temperature for a maximum of two hours, during which food is passed through the primary processing including portion, weighing, and packing. Fish is refrigerated, if it will be sold in lesser time, or will be immediately processed. Fish do not undergo severe structural changes at this temperature and retain their fresh-like properties. Moreover, during refrigeration, fish may undergo *rigor mortis* and conditioning at low temperature, which ultimately improves the quality of fish meat. Refrigeration can be used as the sole preservation method, as most customers prefer seeing the "Fresh" tag in modern retail outlets. The shelf life of frozen fishes can be 3–7 days, depending upon the origin, as well as mode of chemical, biochemical, and enzymatic reactions taking place in the muscles. In most retail stores, whole fish is kept on ice flakes. Refrigeration can also be taken as initial temperature reduction tool required prior to freezing, in which case it is termed as pre-cooling. Fish and its products are allowed to drop to just above freezing temperature (0°C–4°C) in a few hours prior to transferring into the blast freezers, which drop the temperature of fish below zero (almost −9°C to −10°C). In addition, refrigeration can also be taken as a preliminary treatment prior to further processing and value addition.

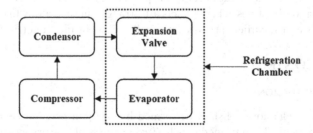

FIGURE 7.9 Refrigeration cycle.

7.9.2 FREEZING

Freezing is the most widely adopted fish preservation method. This method has been used by humans since historic times. With the advent of refrigeration systems, freezing began being used for the storage of foods. Storage of fish and meat products at freezing temperatures (below −18°C) result in long term storage with the highest shelf life. All the microbial activities cease below −8°C, whereas only slow enzymatic activities keep going, and they do not cause serious damage to frozen fish products. Meat should be sealed in airtight polyethylene bags prior to freezing. Its temperature is first dropped by chilling at a temperature less than the environmental temperature (below 15°C) in less than two hours, followed by refrigeration (0°C–4°C) for 4–10 hours. The refrigerated fish products are then subjected to blast freezing (below −36°C to −39°C) until the temperature of the core drops below −10°C, then the products are shifted to cold stores, of which temperature is maintained below −24°C. The frozen fish retains most quality and safety attributes for at least 1 year. If the product is directly exposed to storage conditions, the extremely low temperature may damage the external surface of fish meat, resulting in a browning of the exposed surface. This condition is called freeze/freezer burn. Freezer burn may take place because of rupturing of the packaging material during handling, storage, and distribution. It is recommended that fish may be sliced into required portions, because thawing/defrosting will be required to cut and separate the frozen fish pieces from each other.

7.9.3 DEHYDRATION

Drying involves the dehydration (removal of water) of the fish. Sun drying has also been an ancient food preservation technique. Drying inhibits the microbial growth by reducing the availability of available moisture in sea foods. Sun drying is a cheap and effective method, and dried fishes have fairly long shelf lives. These days, sophisticated dryers have been developed that can dry the fish meat faster than by sun drying. The novel drying methods employ hot air ovens. Usually extremely dry air is passed through a chamber containing fish meat, and the dry air takes away the moisture from the fish surface. Moreover, water may also be removed by air drying and smoking. A combination of different drying methods can also be used. Freeze-drying is the most efficient method used for removal of moisture from fish meat without damaging the texture of food, along with the ability of meat to retain original like texture upon rehydration. Freeze drying operate of the function of sublimation. Drying methods decrease the water activity of fish meat, thus reduce the microbial activity and increase shelf life. Dried fish can have shelf lives up to several years.

7.9.4 FIRST-IN-FIRST-OUT

Storage of food products is an extremely intricate process and requires scientific knowledge. The maintenance of storage conditions as well as keeping the record of life of the product is very important. The product brought to the storage sections is properly recorded in the inventory and assigned to appropriate sections of the stores. The products are arranged in such a way that the earlier product coming to the store is issued earlier. The system is called First-in-First-out (FIFO) system.

7.10 QUALITY CONTROL

7.10.1 SENSORY EVALUATION

Sensory/organoleptic evaluation of fish is performed based upon perceptions of color, odor, and texture of fish by experienced and trained panels. Two methods of sensory evaluation including the European Union (EU) scheme and Quality Index Method (QIM) are usually employed for quality determination of fish [62]. The EU scheme evaluates the whole fish into E, A, B/unfit categories. QIM quantifies the fish quality by giving scores from 0 to 3 for various quality attributes.

7.10.2 Microbial Inspection

Total viable counts (TVC, TPC) represent the number of microorganisms flourishing on the fish. Just after capturing, the TVC range from 100 to 10,000 CFU/g for normal fish. Microbial deterioration keeps increasing during postmortem, *rigor mortis*, and processing. It is the most accurate method of determining fish quality but it is time consuming. Recently, hyperspectral imaging measurements [63] have been reported to be a rapid prediction tool for fish freshness quality, while its results have been reported to correlate highly with TVC.

7.10.3 Chemical Analysis

Postmortem fish muscle undergoes several unavoidable chemical changes, which can be measured in terms of moisture content, volatile compounds, lipid and protein degradation, and depletion of ATP and K value measurement.

7.10.3.1 Moisture Measurement

Fish muscle contains 60%–75% moisture, which affects its texture. Destructive moisture analytical methods, such as the traditional oven-drying method, have been widely used for the determination of moisture content, but they are time consuming and less environmentally sustainable. Novel methods, such as NIR spectroscopy [64] and low-field nuclear magnetic resonance (LF-NMR), are nondestructive methods and can also be used for distribution and compartmentalization of chemically bound, bulk, and free water in fish muscle. Moreover, the water bound by three-dimensional matrix developed by denaturation of fish proteins can also be determined using LF-NMR [65].

7.10.3.2 Protein Degradation and Oxidation

Fish contain approximately 15%–20% proteins, which may undergo degradation and decomposition during postmortem, handling, and processing; thus, causing microorganisms and enzymes to affect their quality attributes and shelf life by altering physical and chemical structures and properties. The degradation and oxidation products of these proteins contribute to characteristic taste and aroma of fish products. Moreover, proteins hold water that is very important in terms of products yield, quality, and safety. Changes in protein contents can be determined by conventional methods, as well as sodium dodecyl sulfate-polyacrylamide gel electrophoresis (SDS-PAGE) and Raman spectroscopy [66]. SDS-PAGE can be used to determine overall changes in protein contents, whereas Raman spectroscopy can be used to monitor changes in secondary protein structures. Moreover, oxidation of fish hemoglobin and myoglobin can be determined by VIS/NIR spectroscopy [67]. Carbonyl contents, active sulfhydryl groups, total sulfhydryl groups, disulfide bonds, and thiol contents are considered the indices of protein quality and oxidation in fish muscle.

7.10.3.3 Lipid Oxidation

Lipid oxidation is affected by enzymes, the degree of saturation, as well as abiotic conditions, such as light and temperature. The presence of unsaturated fatty acids, such as tetradecene acid, palmitoleic acid, EPA, and DHA, in fish make them a useful source of nutrition for humans. However, oxidation of these fatty acids under the influence of light and high temperature breaks them down into the lower molecular weight compounds, including aldehydes, ketones, and alcohols. The changes in these volatile compounds affect the aroma, texture, color, and nutritional value of fishes. The thiobarbituric acid (TBA) value expressed as mg of malonaldehyde (MDA) per kg muscle is a useful indicator of lipid oxidation [68]. Moreover, peroxide value (PV) also indicates the extent of lipid oxidation [68], which could be determined using traditional methods, as well as Raman spectroscopy and proton NMR of lipids.

7.10.3.4 Stage of *Rigor Mortis* and ATP Decomposition

Fish muscles undergo *rigor mortis* after death. During postmortem, the biochemical and physiochemical reactions continue in the same manner, as in the living organisms, but due to the lack of oxygen, muscle ATP starts depleting. The ATP content of the muscle can be taken as a degree of freshness of fish muscle. ATP decomposes to produce several metabolites, which can be determined individually and expressed in terms of K and K1 values [69].

7.10.3.5 Volatile Compounds Measurements

Microorganisms and endogenous enzymes cause changes in the composition of fish constituents and produce volatile compounds, including alcohols, aldehydes, ketones, nitrogen containing compounds (such as ammonia and trimethylamine), sulfur-containing compounds (such as hydrogen sulfide), and methyl mercaptan. These volatile compounds are the degradation and oxidation products of proteins (structural proteins, enzymes, and amino acids) and lipids, which contribute to the characteristic flavor of fish. The microbial and enzymatic deterioration can be estimated in terms of volatile compounds, mainly three groups of chemicals, namely C6-C9 alcohols and carbonyl compounds; ammonia and trimethylamine (related to microbial action); and lipid oxidation products. The extraction of the volatile components is performed by solid-phase micro-extraction headspace analysis and subjected to quantification by gas chromatography (GC) [70], gas chromatography mass spectrometry (GC-MS) [71], and Fourier transform infrared spectroscopy (FT-IR) [72]. Total volatile basic nitrogen (TVB-N) and TMA are used as indicators of fish freshness.

7.10.4 Physical Properties Measurements

The chemical and microbial changes taking place in fish cause several changes in the physical attributes, thus affecting fish quality. The important factors include changes in fish pH, color, texture, and rheological attributes. Reduction in pH has been associated with loss of water-holding capacity, which ultimately results in significant monetary loss during storage, as well as during processing. In addition, color of seafoods is also considered an important indicator of seafood quality.

7.11 CONCLUSION

Fish products are not only important contributor to health and nutrition of human beings, but also an import source of income generation worldwide. Classification of the fishes is done on the basis of similar characteristics, as well as economic value. The fish muscles are slightly different from those of other animals in term of structure, however, in terms of components and nutritional value, they are almost similar. Judicious use of fish is useful for health; however, a few drawbacks of fish consumption have also been known. Fish are not only reared in natural habitats, such as marine environment, rivers, tributaries, and canals, but also in fish farms and fish ponds. However, the nutritional value and quality characteristics of fish vary from environment to environment for each species. Fish are usually transported live to processing plants, as well as retail stores, after harvesting from their habitat, during which quality of the fish is susceptible to deterioration. Processing is a highly economic activity, which involves intensive use of labor and machinery to convert the intact fish into valuable portions or value-added products. Fish undergoes antemortem inspection upon reaching the processing plants, after which it is processed via various unit operations. The nutritional value and sensory quality, which are preserved using either refrigeration, freezing, or dehydration, is of the utmost importance for the consumer. Secondary products development offers greater profitability than that of primary processing. During the storage and dispatch of fish and fish products, a first-in-first-out system is followed. Since, higher quality is desired for greater profitability, the quality of fish and fish products are assessed in terms of organoleptic evaluation, microbial inspections, chemical analyses, and measurement of physical attributes.

REFERENCES

1. FAOSTAT. Global production. in *Fishery Statistical Collections*. 2018. Assessible at: http://www.fao.org/fishery/statistics/global-production/query/en. Accessed on: 27/09/2018.
2. FAOSTAT. Global capture production. in *Fishery Statistical Collections*. 2018. Assessible at: http://www.fao.org/fishery/statistics/global-capture-production/query/en. Accessed on: 27/09/2018.
3. Martin B. What are Fish? *in* Davis B. *Let's Find Out! Marine Life*. 2017. Britannica Educational Publishing Inc., pp 1–32. Assessible at: http://eb.pdn.ipublishcentral.com/product/what-are-fish. Accessed on: 27/09/2018.
4. Sundby, S. and T. Kristiansen, The principles of buoyancy in marine fish eggs and their vertical distributions across the world oceans. *PLoS One*, 2015. **10**(10): e0138821.
5. Eaton, J.G. and R.M. Scheller, Effects of climate warming on fish thermal habitat in streams of the United States. *Limnology and Oceanography*, 1996. **41**(5): 1109–1115.
6. Emoto, A., S. Ishizaki, and K. Shiomi, Tropomyosins in gastropods and bivalves: Identification as major allergens and amino acid sequence features. *Food Chemistry*, 2009. **114**(2): 634–641.
7. Alami-Durante, H. et al., Skeletal muscle growth dynamics and expression of related genes in white and red muscles of rainbow trout fed diets with graded levels of a mixture of plant protein sources as substitutes for fishmeal. *Aquaculture*, 2010. **303**(1–4): 50–58.
8. Kobayashi, A. et al., Comparison of allergenicity and allergens between fish white and dark muscles. *Allergy*, 2006. **61**(3): 357–363.
9. Anttila, K., M. Jäntti, and S. Mänttäri, Effects of training on lipid metabolism in swimming muscles of sea trout (*Salmo trutta*). *Journal of Comparative Physiology B*, 2010. **180**(5): 707–714.
10. Videler, J.J. and P. He, Swimming in marine fish. *Behavior of Marine Fishes: Capture Processes and Conservation Challenges*, 2010: 3–24.
11. Latif, M.S., Influence of nutritional factors on muscle development and texture of Atlantic salmon (*Salmo salar* L.). In vivo and in vitro studies. Master thesis, 2010.
12. Pavelka, M. and J. Roth, Skeletal muscle, dystrophy and myopathy, in *Functional Ultrastructure*. 2015, Springer, Vienna, Austria. pp. 340–349.
13. Waritthitham, A. et al., Muscle fiber characteristics and their relationship to water-holding capacity of Longissimus dorsi muscle in Brahman and Charolais crossbred bulls. *AJAS*, 2010. **23**: 665–671.
14. Yang, H. et al., Effect of protein structure on water and fat distribution during meat gelling. *Food Chemistry*, 2016. **204**: 239–245.
15. Tahmasebi, A. et al., A differential scanning calorimetric (DSC) study on the characteristics and behavior of water in low-rank coals. *Fuel*, 2014. **135**: 243–252.
16. Yao, Y. et al., Assessing the water migration and permeability of large intact bituminous and anthracite coals using NMR relaxation spectrometry. *Transport in Porous Media*, 2015. **107**(2): 527–542.
17. Ali, S. et al., Effect of freeze-thaw cycles on lipid oxidation and myowater in broiler chickens. *Revista Brasileira de Ciência Avícola*, 2016. **18**(1): 35–40.
18. Khan, M.I.H. et al., Investigation of bound and free water in plant-based food material using NMR T2 relaxometry. *Innovative Food Science & Emerging Technologies*, 2016. **38**: 252–261.
19. Schmidt, J.A. et al., Plasma concentrations and intakes of amino acids in male meat-eaters, fish-eaters, vegetarians and vegans: A cross-sectional analysis in the EPIC-Oxford cohort. *European Journal of Clinical Nutrition*, 2016. **70**(3): 306.
20. USDA-FSIS, Basic Report: 15236, Fish, salmon, Atlantic, farmed, raw 2018.
21. Hoffman, J.R. and M.J. Falvo, Protein–which is best? *Journal of Sports Science & Medicine*, 2004. **3**(3): 118.
22. Hosomi, R. et al., Effects of dietary fish protein on serum and liver lipid concentrations in rats and the expression of hepatic genes involved in lipid metabolism. *Journal of Agricultural and Food Chemistry*, 2009. **57**(19): 9256–9262.
23. Hughes, J. et al., A structural approach to understanding the interactions between colour, water-holding capacity and tenderness. *Meat Science*, 2014. **98**(3): 520–532.
24. Lábas, A. et al., First principles calculation of the reaction rates for ligand binding to myoglobin: The cases of NO and CO. *Chemistry–A European Journal*, 2018. **24**(20): 5350–5358.
25. Zhou, C.-Y. et al., The changes in the proteolysis activity and the accumulation of free amino acids during Chinese traditional dry-cured loins processing. *Food Science and Biotechnology*, 2017. **26**(3): 679–687.

26. Delgado, A.M., S. Parisi, and M.D.V. Almeida, Fish, meat and other animal protein sources, in *Chemistry of the Mediterranean Diet*. 2017, Springer, Cham, Switzerland. pp. 177–207.

27. Vandal, M. et al., Reduction in DHA transport to the brain of mice expressing human APOE4 compared to APOE2. *Journal of Neurochemistry*, 2014. **129**(3): 516–526.

28. Rhoades, W., L. Kump, and E. Margalit, Anterior chamber and retina (structure, function and immunology), in Ikezu, T., and Gendelman, H. (Eds.), *Neuroimmune Pharmacology*. 2017, Springer. pp. 39–54.

29. Simopoulos, A.P., An increase in the omega-6/omega-3 fatty acid ratio increases the risk for obesity. *Nutrients*, 2016. **8**(3): 128.

30. Bilandžić, N. et al., Metal content in four shellfish species from the Istrian coast of Croatia. *Bulletin of Environmental Contamination and Toxicology*, 2015. **95**(5): 611–617.

31. Hoffman, R., Can the paleolithic diet meet the nutritional needs of older people? *Maturitas*, 2017. **95**: 63–64.

32. Siscovick, D.S. et al., Omega-3 polyunsaturated fatty acid (fish oil) supplementation and the prevention of clinical cardiovascular disease: a science advisory from the American Heart Association. *Circulation*, 2017. **135**(15): e867–e884.

33. Dyall, S.C., Long-chain omega-3 fatty acids and the brain: A review of the independent and shared effects of EPA, DPA and DHA. *Frontiers in Aging Neuroscience*, 2015. **7**: 52.

34. Appleton, K.M. et al., ω-3 Fatty acids for major depressive disorder in adults: An abridged Cochrane review. *BMJ Open*, 2016. **6**(3): e010172.

35. Bi, X. et al., ω-3 polyunsaturated fatty acids ameliorate type 1 diabetes and autoimmunity. *The Journal of Clinical Investigation*, 2017. **127**(5): 1757–1771.

36. Fu, Z. et al., Dietary ω-3 polyunsaturated fatty acids decrease retinal neovascularization by adipose–endoplasmic reticulum stress reduction to increase adiponectin–. *The American Journal of Clinical Nutrition*, 2015. **101**(4): 879–888.

37. Yanai, R., K.-H. Sonoda, and K.M. Connor, An invited review following the Soujinkai Award: Cytochrome P450l Generated metabolites of ω-3 fatty acids ameliorate choroidal neovascularization. *The Bulletin of the Yamaguchi Medical School*, 2015. **62**(3): 29–36.

38. Calder, P.C., Marine omega-3 fatty acids and inflammatory processes: Effects, mechanisms and clinical relevance. *Biochimica et Biophysica Acta (BBA)-Molecular and Cell Biology of Lipids*, 2015. **1851**(4): 469–484.

39. Christian, L.M. et al., Polyunsaturated fatty acid (PUFA) status in pregnant women: Associations with sleep quality, inflammation, and length of gestation. *PLoS One*, 2016. **11**(2): e0148752.

40. Vladau, V., I. Bud, and R. Stefan, Nutritive value of fish meat comparative to some animal meat. Bulletin of University of Agricultural Sciences and Veterinary Medicine Cluj-Napoca. *Animal Science and Biotechnologies*, 2008. **65**(1–2): 301–305.

41. Marty, G.D., Anisakid larva in the viscera of a farmed Atlantic salmon (Salmo salar). *Aquaculture*, 2008. **279**(1–4): 209–210.

42. Arizono, N. et al., Diphyllobothriasis associated with eating raw pacific salmon. *Emerging Infectious Diseases*, 2009. **15**(6): 866.

43. Choi, A.L. et al., Negative confounding in the evaluation of toxicity: The case of methylmercury in fish and seafood. *Critical Reviews in Toxicology*, 2008. **38**(10): 877–893.

44. Eto, K., M. Marumoto, and M. Takeya, The pathology of methylmercury poisoning (Minamata disease). *Neuropathology*, 2010. **30**(5): 471–479.

45. Moro, M.M. et al., Incidence of anaphylaxis and subtypes of anaphylaxis in a general hospital emergency department. *Journal of Investigational Allergology and Clinical Immunology*, 2011. **21**(2): 142–149.

46. Kono, M. et al., Examination of transformation among tetrodotoxin and its analogs in the living cultured juvenile puffer fish, kusafugu, Fugu niphobles by intramuscular administration. *Toxicon*, 2008. **52**(6): 714–720.

47. Laser, E.D. and P.D. Shenefelt, Hypnosis to alleviate the symptoms of ciguatera toxicity: A case study. *American Journal of Clinical Hypnosis*, 2012. **54**(3): 179–183.

48. Botana, L.M. et al., Functional assays for marine toxins as an alternative, high-throughput-screening solution to animal tests. *TrAC Trends in Analytical Chemistry*, 2009. **28**(5): 603–611.

49. Munday, R. and J. Reeve, Risk assessment of shellfish toxins. *Toxins*, 2013. **5**(11): 2109–2137.

50. Humpage, A., V. Magalhaes, and S. Froscio, Comparison of analytical tools and biological assays for detection of paralytic shellfish poisoning toxins. *Analytical and Bioanalytical Chemistry*, 2010. **397**(5): 1655–1671.

51. He, Y. et al., Analytical approaches for an important shellfish poisoning agent: Domoic acid. *Journal of Agricultural and Food Chemistry*, 2010. **58**(22): 11525–11533.

52. Hungerford, J.M., Scombroid poisoning: A review. *Toxicon*, 2010. **56**(2): 231–243.

53. Bejarano, A.C. et al., Production and toxicity of the marine biotoxin domoic acid and its effects on wildlife: A review. *Human and Ecological Risk Assessment*, 2008. **14**(3): 544–567.

54. Waagbø, R. et al., Short-term starvation at low temperature prior to harvest does not impact the health and acute stress response of adult Atlantic salmon. *PeerJ*, 2017. **5**: e3273.

55. Vanderzwalmen, M. et al., The use of feed and water additives for live fish transport. *Reviews in Aquaculture*, 2018: 1–16.

56. Van Neer, W., Fish remains from late Pleistocene and Holocene archaeological sites near Khashm el Girba, Sudan. *Archaeofauna*, 2017. **3**: 115–126.

57. Lines, J. et al., Electric stunning: A humane slaughter method for trout. *Aquacultural Engineering*, 2003. **28**(3–4): 141–154.

58. Singh, R. et al., Fluoride exposure abates pro-inflammatory response and induces in vivo apoptosis rendering zebrafish (*Danio rerio*) susceptible to bacterial infections. *Fish & Shellfish Immunology*, 2017. **63**: 314–321.

59. Gräns, A. et al., Stunning fish with CO_2 or electricity: Contradictory results on behavioural and physiological stress responses. *Animal*, 2016. **10**(2): 294–301.

60. Si, J.L. et al., Effect of salt content on the denaturation of pike eel (*Muraenesox cinereus* Forsskål, 1775) actomyosin. *Journal of Applied Ichthyology*, 2015. **31**(4): 767–770.

61. Devaraj, S. et al., Toxicological effects of ammonia on gills of *Cyprinus carpio* var. *communis* (Linn.). *Journal of Coastal Life Medicine*, 2014. **2**(2): 94–98.

62. Cheng, J.-H. et al., Recent advances in methods and techniques for freshness quality determination and evaluation of fish and fish fillets: A review. *Critical Reviews in Food Science and Nutrition*, 2015. **55**(7): 1012–1225.

63. Cheng, J.-H. and D.-W. Sun, Hyperspectral imaging as an effective tool for quality analysis and control of fish and other seafoods: Current research and potential applications. *Trends in Food Science & Technology*, 2014. **37**(2): 78–91.

64. Nilsen, H. et al., Visible/near-infrared spectroscopy: A new tool for the evaluation of fish freshness? *Journal of Food Science*, 2002. **67**(5): 1821–1826.

65. Heude, C. et al., Rapid assessment of fish freshness and quality by 1 H HR-MAS NMR spectroscopy. *Food Analytical Methods*, 2015. **8**(4): 907–915.

66. Cheng, J.-H. et al., Applications of non-destructive spectroscopic techniques for fish quality and safety evaluation and inspection. *Trends in Food Science & Technology*, 2013. **34**(1): 18–31.

67. Sivertsen, A.H., T. Kimiya, and K. Heia, Automatic freshness assessment of cod (*Gadus morhua*) fillets by Vis/Nir spectroscopy. *Journal of Food Engineering*, 2011. **103**(3): 317–323.

68. Özogul, Y. et al., Freshness assessment of European eel (*Anguilla anguilla*) by sensory, chemical and microbiological methods. *Food Chemistry*, 2005. **92**(4): 745–751.

69. Niu, J. and J. Lee, A new approach for the determination of fish freshness by electrochemical impedance spectroscopy. *Journal of Food Science*, 2000. **65**(5): 780–785.

70. Wang, P. et al., Ionic liquid-assisted synthesis of α-Fe_2O_3 mesoporous nanorod arrays and their excellent trimethylamine gas-sensing properties for monitoring fish freshness. *Journal of Materials Chemistry A*, 2017. **5**(37): 19846–19856.

71. Dehaut, A. et al., Development of an SPME-GC-MS method for the specific quantification of dimethylamine and trimethylamine: use of a new ratio for the freshness monitoring of cod fillets. *Journal of the Science of Food and Agriculture*, 2016. **96**(11): 3787–3794.

72. Hernández-Martínez, M. et al., Application of MIR-FTIR spectroscopy and chemometrics to the rapid prediction of fish fillet quality. *CyTA-Journal of Food*, 2014. **12**(4): 369–377.

8 Animal Origin Foods as Functional Foods

Faqir Muhammad Anjum, Fakiha Mehak, and Asna Zahid

CONTENTS

8.1 INTRODUCTION

Diet-based therapies are gaining attention in the domain of disease prevention and cure. Functional foods are now gaining a dominant position and popularity among the scientific community due to their biosafety aspects and cost-effectiveness regarding socio-economic changes in the community. Recently, there has been an increasing consumer interest in the health enhancing specific foods known as functional food, nutraceutical and designer food that contains physiologically active ingredients [1]. Clearly, functional foods are those that provide additional health benefits besides the basic nutrients and nutritional need of the body [2]. Although, there is no precise and ubiquitous definition of functional food. However, it can be defined as an ideal food that is considered to be: (a) an everyday food; (b) consumed as part of a conventional diet; (c) formed of natural components; (d) provide extra health benefit beyond its basic nutritive value; (e) reduce the risk of diseases; and (f) have sound, scientifically-based and verified claims [3–6]. The food industry is progressing by leaps and bounds, and now paying more attention to consumer demand for a healthy food supply, especially on a variety of functional foods. Therefore, tremendous amounts of functional foods are easily available for the consumer. Functional food should have pre-approved health claims by the Food and Drug Administration (FDA), according to scientific evidence and agreement among scientists of food and nutrition, and have a market label with reliable nutrition information for consumer [7].

Evidence has showed that physiologically active components of functional foods are classified into four categories: clinical trials; animal studies; experimental *in vitro* laboratory studies;

and epidemiological studies [1]. Current evidence lack clinical trials; whereas, other types of scientific investigations are substantial for functional food and their health promoting components. Functional food plays an important role in health promotion, reducing health care costs, and mitigating diseases [1]. According to the American Dietetic Association (ADA), functional food includes whole foods, fortified foods, enriched foods, and enhanced foods that have positive effects on health when consumed as a part of varied diet on regular basis. The ADA also claims that physiological active components in plant and animal food change the role of diet in human health. The potential of functional food has evolved from the treatment of nutrients deficiencies to the reduction and treatment of diseases [8]. With the advancement in research, the real worth of food is recognized in a better way. Thereby, food cannot evaluate only for its micronutrient and macronutrient contents, but analysis of physiological components is also essential to identify the real worth of food [8]. For instance, animal-sourced food contains several potential components that help in health promotion and diseases prevention. In this chapter, we focus on the value of animal food and their physiological health benefits to the human body. It is important to address the positive role of animal food to increase the consumption. Improving animal nutrition and food processing is crucial to optimizing public health; and to spread education among veterinarians, food scientists, nutritionists, and public awareness about the functionality of animal food.

8.2   ORIGIN OF THE CONCEPT OF "FUNCTIONAL FOOD"

The concept of functional food was first introduced in Japan in 1984. In Japan, functional food has been categorized as Food for Specific Health Uses (FOSHU). It is defined as food products fortified with special constituents that possess advantageous physiological effects [6]. Until now, a specific regulatory approval process for functional food had been only formulated in Japan [9]. In addition, the International Food Information Council (IFIC) defines "functional food as food that provides health benefits beyond basic nutrition" [10]. This definition is similar to the definition of the International Life Sciences Institute of North America (ILSI) that describes "functional food as food that by virtue of physiologically active components, provide health benefits beyond basic nutrition" [11]. In the US and Europe, the functional food category is still unrecognized and does not have a legislative definition. A consistent definition is still missing among countries and has led to the unregulated publishing of health claims in some countries and has limited production of functional food in other countries. Lacking a standard definition, scientists hesitate to promote functional food to the seriously ill populations. It is important to differentiate between functional foods and nutraceuticals, because these compounds have a positive potential in the prevention, management, and treatment of diseases. Besides, functional food scientists should promote a single, proper definition globally that will clarify and improve communication between food and nutrition scientists, policy makers, researchers, and the public. Therefore, it will help to improved public health and decrease the risk of diseases [12].

According to the wide definition, the simplest example of unmodified whole food are fish and beef because they are rich in omega-3 and conjugated linoleic acid, respectively. However, modified food also falls in the realm of functional food because physiologically they are enhanced with active components; for instance, plants with phytochemicals and animal with zoochemicals. Moreover, food biotechnology also provides a trend for functional food development [10].

8.3   FUNCTIONAL INGREDIENTS OF DAIRY PRODUCTS

Undoubtedly, dairy production acts as a functional food because it is the best source of calcium; an important nutrient that prevents osteoporosis and other calcium-related diseases. In addition to calcium, dairy products contain other beneficial components, known as probiotics, which are particularly present in fermented dairy products. Probiotics are live microbial feed supplements that have beneficial effects on the intestinal microbial balance of host [13]. According to an estimate, about 400 species of bacteria

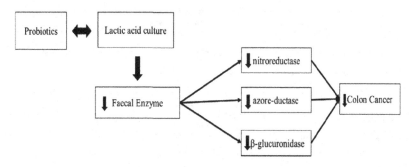

FIGURE 8.1 Mechanistic approach of probiotic to reduce colon cancer. (From Mitall, B.K., and Garg, S.K., *Crit Rev Microbiol.*, 21, 175–86 214; Talamini, R. et al., *Br. J. Cancer.*, 49, 723–729; Van't Veer, P. et al., *Cancer Res.*, 49, 4020–4023.)

are present and divided into two broad categories: beneficial bacteria, such as *Bifidobacterium* and *Lactobacillus*, and detrimental bacteria, such as *Enterobacteriaceae* and *Clostridium* spp. Among the beneficial bacteria that were used in fermentation, lactic acid bacteria have gained more attention [14]. Although, probiotics many attributed health benefits, such as anticarcinogenic, hypocholesterolemic, and antagonistic properties against other harmful pathogens [15], research has shown that probiotics has positive potential benefits against breast and colon cancer, intestinal tract function, immune function, allergy, stomach health, urogenital health, and reducing cholesterol level and blood pressure [16]. The mechanism proposed by probiotic in cancer reduction is shown in Figure 8.1.

Generally, fermented dairy products are the best sources of probiotics and calcium. However, probiotic cultures have been exploited by the dairy industry as a tool for the production of functional food and about 70 probiotic containing products are marketed worldwide; for instance, yogurt, mayonnaise spread, cheese, milk, sour milk, ice cream and so forth [16]. In addition to probiotics, fermented carbohydrates that feed gut microflora are known as prebiotics. It is undigestible food ingredients that stimulate the growth and activity of bacteria to improve colon and host health [19]. It includes starches, dietary fiber, sugar alcohol, oligosaccharides, and other non-absorbable sugar, and, among these, oligosaccharides gained attention because of their positive impact on health [20].

Furthermore, milk also contains specific protein fragments that have a positive impact on body functions and ultimately influences health [21]. Bioactive peptides affect major systems of the body including cardiovascular, digestive, endocrine, immune, and nervous systems. Distinct dietary peptide sequences have the potential to promote health and combat chronic diseases because it exhibits antimicrobial, antioxidative, antithrombotic, antihypertensive, immune-modulatory, and opioid activity [22]. Moreover, milk peptides are promising candidates for numerous health promoting functional foods and has an impact on bones, heart, and the digestive system, as well as improve mood, stress, and weight as shown in Figure 8.2. Recent evidences have proved that bioactive peptides reduce the risk of obesity and type 2 diabetes.

Bioactive peptides are generated during milk fermentation with a dairy starter culture. Peptides have shown different bioactivities in various dairy products, such as cheese and fermented milk. According to research, bioactive peptides exhibit angiotensin-converting enzyme (ACE)-inhibitory activity but it has a varying degree of proteolysis. For instance, ACE-inhibitory activity was low in products with a low degree of proteolysis, including yogurt, fresh cheese, and quark [24,28]. Whereas, ACE-inhibitory activities were detected in higher amounts in middle-aged Gouda cheese, as compared to the short- and long-term ripened cheese [27]. ACE inhibitors are agents that are used for the relaxation of blood vessels and reduce blood pressure. Thus, they help in preventing the production of an enzyme from angiotensin 2, which narrows vessels and raises blood pressure [23]. However, some milk bioactive peptides act as ACE- inhibitors and make milk a functional food [22]. Bioactive peptide in yogurt is unidentified, whereas dahi has active peptides; Ser-Lys-Val-Tyr-Pro and but both act as ACE inhibitors. Likewise, sour milk also contains antihypertensive property [22,28].

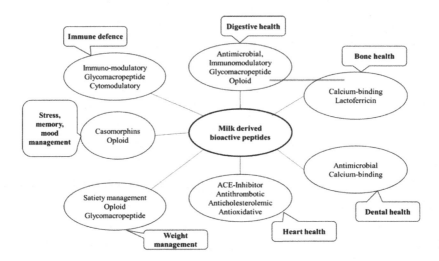

FIGURE 8.2 Functionality of milk protein-derived bioactive peptides and their health benefits. (From Haque E, Chand R *Eur Food Res Technol 227*:7–15; Erdmann K et al., *J Nutr Biochem 19*:643–654; Möller NP, et al., *Eur J Nutr 47*:171–182; Zimecki M, Kruzel ML, *J Exp Ther Oncol 6*:89–106.)

8.4 NOVEL FUNCTIONAL FOOD FROM MARINE SOURCES

Recently, seafood consumption has increased in many countries, and it has led to a better understanding of the health benefits of seafood. According to the Food and Agriculture Organization (FAO), fisheries reached a total of up to 148.5 million metric tons in 2010. Approximately 50%–60% of marine landing is directly used by humans and a large proportion of discard is used for other purposes, like animal feed production, fish meal, and fertilizers [29]. Thousands of new marine natural products possess potent bioactive ingredients that boost human health (Table 8.1). Omega-3 fatty acid, which is classified as eicosapentanoic acid (EPA) and docosahexaenoic acid (DHA) and α-linolenic acid, is one of the most important bioactive components of fish. To some extent, α-linolenic acid is converted to EPA and DHA in the human body. Otherwise, seafood is the best source of polyunsaturated fatty acid (PUFA). Basically, PUFA is formed in unicellular and multicellular marine plants, including phytoplankton and algae, and eventually incorporated into the lipids of marine species [30]. PUFA is present in a rich amount of fatty fish: mackerel, herring, salmon; the liver of white lean fish—cod and halibut; and the blubber of marine mammals—seals, whales, and krill [30].

Scientific studies have proven that omega-3 exhibits various health benefits by improving blood lipid profile, cardiovascular health, membrane lipid composition, eicosanoid biosynthesis, cell signaling, and gene expression. Moreover, it helps in the reduction of inflammation, improves the immune system, reduces the risk of gastrointestinal tumors, decreases allergy disease and blood pressure, prevents diabetes and depression, and is also good for the retinas [16]. Among all the aforementioned diseases and conditions, omega-3 is particularly important for cancer and cardiovascular diseases [10]. Besides health benefits, the FDA recommends DHA and EPA about 3g/day, which is generally recognized as safe (GRAS) [31].

In addition to omega-3 fatty acid, chitosan is present in aquatic animals. Chitin and chitosan polymers are the natural amino polysaccharides with unique structures and properties. Chitin can be deacetylated into various derivatives like chitosan, chitosan oligosaccharides, and glucosamine. Zhang et al. [32] demonstrated that chitosan with low-molecular weight reduces total cholesterol, low-density lipoprotein (LDL), and liver triacylglycerol in rats. Admittedly, chitosan derivatives are more advantageous as nutraceutical agents owing to water solubility. Chitosan oligosaccharides (COS), especially pentamers and hexamers, have antibacterial, antitumor, and immune-enhancing properties.

TABLE 8.1
Health Benefits of Marine Functional Food

Marine Source	Functional Components	Health Benefits
Fish (sardine, macherel, herring, fresh water fish, tuna, salmon, krill, cod) Marine mammals (seal, blubber and whale)	Omega-3 fatty acid (EPA, DPA, DHA)	Has positive effect against various diseases including cardiovascular diseases, high blood pressure, diabetes, inflammatory diseases like arthritis, autoimmune disorder, and cancer. Important for the growth and development of brain and retina of eye.
Oyster, crab, shrimps, crawfish, prawn, squid pen and krill	Chitin/ chitosan (LMW chitosan/ LMW chitin, Chitosan Oligosaccharide COS), Heterochitosan/Hetero-COS, sulphated hetero-COS, Glucosamine	Possess properties like antimicrobial, anti-inflammatory, antioxidant, anti-cancerous. Also good for renal disease, diabetes type 2, weight reduction, and reduce serum lipids level.
Shrimp, lobster, crab, crayfish, trout, salmon, redfish, red snapper, tuna, mussel, squid, octopus, sea cucumber, atlantic herring, pacific herring, pink salmon Fish, crustacean, mollusk	Carotenoids (α,β,ε-Carotene, lycopene and xanthophylls [cryptoxanthin, lutein, zeaxanthin, rhodovibrin, capsanthin, rhodoxanthin, violaxanthin, flavoxanthin, luteochrome, bixin and crocetin)	Act as anti-inflammatory, anti-oxidative, immune-modulatory, anti-cancerous agent. Help to prevent cardiovascular disease and neurodegenerative diseases.
	Protein (protein hydrolysates, bioactive peptides, enzymes)	Has properties of antioxidant, ACE inhibitory activity, anti-inflammatory, anti-coagulant, anti-tumor, immune-modulatory, antithrombotic and anti-hypertensive.

Source: Norris, R. et al., John Wiley & Sons Ltd., Chichester, UK; Zhang, J. et al., *Int J Biol Macromol.*, 51, 504–508; Matsumoto, M. et al., *Eur J Nutr.*, 49, 243–249; Grienke, U. et al., *Food Chem.*, 142, 48–60; Hoffman, D.R. et al., *Prostaglandins Leukot Essent Fatty Acids 81,* 151–158; Raafat, D., Sahl, H.G., *Microbial Biotechnol.*, 2, 186–201; Arihara, K. *Meat Sci.*, 74, 219–229.

Furthermore, low-molecular weight COS also possess antioxidative potential and scavenge free radicals [33]. Although, glucosamine as glycosaminoglycans is a component of connective and cartilage tissues, it is used to treat joint disease, named osteoarthritis. Recent evidence has been reported that it is not only a chondroprotective agent, but also act as anti-inflammatory agent [34].

Furthermore, carotenoids give a yellow, orange, and red color to the skin, shell, and exoskeleton of sea animals. Carotenoids (beta-carotene) act as vitamin A precursors. Marine carotenoids inhibit lipase activity in gastrointestinal lumen and suppress triacylglycerol absorption [35]. Moreover, Fucoxanthin is an example of a marine carotenoid that reduces blood glucose levels and improves insulin resistance. Fucoxanthin and its metabolites have a protective effect against cancer by inhibiting growth of human leukemia cells and human breast cancer and colon cancer cells [36].

8.5 ATTRACTIVE MEAT-BASED BIOACTIVE COMPONENTS

Meat is the fleshy part of animals and an excellent source of protein and other valuable nutrients (iron, vitamin B12, folic acid). Despite of that, meat is associated with a negative image that it can cause cancer and heart diseases because of the high amount of saturated fats [40]. But recent evidence shows that there is some natural substances in meat, such as conjugated linoleic acid, carnosine, anserine, L-carnitine, glutathione, taurine, and creatine, that make meat an attractive food full of health benefits [40]. Moreover, scientific evidence has proved that meat, itself, is not associated with the risk of cardiovascular diseases but the amount of saturated fats in the Western diet is not good for health. Likewise, Mann [41] has described that lean red meat is positively associated with lowering plasma cholesterol, and it is rich in iron, zinc, and vitamin B12. Therefore, we can say that lean meat is good for health because of its numerous bioactive components along with well balance dietary components. Trimming extra fat is necessary to enhance meat quality.

Additionally, in 1987, Ha et al. [43] identified the anticarcinogenic substance from grilled beef meat known as conjugated linoleic acid (CLA). CLA is a mixture of positional and geometric isomers of linolenic acid. There are nine different isomers of CLA in food; it is unique in its characteristics and ruminant animals (beef dairy and lambs) are the best source. In addition to anticarcinogenic properties, CLA possess antioxidative and immunomodulative properties, helps to reduce the risk of diabetes and control obesity [42]. Evidence shows that CLA has a protective effect against atherosclerosis [44]. However, 0.5% CLA supplement on mice showed 60% reduction in body fat and an increase in lean body mass by 14%, as compared to the control, thereby, reducing fat deposition and increasing lipolysis in adipocytes [45].

Meat contains attractive bioactive peptides, which provide additional health benefits beyond basic nutrition. Food protein is used for the synthesis of bioactive peptides either during gastrointestinal proteolysis or by the meat fermentation process. Similarly, various enzymes (pepsin, trypsin, chymotrypsin, elastase, and carboxypeptidase) attacked ingested protein [46]. Furthermore, peptide content in meat also increases during postmortem aging and proteolytic reaction during fermentation. Bioactive peptides of meat and meat products provide them a unique functionality and help to reduce the risk of various chronic disorders as described in Table 8.2.

TABLE 8.2
Functionality of Meat Bioactive Peptide

Bioactive Peptides	Sources	Production Process	Health Benefits
Oligopeptide [47]	Beef, pork, chicken	Aging, storage	ACE-inhibitory effect
• Asp-Leu-Tyr-Ala	Pork	Papain- treated hydrolyzate	Anti-oxidative, anti-fatigue
• Ser-Leu-Tyr-Ala			
• Val-Trp [40]			
• Leu-Lys-Ala	Chicken	Thermolysin treatment	ACE-inhibitory
• Leu-Lys-Pro			
• Leu-Ala-Pro			
• Phe-Gln-Lys-Pro-Lys-Arg			
• Ile-Val-Gly-Arg-Arg-Arg-His-Gln-Gly			
• Phe-Lys-Gly-Arg-Tyr-Tyr-Pro			
• Ile-Lys-Trp) [49]			
Opioid peptide (endorphins, enkephalin, and prodynorphin) [48]	Meats muscles, hemoglobin	Proteolytic treatment	Opiate like effect, positive effect on good for mental health and nerve system, influence gastrointestinal function
Carnosine and anserine (dipeptide) [40]	Skeletal muscle	Enzymatic digestion	Antioxidative

Source: Larsson, S.C. et al., *Am. J. Clin. Nutr.,* 1, 1–7, 2015; Sparks, N., *Worlds Poult. Sci. J.,* 62, 308–315, 2006; 110–113; Nishimura T, et al., *Agric Biol Chem* 52:2323–2330; Pihlanto-Leppälä A, *Trends Food Sci Technol* 11:347–356; Arihara K, et al., *Meat Sci* 57:319–324.

8.6 FUNCTIONAL PROPERTIES OF EGG

Traditionally, eggs were not considered as functional food, and, according to some schools of thought, it has adverse effect on serum cholesterol level. But later, it came under the category of a functional food because it contains various attractive components, including bioactive lipids, vitamins, minerals, and, most important, high biological protein. The consumption of eggs is important because it is rich in biological protein and, hence, one can have an extensive range of important nutrients and bioactive compounds. It is known to carry bioactive lipids (phospholipids), carotenoids (lutein and zeaxanthin), some fat-soluble vitamins, vitamin B complex, and minerals [50]. Egg contributes to 3%–4% of adults' energy requirements and contains 17% water, 11% fats, which are mostly present in the yolk [51]. Egg yolk is a reservoir of nutrients like vitamin A, D, E, K, iron, phosphorous, lipids, and oleic acid that is essential for growth and development of the body [52]. A minor amount of carbohydrates, like glucose, sucrose, maltose fructose, lactose, and galactose, are present. Further, 30%–38% of fatty acids are present in yolk lipid and comprises of stearic acids and palmitic acids. The rest of the one-third of the fatty acids are either polyunsaturated or monounsaturated [53]. Moreover, about 66% triacylglycerol, 28% phospholipids, and 6% cholesterol are the most common lipid contents in egg yolk [54]. Nimalaratne et al. [55] demonstrated the property of eggs and noted certain compounds in eggs exhibit anti-inflammatory, antimicrobial, antioxidant and immunomodulatory properties.

The positive effect of eggs is supposed to be associated with phospholipids: lipids containing phosphorus that are surface active, amphiphilic molecules, contain polar head, and lipophilic tail. It has functional characteristics in cell membranes and has metabolic role in bile, so helps in solubilization of cholesterol and fat food [56]. It also acts as lipoprotein for the transportation of fats between gut and liver. The body utilizes phospholipids as an emulsifier, which works with cholesterol and bile acid to form mixed mixelles in the gall bladder to increase the absorption of fat-soluble substances [57]. However, one large egg can contribute about 13 g phospholipids. Approximately, we consume 3–6 g of lecithin (Phosphatidylcholine) in a day through different food sources like eggs, soy, and meat [58]. Admittedly, egg yolk phospholipids help in the inhibition of cholesterol absorption. Additionally, egg yolk phospholipids, especially phosphatidylethanolamine and phosphatidylcholine, decrease serum cholesterol and apoprotein A-1 and increase serum apoprotein B and liver cholesterol [59] (Table 8.3).

Eggs can be modified by the addition of omega-3 fatty acids that aid in the prevention of cardiovascular diseases and inflammation [61]. The incorporation of flaxseed, fish oil, and marine microalgae into a hen's diet elevates omega-3 fatty acid in eggs [62]. Omega-3 enriched eggs have a positive effect on serum lipid profile. Therefore, it is considered to be good for

TABLE 8.3
Percentages of Egg Phospholipids

Types of Phospholipids	Percentages
Glycerophospholipi and phosphatitidylcholine	72%
Phosphatidylethanolamine	20%
Lysophosphatidylcholine	3%
Sphingolipidsphingomyelin (SM)	3%
Phosphatidylinositol (PI)	2%

Source: Blesso, CN., *Nutrition.*, 7, 2731–2747.

heart health [63]. Moreover, Oh et al. [64] showed that intake of four eggs decreased plasma triacylglycerol concentration and blood pressure, whereas cholesterol level in plasma was not changed.

8.7 OTHER FUNCTIONAL COMPONENTS OF ANIMAL SOURCED FOOD

Although the aforementioned components provide functionality to animal food but in addition to these compounds, some other biologically active substances like L-carnitine, coenzyme Q10, α-lipoic acid, taurine, and choline that play an important role in getting rid of various health ailments.

8.7.1 L-CARNITINE

L-carnitine present in our body is betaine derivative of β-hydroxybutyrate that most commonly found in our liver, as well as in muscle tissues, and accounts for 98% of the total body carnitine concentration [65]. The liver is the main site of synthesis, and, from there, carnitine is transported to skeletal muscles. Therefore, animal foods are a major source of carnitine and skeletal muscles are the main reservoir that contain 200 times more carnitine as compared to blood plasma [66]. It was also isolated from muscle tissue for the first time in 1905. Later in 1927, the structure of carnitine was established. Another name for carnitine is BT, and it is considered an important nutrient for a meal worm (*Tenebrio molitor*). However, it is not a true vitamin but only considered a vitamin-like compound due to its action similar to certain vitamins.

Biosynthesis of carnitine needs two main essential amino acids that make the backbone of the structure and some other micronutrients, such as vitamin B_6, vitamin C, niacin, as well as iron, which together constitute carnitine shown in Figure 8.3. This shows the importance of these micronutrients as if only one of these is missing, stopping carnitine synthesis, and thereby resulting in poor muscle function and fatigue. Hence, the need for foods that are good sources of carnitine should increase in order to prevent its deficiency [65]. Luckily, animal-sourced milk and meat is best for carnitine intake [73].

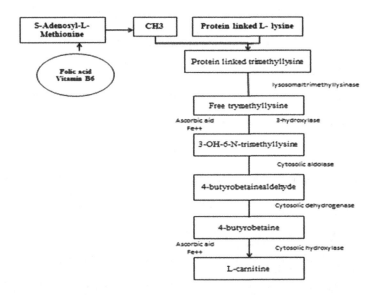

FIGURE 8.3 Biosynthesis of carnitine. (From Walter, P. et al., *Ann NutrMetab.*, 44, 75–96.)

Moreover, carnitine becomes conditionally essential in certain conditions when the body demands spurts of energy, like during pregnancy and breast feeding, and an essential requirement during infancy [10]. The human body contains about 20–25 g of L-carnitine and, apart from that, 100–300 mg of dietary carnitine can be taken per day [65]. L-carnitine abundance in animal tissues reflects its role in energy metabolism, especially carbohydrate and lipid metabolism. However, it ensures the transportation of long-chain fatty acids into the mitochondrial matrix (ß-oxidation site) across the inner mitochondrial membrane and impaired oxidation of fatty acids and myopathy [69]. The other important role of carnitine is its coupling with buffering acyl-CoA that confers its promising therapeutic use. Diet, body composition, and gender are those factors that affect the carnitine status in our body and vary correspondingly [66]. In addition, carnitine also performs as a putative antioxidant as it has shown significant free radical scavenging activity in many in vitro studies [67].

Animal products including meat, poultry, fish, and milk are the best sources of carnitine. Despite these, many brain food products also contain an active metabolite of carnitine; for example, acetyl-L-carnitine that boosts the nervous system and acts as precursor of acetylcholine. Therefore, it plays an important role in many mental illnesses, such as Alzheimer's disease, due to its cholinergic properties [70] and improves the memory as well as decreases depression in the elderly [71]. Carnitine, as a part of carnitine palmitoyltransferase-1enzyme, also helps in energy balance by regulating lipid oxidation as it affects food intake and endogenous glucose production [68].

Primary carnitine deficiency includes the reduction in tissue carnitine concentrations, while secondary carnitine deficiency impairs the lipid oxidation as a result of deficiency of acyl-CoA dehydrogenase. The former one is corrected upon restoration of carnitine level. This indicates the problem in synthesis of carnitine as a result of its renal conservation [69]. Similarly, low levels of carnitine were observed in children with autism [72]. Nevertheless, carnitine deficiency also accounts for its recessive genetic mutation of the sodium dependent carnitine transporter (*OCTN2* or *SLC22A5*) of the plasma membrane, as well as enzyme defect of genetic fatty acid oxidation causes abnormalities in plasma and tissue carnitine level. Apart from this, the use of chronic pivalate-conjugated antibiotics also causes carnitine depletion [73] Likewise, deficiency of carnitine in cancer patients is obvious because it contributes to fatigue. However, supplementation at doses up to 3000 mg/day of carnitine provides the positive results in a placebo-controlled study that effectively ameliorate the cancer-related fatigue [74].

8.7.2 Coenzyme Q10

Coenzyme Q10 is a lipophilic high-molecular weight compound consisting of 10 isoprenoid units attached to substituted benzoquinone moiety. It is also known as ubiquinone due to its ubiquitous occurrence in nature as they are present in every cell of human body. In 1957, coenzyme Q10 was first isolated during mitochondria electron transport system investigation from mitochondria of beef heart [75]. It plays an important role in the generation of cellular energy, as well as is helpful in free radical scavenging activity. At the age of 20 years, the concentration of CoQ10 reaches its highest value and then with the passage of time starts declining progressively, and a reduced ability to synthesize coenzyme Q10 from food after the age of 35–40 results in its deficiency [77]. Aging, stress, poor eating habits, and infection affects one's ability to provide adequate amounts of coenzyme Q10 [10]. Common sources of coenzyme Q10 include the most active organs, such as the kidney, heart, and liver (Table 8.4). The distribution of coenzyme Q10 in human cells suggests that cytosol contains only 10% of the total CoQ10, while mitochondria accounts for up to 50% making it more prone towards free radicals and increasing the chances of accessibility especially during the phosphorylation process [76].

Coenzyme Q10 synthesis takes place in a series of eight steps through various precursors, which also require different vitamins (B2, B3, B5, B6, B12, and folic acid) and minerals in this pathway of CoQ10 biosynthesis, and all these steps take place intracellularly [77]. Tyrosine is an amino acid that goes through various pathways to form CoQ10 as shown in Figure 8.4. During the biosynthesis of CoQ10, its precursor Mevalonate forms that further forms cholesterol,

TABLE 8.4

Food Sources of CoQ10 [77]

Food Sources	Amount of CoQ10 (mg/kg)
Reindeer	157.9
Beef heart	113.3
Chicken heart	92.3–192
Chicken liver	116.2–132.2

Source: Santos, GCD., *Braz J Pharm Sci.,* 45, 607–618.

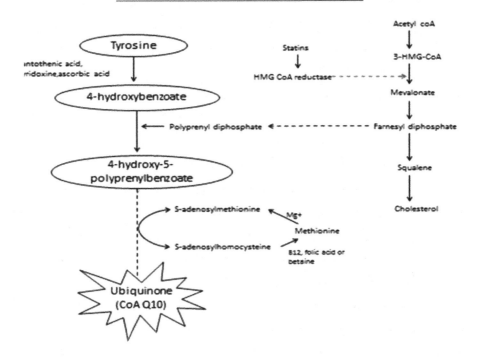

FIGURE 8.4   Synthesis of CoQ10. (From Yang, Y.K. et al. Clin. Chim. Acta., 450, 83–89.)

and, thus, the cholesterol-lowering drugs, such as statins, affect its synthesis and inhibit its reaction. This aggravates the need of CoQ10 supplementation in those drug users to carry out its normal functioning [79].

The three most approved health claims of CoQ_{10} have been studied in various clinical investigations and findings of this extensive scientific work are in agreement of the proposals that say it plays an important role in energy metabolism, improving heart health, and possesses significant antioxidant properties, as well as helps in slowing down the neurodegenerative diseases. This wide range of health benefits suggests its fortification in foods and dairy products are the most appropriate products for this purpose without leaving any deteriorating effect on taste and its stability [75].

As coenzyme Q_{10} presents in all living cells as an essential natural component, it acts as a cofactor in ATP production as well as performs vital antioxidant properties. Various health promoting effects make it a potential ingredient as a supplement to ameliorate different health ailments. Data from various animal and human studies suggest that CoQ_{10} has low toxic effects and has not shown any serious health hazard. The acceptable daily intake is 12mg/kg/day, calculated from the no-observed-adverse-effect level of 1200 mg/kg/day resulting from a 52-week chronic toxicity study in rats; that is, 720 mg/day for a person weighing 60 kg [83].

As coenzyme Q_{10} addresses a wide range of disorders, it requires new insights in its biochemical mechanisms to make it more imperative in therapeutic approach for a patient's treatment, particularly in end-stage heart failure, myocardial protection, pediatric cardiomyopathy, as well as in cardiopulmonary resuscitation. Besides, it also helps in recovering from mitochondrial encephalomyopathies by coupling with vitamin B2. It provides neuroprotection function and repairs oxidative damage in Parkinson's disease as well as protects from ischemia and lesions produced by mitochondrial toxins. Impaired mitochondrial diseases, like Friedreich's ataxia and age-related macular degeneration, have also shown improved results by using CoQ_{10} (400 mg/day) with vitamin E and combination of acetyl-L-carnitine, n-3 fatty acids with coenzyme Q_{10}, respectively, as a result of improved bioenergetics of the photoreceptor complex [84] Cardiovascular diseases are a major cause of mortality worldwide, and CoQ_{10} is present in a high quantity in myocardial tissues. That is why low levels of CoQ10 have been reported in cardiac patients in different research studies as myocardial levels of CoQ10 tends to decline with increasing severity of heart failure [85]. Consequently, utilization of CoQ10 by patients with endothelial dysfunction, heart failure, and hypertension [82] has been considered as an effective therapy, as well as safe and well tolerable [78,79]. Its long-term use may prevent adverse cardiovascular events in patients with chronic heart failure [80]. CoQ_{10} has also been found as anti-aging, and its supplementation showed significant results in a double-blind, placebo-controlled experiment as reducing some visible signs of aging [81].

8.7.3 α-Lipoic Acid

Lipoic acid is covalently bound to the amino group of lysine residues and functions as a cofactor for mitochondrial enzymes by catalyzing the oxidative decarboxylation of pyruvate, α-ketoglutarate and branched-chain α-keto acids [86]. Food sources of lipoic acid are heart, liver, kidney, and red meat and first time isolated from bovine liver. A fat or water-soluble sulfur containing coenzyme, α-Lipoic acid is considered to have an important part in mitochondrial dehydrogenase reactions and is involved in energy metabolism of carbohydrates, proteins, and fats. It performs various physiological functions, such as blood glucose disposal as well as scavenging free-radical activity [10].

Lipoate or lipoic acid being a potential antioxidant assists in various conditions involving oxidative stress, such as diabetes polyneuropathies, neurodegeneration, vascular disease, ischemia-reperfusion injury, HIV, inflammation, radiation injury, hypertension, and cataract formation, as well as restores intracellular glutathione levels [87] as shown in Figure 8.5. These wide ranges of health benefits make animal foods functional foods due to the presence of these essential health promoting ingredients. Furthermore, lipoic acid is also known as the antioxidant of antioxidants as it has the ability to

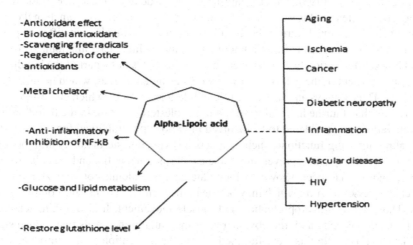

FIGURE 8.5 Functions and uses of lipoic acid. (From Gorąca, A. et al., Pharmacol. Rep., 63, 849–858, 2011.)

regenerate other antioxidants. Likewise, it plays an influential role in attenuating the cytotoxic cytokines, release of free radicals, and second messenger nuclear factor kB (NF-kB) [87].

8.7.4 CHOLINE

Choline is a well-known essential nutrient for human beings. It is an important constituent of a number of compounds including lecithin, sphingomyelin, membrane phospholipids, and plasmalogen. It helps in maintaining the cell integrity [10] and is involved in transmembrane signaling, methyl metabolism, cholesterol transport, cholinergic neurotransmission, and lipid metabolism. Thus, its deficiency can lead to many associated complications, including liver injury, fatty liver, as well as muscle damage [88]. Choline is found in a variety of food products, and the USDA has given the choline content in its updated food database including more than 630 foods. Dietary choline is most abundantly found in eggs, liver, and wheat germ. Choline exists in both free and esterified forms, like phosphatidylcholine, glycerophosphocholine, phosphocholine, and sphingomyelin. Moreover, human milk is a rich source of choline in contrast to bovine milk derived formulas or soy infant formulas [88].

Nonetheless, it can be synthesized by *de novo*, but human requirement is more than this synthesis. Consumption of animal foods provides dietary choline that is mediated by choline transporters after its absorption in the intestine. After its absorption in the small intestine, choline is metabolized immediately, phosphorylated to phosphocholine, and oxidized to betaine in hepatocytes. Betaine helps in the donation of methyl groups to homocysteine to form methionine an essential amino acid and then finally converts into lecithin in all nucleated cells [91]. Betaine acts as a methyl-group donor as homocysteine is converted to methionine by acquiring a methyl group and folate can donate a methyl group to homocysteine. On the other hand, choline is transformed to betaine, which in turn can donate a methyl group to homocysteine.

Choline has been known to help in the development of brain and, subsequently, memory and cognitive functions of the fetus and, thus, decrease the risk of neural tube defects. Its importance in diet increases during pregnancy and old age. Furthermore, consumption of animal-origin food contributes to high choline in diet that improves various complications, including breast cancer, inflammation, heart disease, memory development, and neural tube defects [89,90].

8.7.5 TAURINE

Taurine is a free amino acid, and mammals have an ability to synthesize it endogenously. However, humans require taurine from dietary sources as well. Rich food sources for taurine comprise of shellfish, fish, and seaweed [93]. Though, taurine is not a true amino acid due to the lack of a carboxyl group, but it instead holds a sulfonated acid group. Taurine acts as a functional component in our body as it helps to diminish various health disorders. It is also involved in different physiological functions, like neurotransmission, immunomodulation, intracellular calcium homeostasis, osmoregulation, and bile salt formation [93]. However, this amino acid is not a part of the building blocks of proteins, but it is present in the gall bladder and works as an emulsifier, which helps in binding and uptake of lipids. Thus, it plays an imperative role in bile formation by which cholesterols are bound. This is the reason that Taurine helps in lowering the cholesterol content in the blood of humans.

Moreover, Taurine is considered to be involved in various physiological functions as it performs different health-enhancing functions, such as it acts as hypocholesterolemic, antihypertensive, and antioxidant; thus, subsequently, preventing diabetes, chronic hepatitis, and vascular diseases [93]. Furthermore, Taurine has been shown to modulate several calcium-ion and zinc-ion dependent physiological processes in vitro, which may be due to the formation of taurine complexes with these metal ions. Thus, helps in neuroprotection and muscle movement. It also minimizes the effect of toxic metal ions in our body and, thereby, increases the glutathione levels that reduce significantly because of lead exposure. In this way, Taurine helps in the prevention from neurodegeneration as a result of heavy metal complex formation [94].

8.8 SAFETY ISSUES

In the modern era, the focus on health is increasing as consumer awareness about healthy diet is more in contrast to previous years. Animal foods as functional foods have various health benefits, indeed, yet the safety issue is the most serious concern. Although, the recommended dietary allowances of the majority of the biologically active components have not been decided yet, there is a dire need for new clinical trials to establish the correct daily intake dosage levels. As these biologically active components are a part of foods and make them a functional food, the can also make these foods hazardous if there are definite amounts of safe intake. That is why FDA approved health claims are required for functional foods from animal sources. However, some of the scientific evidence has been available for different functional foods from animal source.

8.9 CONCLUSION

The forecast of animal product consumption was mainly linked with high income levels, but now the trend of animal food consumption is increasing due to its functionality. Increasing evidence supports the argument that the physiological component present in animal food can boost human health and reduce the risk of diseases. These biologically active components include calcium, probiotics, whey proteins, bioactive peptides, n-3 fatty acids, conjugated linoleic acid, sphingolipids, and the conditionally-essential nutrients of L-carnitine, coenzyme Q 10, α-lipoic acid, choline, and Taurine, all widely found in animal products. These components enhance the functionality of animal foods and provide protection against various health disorders. Still, there are some factors that hinder the development and marketing of novel functional food of animal sources because in some regions animal food is considered to be bad due to high saturated contents. But recent research has support the positive relationship between animal food and health. Undoubtedly, the intake of animal food can be enhanced by increasing its availability and targeting functional ingredients to reduce the risk of diseases in ill populations.

REFERENCES

1. Hasler CM (1998) Functional foods: Their role in disease prevention and health promotion. *Food Technol* 52:57–62.
2. Hasler CM (1998) A new look at an ancient concept. *Chem Industry* 2:84–89.
3. Bellisle F, Diplock AT, Hornstra G, Kolezko B, Roberfroid MB, Salminen S, Saris WHM (1998) Functional food science in Europe. *Br J Nutr 80*:1–193.
4. Diplock AT, Aggett PJ, Ashwell M, Bornet F, Fern EB, Roberfroid MB (1999) Scientific concepts of functional foods in Europe: Consensus document. *Br J Nutr 81*:1–27.
5. Roberfroid M (2000) Concepts and strategy of functional food science: The European perspective. *Am J Clin Nutr 71*:1660–1664.
6. Hardy G (2000) Nutraceuticals and functional foods: Introduction and meaning. *Nutrition 16*:688–697.
7. Brody AL, Connor JM, Lord JB (2000) *The United States' Food Industry and its Imperative for New Products. Developing New Food Products for a Changing Marketplace.* CRC Press, Boca Raton, FL.
8. Thomson C, Bloch AS, Hasler CM, Kubena K, Earl R, Heins J (1999) Position of the American Dietetic Association: Functional foods. *J Am Diet Assoc 99*:1278–1285.
9. Arai S (1996) Studies on functional foods in Japan—state of the art. *Biosci Biotechnol Biochem 60*:9–15.
10. Prates JM, Mateus CMRP (2002) Functional foods from animal sources and their physiologically active components. *Rev Méd Vét 153*:155–160.
11. Clydesdale FM (1999) ILSI North America food component reports. *Crit Rev Food Sci Nutr 39*:203–316.
12. Martirosyan DM, Singh J (2015) A new definition of functional food by FFC: What makes a new definition unique? *Funct Foods Health Dis 5*:209–223.
13. Fuller R (1994) History and development of probiotics. In: R. Fuller (Ed.), *Probiotics*. Chapman & Hall, New York.
14. Sanders ME (1994) Lactic acid bacteria as promoters of human health. In: I. Goldberg (Ed.), *Functional Foods*. Springer, Boston, MA.

15. Mitall BK, Garg SK (1995) Anticarcinogenic, hypocholesterolemic, and antagonistic activities of Lactobacillus acidophilus. *Crit Rev Microbiol 21*:175–214.

16. Vass N, Czegledi L, Javor A (2008) Significance of functional foods of animal origin in human health. *Scientific Papers Anim Sci Biotechnol 41*:263–270.

17. Talamini R, La Vecchia C, Decarli A, Franceschi S, Grattoni E, Grigoletto E, Tognoni G (1984) Social factors, diet and breast cancer in a northern Italian population. *Br J Cancer 49*:723–729.

18. Van't Veer P, Dekker JM, Lamers JW, Kok FJ, Schouten EG, Brants HA, Hermus RJ (1989) Consumption of fermented milk products and breast cancer: A case-control study in the Netherlands. *Cancer Res 49*:4020–4023.

19. Gibson GR, Roberfroid MB (1995) Dietary modulation of the human colonic microbiota: Introducing the concept of prebiotics. *J Nutr 125*:1401–1412.

20. Wilson B, Whelan K (2017) Prebiotic inulin-type fructans and galacto-oligosaccharides: Definition, specificity, function, and application in gastrointestinal disorders. *J Gastroenterol Hepatol 32*:64–68.

21. Kitts DD, Weiler K (2003) Bioactive proteins and peptides from food sources. Applications of bioprocesses used in isolation and recovery. *Curr Pharm Des 9*:1309–1323.

22. Korhonen H (2009) Milk-derived bioactive peptides: From science to applications. *J Funct Foods 1*:177–187.

23. Okuda T, Okamura K, Shirai K, Urata H (2018) Effect of angiotensin-converting enzyme inhibitor/calcium antagonist combination therapy on renal function in hypertensive patients with chronic kidney disease: Chikushi anti-hypertension trial-benidipine and perindopril. *J Clin Med Res 10*:117–124.

24. Haque E, Chand R (2008) Antihypertensive and antimicrobial bioactive peptides from milk proteins. *Eur Food Res Technol 227*:7–15.

25. Erdmann K, Cheung BW, Schröder H (2008) The possible roles of food-derived bioactive peptides in reducing the risk of cardiovascular disease. *J Nutr Biochem 19*:643–654.

26. Möller NP, Scholz-Ahrens KE, Roos N, Schrezenmeir J (2008) Bioactive peptides and proteins from foods: Indication for health effects. *Eur J Nutr 47*:171–182.

27. Zimecki M, Kruzel ML (2007) Milk-derived proteins and peptides of potential therapeutic and nutritive value. *J Exp Ther Oncol 6*:89–106.

28. Chobert JM, El-Zahar K, Sitohy M, Dalgalarrondo M, Métro F, Choiset Y, Haertlé T (2005) Angiotensin I-converting-enzyme (ACE)-inhibitory activity of tryptic peptides of ovine beta $-lactoglobulin and of milk yoghurts obtained by using different starters. *Le Lait 85*:141–152.

29. Norris R, Harnedy PA, FitzGerald RJ (2014) Antihypertensive peptides from marine sources. In: B. Hernandez-Ledesma and M. Herrero (Eds.), *Bioactive Compounds From Marine Foods: Plant and Animal Sources*. John Wiley & Sons Ltd., Chichester, UK.

30. Shahidi F, Ambigaipalan P (2015) Novel functional food ingredients from marine sources. *Curr Opin Food Sci 2*:123–129.

31. Pietrowski BN, Tahergorabi R, Jaczynski J (2012) Dynamic rheology and thermal transitions of surimi seafood enhanced with ω-3-rich oils. *Food Hydrocoll 27*:384–389.

32. Zhang J, Zhang W, Mamadouba B, Xia W (2012) A comparative study on hypolipidemic activities of high and low molecular weight chitosan in rats. *Int J Biol Macromol 51*:504–508.

33. Ngo DN, Kim MM, Qian ZJ, Jung WK, Lee SH, Kim SK (2010) Free radical-scavenging activities of low molecular weight chitin oligosaccharides lead to antioxidant effect in live cells. *J Food Biochem 34*:161–177.

34. Nagaoka I., Igarashi M, Hua J, Ju Y, Yomogida S, Sakamoto K (2011) Recent aspects of the anti-inflammatory actions of glucosamine. *Carbohydr Polym 84*:825–830.

35. Matsumoto M, Hosokawa M, Matsukawa N, Hagio M, Shinoki A, Nishimukai M, Hara H (2010) Suppressive effects of the marine carotenoids, fucoxanthin and fucoxanthinol on triglyceride absorption in lymph duct-cannulated rats. *Eur J Nutr 49*:243–249.

36. Miyashita K, Nishikawa S, Beppu F, Tsukui T, Abe M, Hosokawa M (2011) The allenic carotenoid fucoxanthin, a novel marine nutraceutical from brown seaweeds. *J Sci Food Agric 91*:1166–1174.

37. Grienke U, Silke J, Tasdemir D (2014) Bioactive compounds from marine mussels and their effects on human health. *Food Chem 142*:48–60.

38. Hoffman DR, Boettcher JA, Diersen-Schade DA (2009) Toward optimizing vision and cognition in term infants by dietary docosahexaenoic and arachidonic acid supplementation: A review of randomized controlled trials. *Prostaglandins Leukot Essent Fatty Acids 81*:151–158.

39. Raafat D, Sahl HG (2009) Chitosan and its antimicrobial potential–a critical literature survey. *Microbial Biotechnol 2*:186–201.

40. Arihara K (2006) Strategies for designing novel functional meat products. *Meat Sci 74*:219–229.

41. Mann N (2000) Dietary lean red meat and human evolution. *Eur J Nutr 39*:71–79.
42. Azain MJ (2003) Conjugated linoleic acid and its effects on animal products and health in single-stomached animals. *Proc Nutr Soc 62*:319–328.
43. Ha, YL, Grimm NK, Pariza MW (1987) Anticarcinogens from fried ground beef: Heat-altered derivatives of linoleic acid. *Carcinogenesis 8*:1881–1887.
44. Cannella C, Giusti AM (2000) Conjugated linoleic acid a natural anticarcinogenic substance from animal food. *Ital J Food Sci 12*:123–127.
45. Park Y, Albright KJ, Liu W, Storkson JM, Cook ME, Pariza MW (1997) Effect of conjugated linoleic acid on body composition in mice. *Lipids 32*:853–858.
46. Pihlanto A, Korhonen H (2003) Bioactive peptides and proteins. *Adv Food Nutr Res 47*:175–276.
47. Nishimura T, Ra Rhue M, Okitani A, Kato H (1988) Components contributing to the improvement of meat taste during storage. *Agric Biol Chem 52*:2323–2330.
48. Pihlanto-Leppäla A (2000) Bioactive peptides derived from bovine whey proteins: Opioid and ace-inhibitory peptides. *Trends Food Sci Technol 11*:347–356.
49. Arihara K, Nakashima Y, Mukai T, Ishikawa S, Itoh M (2001) Peptide inhibitors for angiotensin I-converting enzyme from enzymatic hydrolysates of porcine skeletal muscle proteins. *Meat Sci 57*:319–324.
50. Larsson SC, Akesson A, Wolk A (2015) Egg consumption and risk of heart failure, myocardial infarction, and stroke: Results from 2 prospective cohorts. *Am J Clin Nutr 1*:1–7.
51. Sparks N (2006) The hen's egg–is its role in human nutrition changing? *Worlds Poultry Sci J 62*:308–315.
52. Stadelman WJ, Debbie N, Lynne N (1995) *Egg Science and Technology*, 4th ed. CRC Press, Boca Raton, FL.
53. Anton M (2007) Composition and structure of hen egg yolk. In: R. Huopalahti, M. Anton, R. Lopez-Fandino, and R. Schade (Eds.), *Bioactive Egg Compounds*. Springer, Berlin, Germany.
54. Campos AM, Ricardo F, Alves E, Reis A, Couto D, Domingues P, Domingues MRM (2016) Lipidomic investigation of eggs' yolk: Changes in lipid profile of eggs from different conditions. *Food Res Inter 89*:177–185.
55. Nimalaratne C, Bandara N, Wu J (2015) Purification and characterization of antioxidant peptides from enzymatically hydrolyzed chicken egg white. *Food Chem 188*:467–472.
56. Vertzoni M, Markopoulos C, Symillides M, Goumas M, Imanidis G, Reppas C (2012) Luminal lipid phases after administration of a triglyceride solution of danazol in the fed state and their contribution to the flux of danazol across Caco-2 cell monolayers. *Mol Pharm 9*:1189–1198.
57. Li J, Wang X, Zhang T, Wang C, Huang Z, Luo X, Deng Y (2015) A review on phospholipids and their main applications in drug delivery systems. *Asian J Pharmacol Sci 10*:81–98.
58. Sahelian R (2016) Phospholipid supplements and their health benefits. Accessed March 17, 2018. Available at: http://www.raysahelian.com/phospholipids.html.
59. Murata M, Imaizumi K, Sugano M (1982) Effect of dietary phospholipids and their constituent bases on serum lipids and apolipoproteins in rats. *J Nutr 112*:1805–1808.
60. Blesso CN (2015) Egg phospholipids and cardiovascular health. *Nutrition 7*:2731–2747.
61. Holub DJ, Holub BJ (2004) Omega-3 fatty acids from fish oils and cardiovascular disease. *Mol Cell Biochem 263*:217–225.
62. Surai P, Sparks N (2001) Designer eggs: From improvement of egg composition to functional food. *Trends Food Sci Technol 12*:7–16.
63. Lewis NM, Seburg S, Flanagan N (2000) Enriched eggs as a source of n-3 polyunsaturated fatty acids for humans. *Poultry Sci 79*:971–974.
64. Oh SY, Ryue J, Hsieh CH, Bell DE (1991) Eggs enriched in omega-3 fatty acids and alterations in lipid concentrations in plasma and lipoproteins and in blood pressure. *Am J Clin Nutr 54*:689–695.
65. Walter P, Schaffhauser AO (2000) L-Carnitine, a "vitamin-like substance" for functional food. Proceedings of the Symposium on L-carnitine, April 28 to May 1, 2000 Zermatt, Switzerland. *Ann Nutr Metab 44*:75–96.
66. Steiber A, Kerner J, Hoppel CL (2004) Carnitine: A nutritional, biosynthetic, and functional perspective. *Mol Aspects Med 25*:455–473.
67. Gülcin İ (2006) Antioxidant and antiradical activities of L-carnitine. *Life Sci 78*:803–811.
68. Obici S, Feng Z, Arduini A, Conti R, Rossetti L (2003) Inhibition of hypothalamic carnitine palmitoyltransferase-1 decreases food intake and glucose production. *Nat Med 9*:756.
69. Treem WR, Stanley CA, Finegold DN, Hale DE, Coates PM (1988) Primary carnitine deficiency due to a failure of carnitine transport in kidney, muscle and fibroblasts. *N Engl J Med 319*:1331–1336.
70. White HL, Scates PW (1990) Acetyl-L-carnitine as a precursor of acetylcholine. *Neurochem Res 15*:597–601.

71. Salvioli G, Neri M (1994) L-acetylcarnitine treatment of mental decline in the elderly. *Drugs Exp Clin Res 20*:169–176.

72. Filipek PA, Juranek J, Nguyen, MT, Cummings C, Gargus JJ (2004) Relative carnitine deficiency in autism. *J Autism Dev Disord 34*:615–623.

73. Stanley CA (2004) Carnitine deficiency disorders in children. *Ann N Y Acad Sci 1033*:42–51.

74. Cruciani RA., Dvorkin E, Homel P, Malamud S, Culliney B, Lapin J, Portenoy RK, Esteban-Cruciani, N (2006) Safety, tolerability and symptom outcomes associated with L-carnitine supplementation in patients with cancer, fatigue, and carnitine deficiency: A phase I/II study. *J Pain Sympt Manage 32*:551–559.

75. Pravst I, Zmitek K, Zmitek J (2010) Coenzyme Q10 contents in foods and fortification strategies. *Crit Rev Food Sci Nutr 50*:269–280.

76. Kalén A, Appelkvist, EL, Dallner G (1989) Age-related changes in the lipid compositions of rat and human tissues. *Lipids 24*:579–584.

77. Santos GCD, Antunes LMG, Santos ACD, Bianchi MDLP (2009) Coenzyme Q10 and its effects in the treatment of neurodegenerative diseases. *Braz J Pharm Sci 45*:607–618.

78. Yang YK, Wang LP, Chen L, Yao XP, Yang KQ, Gao LG, Zhou XL (2015) Coenzyme Q10 treatment of cardiovascular disorders of ageing including heart failure, hypertension and endothelial dysfunction. *Clin Chim Acta 450*:83–89.

79. DiNicolantonio JJ, Bhutani J, McCarty MF, O'Keefe JH (2015) Coenzyme Q10 for the treatment of heart failure: A review of the literature. *Open Heart 2*:326.

80. Mortensen SA, Rosenfeldt F, Kumar A, Dolliner P, Filipiak KJ, Pella D, Alehagen U, Steurer G, Littarru GP (2014) The effect of coenzyme Q10 on morbidity and mortality in chronic heart failure: results from Q-SYMBIO: A randomized double-blind trial. *JACC: Heart Fail 2*:641–649.

81. Zmitek K, Pogacnik T, Mervic L, Zmitek J, Pravst I (2017) The effect of dietary intake of coenzyme Q10 on skin parameters and condition: Results of a randomised, placebo-controlled, double-blind study. *BioFactors 43*:132–140.

82. Langsjoen P, Willis R, Folkers K (1994) Treatment of essential hypertension with coenzyme Q10. *Mol Aspects Med 15*:265–272.

83. Hidaka T, Fujii K, Funahashi I, Fukutomi N, Hosoe K (2008) Safety assessment of coenzyme Q10 (CoQ10). *Biofactors 32*:199–208.

84. Littarru GP, Tiano L (2010) Clinical aspects of coenzyme Q10: An update. *Nutrition 26*:250–254.

85. Singh U, Devaraj S, Jialal I (2007) Coenzyme Q10 supplementation and heart failure. *Nutr Rev 65*:286–293.

86. Gorąca A, Huk-Kolega H, Piechota A, Kleniewska P, Ciejka E, Skibska B (2011) Lipoic acid–biological activity and therapeutic potential. *Pharmacol Rep 63*:849–858.

87. Shay KP, Moreau RF, Smith EJ, Smith AR, Hagen TM (2009) Alpha-lipoic acid as a dietary supplement: Molecular mechanisms and therapeutic potential. *Biochim Biophys Acta Lipids Lipid Metab 1790*:1149–1160.

88. Vennemann FB, Ioannidou S, Valsta LM, Dumas C, Ocke MC, Mensink GB, Lindtner O et al. (2015) Dietary intake and food sources of choline in European populations. *Br J Nutr 114*:2046–2055.

89. Cho E, Zeisel SH, Jacques P, Selhub J, Dougherty L, Colditz GA, Willett WC (2006) Dietary choline and betaine assessed by food-frequency questionnaire in relation to plasma total homocysteine concentration in the Framingham offspring study. *Am J Clin Nutr 83*:905–911.

90. Zeisel SH, da Costa KA (2009) Choline: An essential nutrient for public health. *Nutr Rev 67*:615–23.

91. Li Z, Vance DE (2008) Phosphatidylcholine and choline homeostasis. *J Lipid Res 49*:1187–1194.

92. Holdt SL, Kraan S (2011) Bioactive compounds in seaweed: Functional food applications and legislation. *J Appl Phycol 23*:543–597.

93. Bouckenooghe T, Remacle C, Reusens B (2006) Is taurine a functional nutrient? *Curr Opin Clin NutrMetab Care 9*:728–733.

94. Della Corte L, Crichton RR, Duburs G, Nolan K, Tipton KF, Tirzitis G, Ward RJ (2002) The use of taurine analogues to investigate taurine functions and their potential therapeutic applications. *Amino Acids 23*:367–379.

9 Bioactive Compounds from Animal Origin Foods

Muhammad Rizwan Tariq

CONTENTS

9.1 INTRODUCTION

A compound that effects a living organism, tissue, or cell is known as a bioactive compound. Bioactive compounds are distinguished from essential nutrients in the field of nutrition. Nutrients are vital for the body's sustainability, while, bioactive compounds are not essential, because nutrients fulfill the same function and the body can function properly in their absence. Bioactive compounds have a great impact on health. Both plant and animal products contain bioactive compounds and they can be produced synthetically. Fatty acids present in milk and fish are examples of bioactive compounds in animal products. Other examples of bioactive compounds are caffeine, carotenoids, flavonoids, carnitine, choline, creatine, coenzyme Q, dithiolthiones, polysaccharides, phytosterols, phytoestrogens, glucosinolates, polyphenols, prebiotics, taurine, and anthocyanins.

9.2 BIOACTIVE COMPOUNDS OF MEAT

Plants, such as fruits and vegetables, contain a variety of biologically active phytochemicals. In addition to plants, meat and cured meats also contain various bioactive compounds with various physiological properties like conjugated linoleic acid (CLA), coenzyme Q10, carnosine, taurine, creatine, melatonin, glutathione, lipoic acid, glucosamine, L-carnitine, chondroitin, and choline.

9.2.1 Conjugated Linoleic Acid (CLA)

Meat also contains trans-fatty acids, which are secreted by the rumen bacteria as a result of bio-hydrogenation reactions. Among them, the most common is CLA, which is a trans-fatty acid and it is associated with several health benefits and used for prevention of diabetes, cardiovascular diseases, and obesity. Around 40 years ago, a substance was discovered in the extracts of roast meat that was able to inhibit the activity of mutagenic substances. Subsequently, it was shown that this substance was, in fact, CLA, which has repeatedly shown strong anti-carcinogenic properties in experimental studies. Meat and milk of ruminants contain CLAs [1–3]. Fats of ruminant animals contain large amount of CLA, and rumen bacteria by their isomerase action convert linoleic acid to CLA. In ruminant, it is conveyed to the muscles and mammary tissue after its absorption. Grilled beef extracts comprise various types of octadecadienoic acid isomers. Concentration of CLA in beef fat is 3–8 mg/g of fat. Factors that affect the CLA content in meat are feed composition, age, and breed [4]. Grass-fed animal products have 3–5 times more CLA content than the hay and silage-fed animals. Remarkably, heating (cooking and processing) also increases the CLA content of foods. Additionally, in fermented milk and meat products, lactic acid bacteria promote CLA formation [5,6]. In beef, the most common and abundant CLA isomer is octadecac9, t11-dienoic acid. This fatty acid has gained importance due to its anticarcinogenic activity. It was proved by recent epidemiological studies that high-fat dairy food products and larger intake of CLA reduces colorectal cancer risks [7]. Besides this, it also possesses antioxidative, immunomodulative, and antiartheriosclerotic properties [8]. It also plays an important role controling obesity, diabetes, and modulation of bone metabolism. Obesity is one of the major causes for the development of type 2 diabetes. Due to its anti-diabetic activity, CLA induces remarkable modifications in the metabolic parameters of a type 2 diabetic subject. In an experimental group of rats, short-term CLA feeding was provided to them, and, as a result, they showed decreased fasting glucose, free fatty acid (FFA) levels, triglyceridemia, insulinemia, and leptinemia as compared to control [9]. In other findings, dietary administration of CLA into rat muscles was accomplished by enhanced glucose uptake and mRNA marker of adipose differentiation. Identical cases were observed in anti-adipogenicity in which enhanced long-time CLA feeding induced lipodystrophy and insulin resistance [10]. When CLA is supplemented to a hypercholesterolemic diet of experimental rabbits and hamsters, it reduces total cholesterol, LDL, serum triglycerides, and atherosclerotic plaque formation. But, its effects on experimental mice show contradictions because CLA stimulates aortic fatty streaks production. So, in different animal models, CLA stimulates differential effects on the lipid profile and on atherogenic markers. That's why use of CLA for prevention of cardiovascular disease and atherosclerosis in humans is still misunderstood and unclear [9,10]. The anticarcinogenic bioactivity of CLA in experimental animals is anticipated based on the inhibition of different kinds of cancer like colon, skin, prostate, mammary, tumorigenesis, and forestomach neoplasia. On its anticarcinogenic effect, previous studies have not generated any reliable results, and it does not prompt tumor. It is assumed that CLA present in diet generally mediates the origination and elevation carcinogenesis. So, CLA may restrain carcinogen metabolism, carcinogen-DNA adduct creation, and free radical-induced oxidation in the origination stage. While in the elevation stage, it initiates control cell proliferation and apoptosis by the regulation of interconnected molecular signaling events of cell cycle. CLA already shows its anticarcinogenic activity at relatively low concentrations, which is in less than 1% of food. This is exciting to note that among the other special effects of CLAs is its ability to influence the metabolism of fats and, in experimental animals, it reduces the amount of body fat [9]. Conjugated linoleic acid in meat and milk of the ruminants is influenced by diet, especially in the concentration of PUFA and by rumen conditions. The intake of dietary CLA in our diet is completely dependent on the assumption of meat and milk from ruminants, particularly from the consumption of fats from milk and meat, with higher values present in animals raised on pasture, which in general have even higher levels of polyunsaturated fats [10].

9.2.2 COENZYME Q10

Coenzyme Q10 is a constituent of mitochondrial electrons transport chain. It is also attributed to having antioxidant properties on fat levels, proteins, and DNA [11]. Meat is a significant cradle of coenzyme Q10, and its content is closely related to the number of mitochondria in muscle cells. The best sources are meat and fish, but cooking can cause a loss of around 15%–32%. Coenzyme Q belongs to group of lipophilic compounds that are found naturally. These compounds contain a common benzoquinone ring structure and differ only in the isoprenoid side chain length. Coenzyme Q10 (2,3-dimethoxy-5-methyl-6-decaprenyl-1,4-benzoquinone) is their group member [12]. In its side chain, it contains 10-repeated isoprene units. In humans and mammals, Q10 is the most predominant form of coenzymes. It is widely present in the form of ubiquinone (oxidized form) or ubiquinol (reduced form) in most tissues. In a normal adult human, total amount of coenzyme Q10 is around 0.5–1.5 g, while tissues have its varying concentrations. Heart, kidney, and liver tissues have higher energy requirements and lipid content. These tissues possess the highest concentrations of coenzyme Q10 i.e., 110, 70, and 60 mg/g tissue, respectively, and lungs possess lower concentration (8 mg/g tissue) of this coenzyme [13]. Mostly, coenzyme Q10 is present in its reduced form, except in brain and lungs. Regarding its subcellular distribution, mitochondrial inner membrane contains its 40%–50% proportion. In human tissues, it is obtained from food supplements, by food intake, or either synthesized endogenously. It is present in abundant amount in heart muscles, but cereals, vegetables, and fruits have it in low concentration (<10 mg/g food). Its concentration varies due to seasonal variations, differences in animal species, and analytical methods [12]. Nowadays, coenzyme Q10 is used as a dietary supplement and, due to its importance in supporting human health, its fame is increasing day by day. It also performs a major role in antioxidation, gene expression, mitochondrial energetic production, and cell signaling. Its supplements are used to treat male infertility, hypertension, heart diseases, cancer, atherosclerosis, diabetes, and neurodegenerative disease [11]. It is crucial for the production of ATP because it is used as a cofactor in the electron transport chain (ETC) of mitochondria and works in transferring protons and electrons in the respiratory chain as a peripatetic redox agent [13]. It is used to treat cardiovascular disease due to its important pathophysiological and therapeutic properties. It has been observed that due to Q10 levels, a negative correlation exists between myocardial tissue and plasma and with the rigorousness of cardiovascular dysfunction and symptoms. In standard medical therapy, Q10 supplementation has been given to heart failure patients, and it is associated with improvement signs in a couple of relevant clinical parameters in heart failure [14,15]. Ubiquinol is the reduced form of coenzyme Q10 [16]. It provides protection to the proteins of mitochondrial membrane, membrane phospholipids, and deoxyribonucleic acid against free radical-induced oxidative mutilation by removing free radicals. In LDL cholesterol, vitamin E and ubiquinol are two endogenous antioxidants and they provide protection against peroxidation of lipids. Hence, coenzyme Q10 is very beneficial in preventing the pathogenesis of atherosclerosis. Q10 supplementation is very essential to elders for the treatment of Parkinson's and Alzheimer's diseases because Q10 level declines with age [15]. It is suggested by substantial evidence that pathogenesis of neurodegenerative disease occurs due to mitochondrial dysfunction and oxidative damage. So, Q10 administration with other antioxidants leads to additive or synergistic beneficial effects that targets oxidative species reduction and mitochondrial uncoupling proteins [17].

9.2.3 CARNOSINE

Carnosine is a dipeptide which contains β-alanine and histidine amino acids. It possesses strong antioxidant and anti-genotoxic activities, even the anti-aging of cells [18]. In studies of mice fed diets supplemented with carnosine, a minor oxidative and inflammatory progression was observed in induced neurodegenerative diseases, from which we can deduce a possible role in the prevention of Parkinson's disease [19]. In muscle tissue, it functions as a buffer and participates in several biological functions. It is found in meat and fish, but not in plants. The cooking of meat reduces the content by 25%–40%. In a recent study, after ingestion of beef, bioavailability of carnosine has been proved by determining its concentration in human plasma [20]. A new sensitive procedure has been developed for the determination of these bioactive compounds, including carnosine, due to increased attention in these meat-based bioactive compounds. A product made from a by-product of corned beef is used as a functional food ingredient in Japan and it contains a good amount of L-carnitine and carnosine [19].

9.2.4 TAURINE

Taurine is a sulphur-containing amino acid that is synthesized from methionine. In liver, it is present in the form of free acid or as a constituent of the protein and is present in high amounts in most animal tissues [21]. Taurine plays an essential role in the synthesis of bile acids, which are derived from cholesterol and facilitate their elimination. Bile is also essential for the absorption of fat-soluble vitamins. During lactation and at times of immune challenges, it acts as an essential amino acid. It also protects our body from oxidative stress. A good dietary source of taurine is meat, which contains 77 mg per 100 g of beef [22]. Together with zinc, taurine is also important for vision. Its critical role was revealed in 1975, when it was discovered that the retinal degeneration occurred in those with taurine deficiency and it was found that the consumption of artificial milk without taurine could cause cardiac and retina dysfunction in preterm infants. Both of these problems can be prevented by the addition of taurine to synthetic artificial milk. It is now recognized that taurine possesses a vital role in human physiology and nutrition. Its positive effects are found in the digestive, endocrine, immune, muscular, neurological, reproductive, cardiovascular systems, and eye levels. Studies on rats subjected to intense physical activity have shown that it reduces oxidative stress in the muscle and, therefore, reduces damage of the muscle cells [21]. Taurine appears to counteract the aging process due to its anti-free radical action. This amino acid is important for the synthesis of nitric oxide, a potent vasodilator; and therefore, appears to stimulate cardiac efficiency and contractility by increasing the blood supply to the myocardium. Taurine is present only in animal foods.

9.2.5 CREATINE: FOR THE IMPROVEMENT OF MUSCLE PERFORMANCE

Beef contains 350 mg/100 g of creatine. In muscle energy metabolism, creatine and creatine-phosphate plays an important role. So, in certain circumstances, adding creatine to the diet promotes muscle performance. Through the removal of water, creatine present in muscles is slowly converted to creatinine with the formation of a ring structure, a phenomenon that is accelerated during the cooking of meat. Not being present in vegetables, those who follow a strict vegetarian diet have lower levels of creatine than non-vegetarians, and this may lower the muscle performance level [22].

9.2.6 MELATONIN (N-ACETYL-5-METHOXY-TRYPTAMINE)

Melatonin is a hormone. In mammals, this hormone is mainly produced by the pineal glands [23]. It is metabolically synthesized in four intracellular enzymatic phases by using plasma tryptophan as a predecessor. These enzymatic phases are catalyzed by aromatic amino acid decarboxylase, tryptophan hydroxylase, hydroxyindole-O-methyltransferase, and arylalkylamine-N-acetyltransferase. Its production is inhibited in the presence of light, so its level is greater at night rather than day. This hormone is also produced in the gastrointestinal tract of vertebrates [24]. Food intake is directly associated with the tissue and plasma melatonin concentrations [25]. In some countries, food stores sell it as a food supplement. It is currently suggested that its use in low amounts is safe due to its beneficial effects. It is also used to treat sleep and psychiatric disorders. Melatonin rhythm and pineal secretion impairment have been observed in various psychiatric disorders, such as unipolar depression, bipolar disorder, and seasonal affective disorder. Due to this impairment, lower melatonin level has been observed in patient's serum. Thus, on the basis of melatonin replacement therapy, the sleep quality of elderly insomniacs can be ameliorated by the replacement of age-associated decline of melatonin with physiological dosages. This hormone is also employed to treat bothered sleep in youngsters with disabilities of neurodevelopmental by reducing the time of sleep inception [26].

9.2.7 GLUTATHIONE

Glutathione is an important anti-oxidative compound. Its function is to provide cellular defense against different pathological and toxicological processes. Red meat is rich in glutathione and contains 12–26 mg/100 g of beef. Inside the cell, glutathione has the ability to inactivate free radicals such as hydrogen peroxide, thus protecting the cell from lipids or oxidized proteins and prevents DNA damage. Glutathione also acts as a detoxifying agent and blocks different heavy metals, such as mercury, lead, cadmium, aluminum, and other toxics (drugs, alcohol, tobacco, etc.), thus makes their elimination easier and quicker and prevents these poisons to bind with -SH groups of tissue proteins and enzymes deteriorating them. It also promotes the bioavailability of iron. Finally, glutathione carries out pro-immune activities and protects the central nervous system. Some fresh vegetables, eggs, and meat, especially pork and beef, have a high content of glutathione [27].

9.2.8 LIPOIC ACID: ANTIOXIDANT MOLECULE

Lipoic acid is an antioxidant molecule. It protects both the membranes and the organelles of the cell. It is present in the mitochondria of animal cells. It is present in larger amounts in the muscles of animals that move more. Lipoic acid is also a powerful chelator and capable of removing iron, copper, lead, cadmium, and mercury metals from the blood.

9.2.9 GLUCOSAMINE (2-AMINO-2-DEOXY-D-GLUCOSE)

Glucosamine is an amino monosaccharide, which is produced endogenously from glucose. Meat, poultry, and fish contain considerable amounts of glucosamine. One of the best forms of nutritional supplements is glucosamine sulfate. Other glucosamine nutritional supplements are glucosamine hydrochloride and N-acetyl-glucosamine. These compounds are produced from chitin. Its supplementation can be taken by oral administration and by intravenous, intra-articular, and intramuscular injections. The absorption of these dietary supplements into the bloodstream is fast by all routes of administration. About 90% of glucosamine taken by oral administration can be enthralled, while nearly 26% is offered for tissue usage. Almost all human tissues contain glucosamine, but liver, kidney, and cartilage contain higher concentrations [28]. In liver, it is reduced into smaller molecules by combining with plasma proteins and used for different biological processes. The presence of glucosamine concentrates in cartilage suggests that it has a major role in the structure and function of cartilage. It is utilized as a substrate during production of glycosaminoglycans and proteoglycans. These compounds are present in extracellular matrix of cartilage. Due to absence of proteoglycans, articular cartilage is degenerated. So, glucosamine is crucial for restoring of proteoglycan-rich matrix. It is also essential for balancing of cartilage metabolism and for protection of damaged cartilage from metabolic impairment. That's why glucosamine has been used to treat osteoarthritis. Over the past 40 years, many studies have shown that glucosamine supplements are proved to be beneficial in treating osteoarthritis [27].

9.2.10 L-CARNITINE

L-carnitine is a small molecule, which is derived from lysine. It performs a vital role in fatty acids metabolism and facilitates their penetration into the mitochondria and their subsequent oxidation. It is produced from methionine and lysine and its synthesis is greatly affected by the bioavailability of these elements. L-carnitine passes into the blood after its biosynthesis and, depending on their energy capacity, it is distributed to organs and tissues, especially in the muscles and heart. L-carnitine and β-hydroxy-γ-trimethyl amino butyric acid are found in the skeletal muscles of different animals. Beef is a rich source of L-carnitine and contains 1300 mg/kg in the thigh. In the human body, it produces energy and lowers cholesterol levels. It also helps in the absorption of calcium and chromium picolinate for improving skeletal strength and the building of lean muscle mass, respectively [29]. L-carnitine also blocks apoptosis and prevents skeletal muscle myopathy in case of heart failure. In the United States (US), L-carnitine containing drink products have been marketed. This product provides various beneficial effects, such as fast recovery from fatigue and maintenance of stamina. Similar types of drink products have been marketed in Japan which contains a good amount of L-carnitine and carnosine. This product is used as a functional food ingredient and it is synthesized from a by-product of corned beef. L-carnitine is provided by foods besides its endogenous origin. In the human body, about 80% of L-carnitine comes from the diet with a regular omnivorous diet. It decreases sharply in vegan diets because most of the L-carnitine is provided by meat, fish, and dairy products. It is considered a nutrient like vitamins, and the lack or insufficient intake of L-carnitine in the muscles and in the cardiac cells can cause myopathies and cardiac disorders [30]. L-carnitine is crucial for fatty acid oxidation because it is a significant component of a transport system. This scheme is used for the transferring of stimulated long-chain fatty acids into the matrix through the inner membrane of mitochondria, where β-oxidation occurs. Therefore, uptake of L-carnitine by cytosol of skeletal and cardiac muscle cells is essential for the energy metabolism of muscles. So, due to its vital role in the metabolism of fatty acid and production of energy, its insufficiency badly affects the functioning of the central nervous system and skeletal/cardiac muscles. Therefore, for treatment of impediments prompted by deficiency of L-carnitine, supplementation of L-carnitine therapy has been used to cure painful neuropathies, Alzheimer's disease, cardiovascular disease, and to improve immune function. Besides these, it has also been proved effective for the management of obesity, total energy expenditure, and improving intolerance of glucose [31].

9.2.11 CHONDROITIN

Chondroitin is a linear polysaccharide, which is formed by combining alternating disaccharide units of D-glucuronic acid and D-N-acetyl-galactosamine. A small proportion of sulfate esters is present in naturally isolated chondroitin [32]. In protein cores, it is attached with serine residues and, due to this attachment, it is an important part of proteoglycans, which have an important role in structural building organization of extracellular matrix. Pig and Ox cartilage contains about 35%–40% chondroitin [33]. It has also been isolated from shark cartilage, crabs, and squid. Clean chondroitin 4-sulfate has also been isolated from trachea and nasal septa of cattle by consuming 1% K_2CO_3 and NaCl. Different methods are used for removing its protein impurities, such as adsorption, proteolytic degradation, and precipitation [32]. Chondroitin sulfate is also used to treat osteoarthritis. It reduces the catabolic activity of chondrocytes by stimulating synthesis of proteoglycans and by inhibiting proteolytic enzyme synthesis. It induces anti-inflammatory action by modulating osteoprotegerin/receptor activator [33]. In this way, chondroitin protects osteoblasts of subchondral bone and matrix of cartilage from damage of cells and death. That's why, a remarkable amount of chondroitin sulfate is essential for cartilage to provide resistance and elasticity against tensile stresses [34].

9.2.12 CHOLINE (TRIMETHYL-β-HYDROXYETHYLAMMONIUM)

Choline is a quaternary ammonium compound. It was first found in the bile isolate of pig. It is also a basic constituent of lecithin phospholipid. Mostly, it enters into human body through the diet. Beef steak, Beef liver, eggs, and bovine milk contain remarkable concentrations of choline, which are 5831, 75, 150, and 42 mmol/kg, respectively It also acts as essential nutrient. Many food sources contain choline, which it plays an important role in the development of the central nervous system [35]. Maternal choline reserves tend to dry up during pregnancy and lactation periods. It was shown by animal studies that the state of choline pre- and post-natal can have long-term effects on the attention and memory of the unborn child. Choline during pregnancy and the early stages of life can alter brain functions, resulting in improved memory for a lifetime [36]. This change in memory function seems to be the cause of changes in the development of the memory center known as hippocampus in the brain which have long-term effects so that the memory in the elderly may, in part, are determined by what the mother ate during the pregnancy. Foods rich in choline are beef liver, chicken liver and eggs, and pork [37]. In the upper small intestine, free choline is directly absorbed. Nearly half of choline before its absorption is metabolized into betaine. When it is ingested in large amounts, then intestinal bacteria metabolize choline into trimethylamine. Enzymes present in pancreatic secretions and intestinal mucosal cells carry out its hydrolysis when it is ingested in the form of lecithin and then after hydrolysis, it is absorbed as lyso lecithin, and lecithin is reformed in the enterocyte. Free choline is released in the tissues and organs by enzymatic cleavage of lecithin. Other choline-containing compounds are phosphoryl choline, glyceryl phosphoryl choline, and sphingomyelin present in human diet in small quantities. All these compounds are cleaved to generate free choline in the enterocyte or in tissues/organs [38].

Deficiency of choline causes various disorders in body systems and organs because it is an indispensable nutrient for human health. In the past it has also been used as a therapeutic agent. In mammalian tissues, choline participates in four major enzymatic reactions—oxidation, phosphorylation, base exchange, and acetylation. Transfer of the phosphate group has been carried from ATP to choline's hydroxyl group by choline phosphotransferase enzyme. Phosphorylated choline acts as an intracellular storehouse of choline. In the phosphatidylcholine synthesis, the first step is the choline phosphorylation. Betaine aldehyde is the oxidation product of choline, which is transformed by choline oxidase enzyme system to betaine. Then, acetylcholine is formed by the reaction of acetyl coenzyme A with choline, and this reaction is catalyzed by choline acetyltransferase. In the final base exchange reaction, choline is reversibly substituted within endogenous phospholipids in the presence of calcium ions for serine, ethanolamine, and inositol [33].

Choline is used as a precursor for the production of phosphatidylcholine via cytidine diphospho-choline pathway. In cell membranes, it accounts for 50% of phospholipids. So, for cell membrane transportation and structural integrity, sufficient amount of choline is essentially required. Apart from this, it is also a significant constituent of very low-density lipoprotein, which is liable for triglycerides secretion from the liver. Therefore, prolonged insufficiency of choline can cause risks of fatty liver and hepatocarcinoma [36]. Its deficiency can cause significant escalation in cell proliferation and synthesis of DNA, and due to this reason various chemical carcinogens can be produced from cells. The oxidized choline metabolite betaine acts as a major methyl donor, and undermethylation of DNA occurs due to choline deficiency. This undermethylation leads to abnormal expression of genetic information and chromosomal instabilities. In liver, deficiency of choline leads to increased lipid peroxidation due to which free radicals are generated. These free radicals can cause carcinogenesis by modification of DNA. As a precursor of acetylcholine, choline is involved in regulating sleep, to control muscle activity, in the regulation of anxiety, learning, and can be connected to a slowdown in the loss of cognitive abilities in the elderly [38].

9.3 BIOACTIVE PEPTIDES OF MEAT

In addition to bioactive compounds in meat, there are peptide derivatives of proteins that are another group of functional compounds with protective activities. When evaluating the quality of a protein, in addition to the composition of amino acids, it is also essential to consider their ability to generate specific bioactive peptides during digestion. Bioactive peptides are sequences of 2–30 amino acids that have a positive good effect on consumer health. They also play an important role in the prevention of various diseases, which are associated with the development of metabolic syndrome and mental illness. Meat contains different proteins and peptides with important physiological activities.

There is still limited information on bioactive peptides of meat origin. However, enzymatic hydrolysates of different food proteins, such as milk and soy proteins, are used for the isolation of various physiologically functional peptides [39]. For the first time, isolation of bioactive peptides from food proteins were described by Mellander in 1950 [40]. Since then, numerous studies have been done on bioactive peptides which can be produced from different food proteins [39].

Extensive studies have been done on angiotensin I-converting enzyme (ACE) inhibitory peptides synthesized from food proteins. These peptides are used in different pharmaceuticals and physiologically functional foods due to their antihypertensive effects [41]. It also plays a vital physiological role in blood pressure regulation. In addition to antihypertensive peptides, food proteins generate various bioactive peptides, such as antimicrobial, antithrombotic, opioid, immuno-modulating, prebiotic, mineral-binding, hypocholesterolaemic, and antioxidative peptides. Milk proteins are a rich source of these bioactive peptides [42]. Opioid peptides affect the nervous system due to their affinity for an opioid receptor [43]. Immuno-modulating peptides trigger the phagocytic activities of macrophages and proliferation of lymphocytes [39]. Growth of pathogenic bacteria is inhibited by antimicrobial peptides [44]. Mineral-binding peptides are produced from milk proteins, such as caseino-phosphopeptides (CPP). These peptides act as a carrier for calcium and other minerals and possess anti-carcinogenic activity [45].

Although the activity of these peptides is latent when they are part of the sequence of the protein, they are released and activated during digestion in the gastrointestinal tract. The same mechanism occurs during fermentation, seasoning, or food processing. The peptides modulate the physiological function through the binding interactions to specific receptors on cells that lead to physiological responses. It has been shown that peptides derived from collagen have a positive effect on bone functionality, but, in general, the beneficial health effects of the peptides from meat include antihypertensive, antioxidant, antithrombotic, modulation of the immune response, and antimicrobial activity. Bioactive peptides are considered to be very important in the prevention of the metabolic syndrome and in the maintenance of mental health [46].

9.4   CONCLUSION

Although extensive research and development has been done on functional foods from the dairy industry, until now, slight attention has been paid to functional meat products. However, efforts are still under progress for the research and development of functional meat products. In developed countries, healthier meat and meat products are important in diet due to their major contribution to human health. So, production and utilization of bioactive compounds of meat origin, including bioactive peptides that can be generated from meat proteins, is a promising means for the development of nutritionally rich functional meat products. Such efforts would help the consumers in taking scientific benefits and advantages of meat and meat components for human health.

REFERENCES

1. Gnadig, S., Xue, Y., Berdeaux, O., Chardigny, J.M., & Sebedio, J.-L. (2000). Conjugated linoleic acid (CLA) as a functional ingredient. In Mattila-Sandholm, T., & Saarela, M. (Eds.), *Functional Dairy Products* (pp. 263–298). Boca Raton, FL: CRC Press.
2. Nagao, K., & Yanagita, T. (2005). Conjugated fatty acids in food and their health benefits. *J Biosci Bioeng* 100:152–157.
3. Watkins, B.A., & Yong, L. (2001). Conjugated linoleic acid: The present state of knowledge. In Wildman, R.E.C. (Ed.), *Handbook of Nutraceuticals and Functional Foods* (pp. 445–476). Boca Raton, FL: CRC Press.
4. Dhiman, T.R., Nam, S.H., & Ure, A.L. (2005). Factors affecting conjugated linoleic acid content in milk and meat. *Crit Rev Food Sci Nutr* 45:463–482.
5. Alonso, L., Cuesta, E.P., & Gilliland, S.E. (2003). Production of free linoleic acid by lactobacillus acidophilus and lactobacillus casei of human intestinal origin. *J Dairy Sci* 86:1941–1946.

6. Xu, S., Boylston, T.D., & Glatz, B.A. (2005). Conjugated linoleic acid content and organoleptic attributes of fermented milk products produced with probiotic bacteria. *J Agric Food Chem* 53:9064–9072.

7. Larsson, S.C., Bergkvist, L., & Wolk, A. (2005). High-fat dairy food and conjugated linoleic acid intakes in relation to colorectal cancer incidence in the Swedish Mammography Cohort. *Am J Clin Nutr* 82:894–900.

8. Azain, M.J. (2003). Conjugated linoleic acid and its effects on animal products and health in single-stomached animals. *Proc Nutr Soc* 62:319–328.

9. Schmid, A., Collomb, M., Sieber, R., & Bee, G. (2006). Conjugated linoleic acid in meat and meat products: A review. *Meat Sci* 73:29–41.

10. Belury, M.A. (2002). Dietary conjugated linoleic acid in health:physiological effects and mechanisms of action. *Annu Rev Nutr* 22:505–531.

11. Overvad, K., Diamant, B., Holm, L., Hulmer, G., Mortensen, S.A., & Stender, S. (1999). Review: Coenzyme Q10 in health and disease. *Eur J Clin Nutr* 53:764–770.

12. Purchas, R.W., & Busboom, J.R. (2005). The effect of production system and age on levels of iron, taurine, carnosine, coenzyme Q10, and creatine in beef muscles and liver. *Meat Sci* 70:589–596.

13. Bhagavan, H.N., & Chopra, R.K. (2006). Coenzyme Q10: Absorption, tissue uptake, metabolism and pharmacokinetics. *Free Radic Res* 40(5):445–453.

14. Sarter, B. (2002). Coenzyme Q10 and cardiovascular disease: A review. *J Cardiovasc Nurs* 16(4):9–20.

15. Singh, U., Devaraj, S., & Jialal, I. (2007). Coenzyme Q10 supplementation and heart failure. *Nutr Rev* 65(6):286–293.

16. Littarru, G.P., & Tiano, L. (2007). Bioenergetic and antioxidant properties of coenzyme Q10: Recent developments. *Mol Biotechnol* 37(1):31–37.

17. Beal, M.F. (2004). Mitochondrial dysfunction and oxidative damage in Alzheimer's and Parkinson's diseases and coenzyme Q10 as a potential treatment. *J Bioenerg Biomembr* 36(4):381–386.

18. Brown, C.E. (1981). Interactions among carnosine, anserine, ophidine and copper in biochemical adaptation. *J Theor Biol* 88:245–256.

19. Mora, L., Sentandreu, M.A., & Toldrá, F. (2007). Hydrophilic chromatographic determination of carnosine, anserine, balenine, creatine, and creatinine. *J Agric Food Chem* 55:4664–4669.

20. Park, Y.J., Volpe, S.L., & Decker, E.A. (2005). Quantitation of carnosine in humans plasma after dietary consumption of beef. *J Agric Food Chem* 53:4736–4739.

21. Bouckenooghe, T., Remacle, C., & Reusens, B. (2006). Is taurine a functional nutrient? *Curr Opin Clin Nutr* 9:728–733.

22. Purchas, R.W., Rutherfurd, S.M., Pearce, P.D., Vather, R., & Wilkinson, B.H.P. (2004). Concentrations in beef and lamb of taurine, carnosine, coenzyme Q10, and creatine. *Meat Sci* 66:629–637.

23. Carrillo-Vico, A., Guerrero, J.M., Lardone, P.J., & Reiter, R.J. (2005). A review of the multiple actions of melatonin on the immune system. *Endocrine* 27(2):189–200.

24. Pacchierotti, C., Iapichino, S., Bossini, L., Pieraccini, F., & Castrogiovanni, P. (2001). Melatonin in psychiatric disorders: A review on the melatonin involvement in psychiatry. *Front Neuroendocrinol* 22:18–32.

25. Bubenik, G.A. (2002). Gastrointestinal melatonin localization, function, and clinical relevance. *Dig Dis Sci* 47(10):2336–2348.

26. Phillips, L., & Appleton, R.E. (2004). Systematic review of melatonin treatment in children with neurodevelopmental disabilities and sleep impairment. *Dev Med Child Neurol* 46:771–775.

27. Olde Rikkert, M.G.M., & Rigaud, A.S.P. (2001). Melatonin in elderly patients with insomnia a systematic review. *Z Gerontol Geriatr* 34:491–497.

28. Anderson, J.W., Nicolosi, R.J., & Borzelleca, J.F. (2005). Glucosamine effects in humans: A review of effects on glucose metabolism, side effects, safety considerations and efficacy. *Food Chem Toxicol* 43:187–201.

29. Shimada, K., Sakura, Y., Fukushima, M., Sekikawa, M., Kuchida, K., Mikami, M. et al. (2005). Species and muscle differences in L-carnitine levels in skeletal muscles based on a new simple assay. *Meat Sci* 68:357–362.

30. Vescovo, G., Ravara, B., Gobbo, V., Sandri, M., Angelini, A., Dalla Libera, L. et al. (2002). LCarnitine: A potential treatment for blocking apotosis and preventing skeletal muscle myopathy in heart failure. *Am J Physiol* 283:C802–C810.

31. Steiber, A., Kerner, J., & Hoppel, C.L. (2004). Carnitine: A nutritional, biosynthetic, and functional perspective. *Mol Aspects Med* 25:455–473.

32. Pigman, W. (Ed.) (2012). *The Carbohydrates: Chemistry and Biochemistry*. Amsterdam, the Netherlands: Elsevier.

33. Asimakopoulou, A.P., Theocharis, A.D., Tzanakakis, G.N., & Karamanos, N.K. (2008). The biological role of chondroitin sulfate in cancer and chondroitin-based anticancer agents. *In Vivo* 22:385–390.

34. Martel-Pelletier, J., Tat, SK., & Pelletier, J.P. (2010). Effects of chondroitin sulfate in the pathophysiology of the osteoarthritic joint: A narrative review. *Osteoarthritis Cartilage* 18:S7–S11.

35. Zeisel, S.H., & Blusztajn, J.K. (1994). Choline and human nutrition. *Annu Rev Nutr* 14:269–296.

36. Sanders, L.M., & Zeisel, S.H. (2007). Choline: Dietary requirements and role in brain development. *Nutr Today* 42(4):181–186.

37. Flanagan, J.L., Simmons, P.A., Vehige, J., Willcox, M.D., & Garrett, Q. (2010). Role of carnitine in disease. *Nutr Metab* 7:30.

38. Zeisel, S.H. (1981). Dietary choline: Biochemistry, physiology, and pharmacology. *Annu Rev Nutr* 1:95–121.

39. Korhonen, H., & Pihlanto, A. (2007). Bioactive peptides from food proteins. In Hui, Y.H. (Ed.), *Handbook of Food Products Manufacturing – Health, Meat, Milk, Poultry, Seafood, and Vegetables* (pp. 5–37). Hoboken, NJ: John Wiley & Sons.

40. Mellander, O. (1950). The physiological importance of the casein phosphopeptide calcium salts II: Peroral calcium dosage of infants. *Acta Soc Med Uppsala* 55:247–255.

41. Meisel, H., Walsh, D.J., Murry, B., & FitzGerald, R.J. (2005). ACE inhibitory peptides. In Mine, Y., & Shahidi, F. (Eds.), *Nutraceutical Proteins and Peptides in Health and Disease* (pp. 269–315). Boca Raton, FL: CRC Press.

42. Gobbetti, M., Minervini, F., & Rizzello, C.G. (2007). Bioactive peptides in dairy products. In Hui, Y.H. (Ed.), *Handbook of Food Products Manufacturing – Health, Meat, Milk, Poultry, Seafood, and Vegetables* (pp. 489–517). Hoboken, NJ: John Wiley & Sons.

43. Guesdon, B., Pichon, L., & Tomé, D. (2005). Opioid peptides. In Mine, Y., & Shahidi, F. (Eds.), *Nutraceutical Proteins and Peptides in Health and Disease* (pp. 367–376). Boca Raton, FL: CRC Press.

44. Chan, J.C.K., & Li-Chan, E.C.Y. (2005). Antimicrobial peptides. In Mine, Y., & Shahidi, F. (Eds.), *Nutraceutical Proteins and Peptides in Health and Disease* (pp. 99–136). Boca Raton, FL: CRC Press.

45. Cross, K.J., Huq, N.L., & Reynolds, E.C. (2005). Anticariogenic peptide. In Mine, Y., & Shahidi, F. (Eds.), *Nutraceutical Proteins and Peptides in Health and Disease* (pp. 335–351). Boca Raton, FL: CRC Press.

46. Bougle, D., & Bouhallab, S. (2005). Mineral-binding proteins and peptides and bioavailability of trace elements. In Mine, Y., & Shahidi, F. (Eds.), *Nutraceutical Proteins and Peptides in Health and Disease* (pp. 29–40). Boca Raton, FL: CRC Press.

10 Bioactive Components from Milk and Milk Products

Saima Rafiq

CONTENTS

10.1 INTRODUCTION

Dietary interventions have gained immense attention due to their health promoting aspects beyond medicinal treatments. Milk is rich source of nutritionally important bioactive components, (Figure 10.1) which play essential roles in human health and nutrition [1]. These components include proteins, peptides, carbohydrates and lipids, glycolipids, and other minor biomolecules. Once these components are liberated from milk and dairy products, they exhibit various physiological functions and health promoting properties. The functional food products are developed and marketed by dairy industries and perform several physiological roles in the body, such as weight management and improved immunity; reduced infections and osteoporosis [2]; controlled blood pressure, cardiovascular disease, and diabetes; and anti-inflammatory and anticancer functions [3,4].

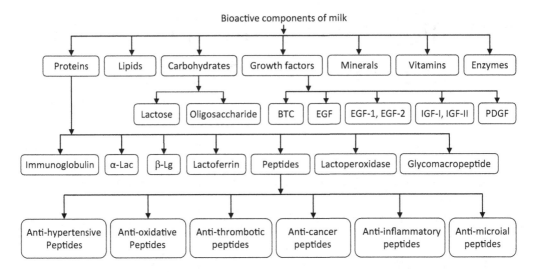

FIGURE 10.1   Bioactive components of milk and milk products.

10.2   BIOACTIVE PROTEINS FROM MILK AND MILK PRODUCTS

At present, the milk proteins are the principal source of bioactive components and, therefore, a well-studied constituent of milk. Milk proteins and peptides have perceived core attention as functional ingredients to combat chronic ailments, such as cardiovascular diseases, obesity, diabetes, and cancer. The nutritional and functional importance of milk proteins is widely recognized [5], and dairy products contribute significantly to daily protein intake, balanced profile of amino acids, structural, and sensorial attributes to dairy products.

The bioactivity of the milk protein is dormant, incomplete, or even absent in the original protein. However, the liberation of bioactivity could be achieved through proteolytic digestion to release the bioactive peptide from native protein [6], food processing, milk fermentation, enzymatic hydrolysis through digestive enzymes in the gastrointestinal tract, and enzymes derived from microorganisms or plants [7]. Digestive enzymes can naturally occur in milk and, therefore, supplement those products with functional characteristics [6]. The production of bioactive peptides from different mechanisms is shown in Figure 10.2.

Major milk protein, caseins, and whey proteins perform different therapeutic and functional roles in the body [5]. Fermented milk products, Calpis®, Evolus®, and other products derived from casein, are given in Table 10.1.

Several physiological and biological functions are provided by the bioactive peptides released by casein and its fractions. The main activities include antioxidant, antithrombotic, antihypertensive, antimicrobial, and opioid-like and cholesterol-lowering properties [4,8].

The total whey protein complexes have been concerned in many health promoting characteristics. These help to improve wound care and repair, anticipation of muscular atrophy, improved

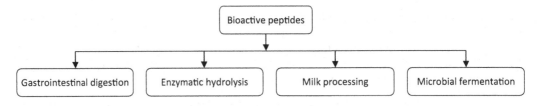

FIGURE 10.2   Different processes for liberation of bioactive peptides from milk native proteins.

TABLE 10.1

Commercial Dairy Products Containing Bioactive Peptides Derived from Casein

Brand Name	Type of Product	Bioactive Peptides	Health/Function Claims	Producer
Calpis	Sour milk	β-CN and κ-CN	Blood pressure reduction	Calpis Co., Japan
Evolus	Calcium enriched fermented milk drink	β-CN and κ-CN	Blood pressure reduction	ValioOy, Finland
BioPUREGMP	Whey protein isolate	κ-CN	Prevention of dental caries, clotting of blood	Davisco, USA
PRODIET F200/ Lactium	Flavored milk drink, capsules	α_{S1}-CN	Reduction of stress effects	Ingredia, France
Festivo	low-fat hard cheese	α_{S1}-CN α_{S1}-CN	No health claim	MTT Agrifood Research, Finland
C12 peptide	Ingredient-hydrolysate	Casein derived Peptide	Reduction of blood pressure	DMV International, Netherlands
Capolac	Ingredient	Casein derived Peptide	Helps mineral absorption	Arla Foods, Sweden
PeptoPro	Ingredient-hydrolysate	Casein derived Peptide	Improves athletic performance and muscle recovery	DMV International, Netherlands

physical performance, recovery after exercise, satiety control and weight management, cardiovascular health [9], anticancer effects [10], healthy aging, managing mucosal inflammation, microbial infections [11], and a hypoallergenic infant diet. The health promoting potential of major whey proteins and their commercial applications are discussed here.

10.2.1 IMMUNOGLOBULINS (IG)

Immunoglobulins are antibodies present in the milk and colostrums of lactating mammals and carry the biological function of antibodies against antigens [12]. Therefore, they play an important role in giving offspring protection from pathogens and infection. The Igs are divided into five different classes (IgA, IgD, IgE, IgG, and IgM) depending on the structure, properties, and biological function. In colostrum, these are 70%–80% of the total protein, while only 1%–2% of milk totals proteins. Globally, the market demand for such products is continuously increasing for dairy animals and as dietary supplements for humans. The several parts of cellular and humoral immune system are connected by these Igs. They have the ability to reduce bacterial metabolism, enhance phagocytosis and destroy bacteria, help to stop microbial adhesion, and deactivate toxins and viruses.

A randomized, double-blind, parallel-group, placebo-controlled study reported that consumption of Ig from bovine milk emerged to have a positive effect on patients suffering from mild hypercholesterolemia. The result showed that both the total cholesterol measured from baseline and LDL-cholesterol decreased [13].

10.2.2 α-LACTALBUMIN (α-LAC)

The α-Lac is the predominant whey protein in human milk and accounts for about 20% of the proteins in bovine whey. It is fully synthesized in the mammary gland where it acts as a coenzyme for biosynthesis of lactose. The peptides of the partly hydrolyzed protein, amino acids of the fully digested protein or whole molecule mechanisms are involved for favorable properties of α-Lac.

The α-Lac is a rich supply of the essential amino acids of methionine, tryptophan, and cysteine, which are precursors of serotonin and glutathion [14,15]. Specific proteins and peptides result from these hydrolysates and contribute different functional and biological roles, including antimicrobial, antioxidant, antihypertensive, anticarcinogenic, immunomodulatory, and opioid. The α-La has a metal-binding protein, specifically for calcium, and exhibits an antiulcer function [16], provides a protective effect against gastric mucosal injury [17], increases the brain tryptophan and serotonin activity, and improves the ability to cope with stress [18].

10.2.3 β-Lactoglobulin (β-Lg)

β-Lg accounts for 50% of the proteins in whey. This protein is absent in human milk. It contains a large amount of sulfur due to its cystein residues [18]. β-Lg has been proven to have many physiological functions, such as control blood pressure, reduce oxidative stress, have antimicrobial and anticarcinogenic capabilities, modulates immune functions, and can lower cholesterol levels. Also, the opioid peptide lactorphin [Tyr-Leu-Leu-Phe; f (102–105)] has been shown to improve arterial functions in SHR rats [19].

10.2.4 Lactoferrin (LF)

The colostrum, milk, and other body secretions and cells have an iron-binding glycoprotein called lactoferrin (LF). This protein acts against microbes (Table 10.2), pathogens, inflammation, and cancer, reduces oxidative processes, and regulates the immune system [20]. The digestive enzyme pepsin can cleave to the LF to produce peptides lactoferricin f (18–36) and lactoferrampin f (268–284) of an antimicrobial nature. The LF contribute its role against microbes due to its iron-binding capacity, attachment to the microbial membrane (lipopolysaccharide), and, thus, inhibiting viral replication; and microbe detachment to epithelial cells or enterocytes. The *in vitro* antimicrobial potential of LF has been established against many pathogens, including enteropathogenic *E. coli; Clostridium perfringens; Candida albicans; Haemophilus influenzae; Helicobacter pylori; Listeria monocytogenes; Pseudomonas aeruginosa; Salmonella typhimurium; S. enteriditis; Staphylococcus aureus; Streptoccccus mutans; Vibrio cholerae;* and hepatitis C, G, and B virus; HIV-1; cytomegalovirus; poliovirus; rotavirus; and herpes simplex virus [21].

The LF can regulate cellular and humoral immune systems by the production of lymphocytes; activation of macrophages, monocytes, natural killer cells, and neutrophils; cytokine and nitric oxide production; and stimulating antibody response [22]. It can also combat against the hepatitis C virus infection and is beneficial for neurodegenerative disorders and treatment of some cancer types. Several products comprised of LF have gained much interest with increased demand worldwide. It is synthesized in many industries as functional foods and pharmaceutical preparations [22,23]. The yogurt products launched in Japan and Taiwan and baby foods and infant formulas marketed in South Korea, Japan, and China.

TABLE 10.2
Bioactive Peptides Derived from Milk Proteins with Specific Functionality

Bioactive Peptides	Precursor Protein	Bioactivity	References
α-Lactorphin, β-lactorphin	α-LA, β-LG	Opioid agonist	[24]
Lactoferroxins	LF	Opioid antagonist	[25]
Lactokinins	α-LA, β-LG	ACE-inhibitory	[26]
Lactoferricin	LF	Antimicrobial	[22]

10.2.5 Lactoperoxidase (LP)

Lactoperoxidase (LP) is a glycoprotein found in colostrum and milk. Different chromatographic techniques can be employed to recover this enzyme in a considerable amount from whey. This enzyme can destroy or reduce the growth of microorganisms (bacteria, viruses, fungi, molds, and protozoa) by oxidation of sulphydryl (SH) groups of microbial enzymes through hypothiocyanate (OSCN-) production. It can kill Gram-negative pathogenic and spoilage bacteria (*E. coli, Salmonella* spp., *Pseudomonas* spp., and *Campylobacter* spp.), Gram-positive bacteria (*Listeria* spp., *Staphylococcus* spp., and *Streptococcus* spp.) and *Candida* spp., and protozoan (*Plasmodium falciparium*), HIV type 1, and polio virus. It can provide a natural method for preserving raw milk due to the presence of all necessary components to make the system ideal and preserving different products, like meat, fish, vegetables, fruits and flowers, dental health care products, and animal feeds [27,28].

10.2.6 Glycomacropeptide (GMP)

Glycomacropeptide (GMP) is mainly produced from cheese whey which accounts for 20%–25% of the proteins. It is a C-terminal glycopeptide f (106–169) released from the κ-casein molecule at 105 Phe–106 Met by the action of chymosin. The molecular weight of GMP is about 8,000 Daltons, and it is comprised of (50%–60%) a carbohydrate (glycoside) fraction. The non-glycosylated type of GMP is referred as caseinomacropeptide (CMP). The biological activities of GMP have received much attention currently because it can inhibit adhesion of cariogenic bacteria, inactivate microbial toxins, and influenza virus, helps immune system modulation and bifidobacteria proliferation, restrains gastric hormone activities, and regulates blood pressure by antihypertensive and antithrombotic mechanism, is anticarcinogenic, and useful for hepatic diseases and phenylketonuria [29,30]. It is valuable for brain development and improvement of learning ability [31], regulates intestines, inhibits gastric secretions, slows down stomach motility, and stimulates the release of cholecystokinin (CKK), thus, controlling food intake, digestion, and weight management, and modulation of gut microflora [29].

10.2.7 Bioactive Peptides

Bioactive peptides are specific protein fragments, which have an affirmative influence on body functions, thereby expressing hormone or drug-like activity [32,33]. They offer therapeutic aids due to high biofunctionality and specificity to targets, low levels of toxicity, structural diversity, and less accumulation in body tissues. Initially, the bioactive peptides were explained by Mellander [34] when he illustrated that the vitamin D independent calcification was enhanced in rachitic infants by the consumption of casein-derived phosphorylated peptides. Later, vital studies explored innovative research allied to the generation of bioactive peptides. Functionalities of bioactive peptides include antihypertensive, antioxidative, antithrombotic, anti-inflammatory, anticancer and antimicrobial, hypocholesterolemic, immunomodulatory, and mineral binding activities [35].

The bioactivity of peptides is based on amino acid composition and sequence. These peptides have been found in enzymatic protein hydrolysates and fermented dairy products, but they can also be released during gastrointestinal digestion of proteins [25,35,36]. Bioactive peptides are inactive within the sequence of the parent protein molecule and can be released from precursor proteins by enzymatic hydrolysis by digestive enzymes, fermentation of milk with proteolytic starter cultures, and proteolysis by enzymes derived from microorganisms or plants. The fermented dairy products (yogurt, sour milk, dahi, and cheese are rich sources of bioactive peptides) [32]. There are different factors affecting the production, release, amount, and functionality of these peptides, which mainly include starter culture, product, duration of fermentation, and storage conditions [37].

10.2.7.1 Antihypertensive Peptides

There is a tremendous increase of several physiological disorders globally, such as hypertension, oxidative stress, hypercholesterolemia, diabetes, and cancer. Hypertension is a significant challenge to public health worldwide, leading to cardiovascular complications including stroke, congestive failure, and coronary heart diseases. It is known as the "silent killer" due to the fact that more than 50% of hypertensive individuals are unaware of the condition [38]. Hypertension affects one in three individuals over the age of 45 years in Pakistan, and there are an estimated 12 million hypertensive people in the country [39].

Hypertension is generally controlled by medications using vasodilators, calcium channel blockers, diuretics, and angiotensinogen-converting enzyme (ACE)-inhibitors. The synthetic ACE-inhibitors (enalapril, alecepril, captopril, lisinopril) are utilized broadly for the treatment regardless of their adverse effects, such as angioedema, hypotension, cough, elevated potassium level, and renal malfunctions [40,41]. In this perspective, the demand and curiosity for natural (food-derived) peptides has increased due to safety and economical value. It has been established that the utilization of dairy products comprising antihypertensive peptides greatly lowers blood pressure.

Pharmaceuticals, including diuretics, calcium channel blockers, vasodilators, and ACE-inhibitors, are broadly utilized to reduce blood pressure. Diuretics work to remove excessive water and sodium from the body. The entry of calcium to heart muscle cells and blood vessels is mainly prevented through calcium channel blockers, which decrease blood pressure. Vasodilators relax blood vessels, while synthetic ACE-inhibitors can hinder the production of angiotensin II, thereby lowering blood pressure. But these antihypertensive medicines have several unwanted effects on the body. Therefore, diet-related preventive measures for hypertension are of great interest. Protein-derived ACE-inhibitory peptides can offer opportunity for the production and development of a novel bifunctional food. Blood pressure is controlled by various biochemical pathways, including rennin-angiotensin-aldosterone system (RAS). ACE, the principal enzyme of this pathway, is widely distributed in mammalian tissues, neuroepithelial, and male germinal cells [42].

Many ACE-inhibitory peptides isolated from different foods, such as casein [43], fermented milk [44], different cheese varieties [45–47], soy [48], egg [49,50], and fish [51,52], have been identified and reported [53]. Meisel et al. [54] compared the ACE-inhibitory potential in water-soluble fractions of several cheese (Roquefort, Camembert, Tilsit, Gouda, Edam, Leerdam, Emmental, Parmesan) varieties. Afterwards, they found the strongest activity in the medium-aged Gouda, as compared to fresh and ripened Gouda cheese [53]. In Festivo cheese, maximum ACE-inhibition was noticed at 13 weeks and decreased thereafter [45]. The ACE-inhibitory activity of control and probiotic Cheddar cheeses increased in the first 6 months of ripening and remained constant in the next 3 months. However, after 9 months of ripening, no considerable difference was observed [54,55]. The proteolytic enzymes, such as alcalase, thermolysin, subtilisin, and the successive treatment with pepsin and trypsin to simulate gastrointestinal digestion also have been employed to release various bioactive peptides of several physiological roles [56,57] (Table 10.3).

Also, yogurt bacteria, cheese starter bacteria, and commercial probiotic bacteria have been demonstrated to produce different bioactive peptides in milk during fermentation [62–64]. It was demonstrated that fermentation of milk with single industrial dairy cultures generated antioxidant activity in the whey fraction [65]. The activity correlated positively with the degree of proteolysis suggesting that peptides were responsible for the antioxidative property. In another study [66], the fermentation of milk with a commercial starter culture mixture of five LAB strains followed by hydrolysis with a microbial protease increased ACE-inhibitory activity of the hydrolysate and two strong ACE-inhibitory tripeptides (Gly-Thr-Trp and Gly-Val-Trp) were identified. The hypotensive effect of the hydrolysate containing these peptides was demonstrated in an animal model study using spontaneously hypertensive rats (SHR).

TABLE 10.3

ACE-Inhibitory Peptides Produced by Various Microorganisms

Culture Used	Parent Protein	Peptide Sequence	Reference
Lb. helveticus CP90 proteinase	ß-casein	Lys-Val-Leu-Pro-Val-Pro-(Glu)	[11]
Lactobacillus helveticus, Saccharomyces cerevisiae	ß-casein, κ-casein	Val-Pro-Pro, Ile-Pro-Pro	[58]
Lb. helveticus ICM 1004 cell free extract	Skim milk Hydrolysate	Val-Pro-Pro, Ile-Pro-Pro	[59]
Lactobacillus GG enzymes + pepsin & trypsin	ß-casein, αs1-casein	Tyr-Pro-Phe-Pro, Ala-Val-Pro-Tyr-Pro-Gln-Arg, Thr-Thr-Met-Pro-Leu-Trp	[60]
Lb. delbrueckii subsp. *bulgaricus* SS1 *Lactococcus lactis* subsp. *cremoris* FT4	ß-casein κ-casein	Multiple fragments	[59,60]
Streptococcus Thermophiles + *Lc. lactis* subsp. *lactis* biovar. *diacetylactis*	ß-casein	Ser-Lys-Val-Tyr-Pro	[42]
Lb. delbrueckii subsp. *bulgaricus*	ß-casein	Ser-Lys-Val-Tyr-Pro-Phe-Pro-Gly Pro-Ile	[42]
Lb. rhamnosus + digestion with pepsin and Corolase PP	ß-casein	Asp-Lys-Ile-His-Pro-Phe, Tyr-Gln-Glu-Pro-Val-Leu, Val-Lys-Glu-Ala-Met-Ala-Pro-Lys	[61]

10.2.7.2   Antioxidative Peptides

Oxidative stress is another important factor responsible for the initiation of cardiovascular diseases [67]. The reactive oxygen species (ROS), such as superoxide anion radicals, hydroxyl radicals, and non-free radical species, are produced during normal body reactions [68,69]. Moreover, some external agents, mainly ultraviolet light, ionizing radiation, environmental toxins, can also trigger the production of ROS.

In the human body, enzymatic antioxidants help to control over oxidation processes [70]. However, when free radicals are produced in excess, they hit biological molecules [71] and enzymes [72] leading to many degenerative ailments [73,74]. In addition, free-radicals also contribute lipolytic and peroxidative changes, which cause deterioration in quality and acceptability of foods during processing and storage [75]. Therefore, it becomes necessary to inhibit the per-oxidation of lipids and the production of free radicals in living cells [76] and food stuffs. This problem makes the use of natural antioxidants for chemotherapeutic and preservation properties with no or little side effects attractive. The derived peptides show the potential of antioxidants without any side effects. The exploitation of protein hydrolysates and peptides in functional foods contributes additional benefits over other natural antioxidants, because of their nutritional value, as well as other desired functional (antioxidant activity) properties [77]. The protein hydrolysates from various foods have been exposed to exert antioxidant and anti-inflammatory effects including pea [78] and fish protein [79] and casein hydrolysates [80,81]. The antioxidant peptides maintain antioxidant defense systems by scavenging free radicals [82] and hindering the production of ROS. The multifunctional character of peptidic antioxidants [83] may have the potential to control oxidative stress in foods. Moreover, these are comparatively safe and healthy compounds with low molecular weight, low cost, high activity, and easy absorption [84]. Recently, great attention has emerged to assess the antioxidative potential of peptides derived from fermented milk products and their promising applications as novel functional foods and nutraceuticals.

Milk fermentation has been described as a strategy to produce antioxidative peptides from proteins [85–90]. Although, the production of these peptides can be influenced by the operational conditions, degree of hydrolysis, type of protease [91,92], peptide structure [93] and peptide concentration [94] molecular weight and the configuration of peptides and strains used in the cheese making [95]. Antioxidative peptides can be released from caseins, soybean, and gelatin in hydrolysis by proteolytic enzymes [8]. Researchers [96,97] have shown that peptides derived from casein have free radical scavenging activity and inhibit enzymatic and nonenzymatic lipid peroxidation.

10.2.7.3 Antithrombotic Peptides

Besides hypertension, the development of thrombus (blood clot) in the circulatory system also causes cardiovascular ailments through vascular blockage, pulmonary embolism, and myocardial infarction [98]. In normal circulation, a healthy haemostatic system suppresses the formation of blood clots and prevents the blood loss in case of vascular injury. Though the intravenous heparin and thrombolytic drugs are used for the treatment, but they may also result in bleeding problems [99]. To tackle such complications, the nutraceutical ingredients, especially peptides with anti-thrombotic potential, may present an attractive approach. Antithrombotic peptides, which show nearly no toxic effect, have broad applications in the prevention and cure of cardiovascular disease [100,101].

The bovine κ-casein fractions (f106–116 and f39–42), named casoplatelins, obtained from tryptichydrolysates show antithrombotic activity by inhibiting fibrinogen binding with blood platelet [102]. The casoplatelin peptides derived from milk proteins have MAIPPKKNQDDK and KRDS sequence of amino acids. KRDS peptide derived from human lactoferrin has similarities to the RGDS peptide derived from the α-fibrinogen chain (f572–575). These two peptides released during gastrointestinal digestion and absorbed intact into the blood exert an antithrombotic effect *in vivo* [103]. The behavior of κ-casein f106–f116 is similar to that of the C-terminal peptide of the human fibrinogen γ-chain [104]. The other two smaller tryptic peptides (f106–112 and f113–116) derived from κ-casein exerted a minimum effect on platelet aggregation and did not inhibit fibrinogen binding [105].

10.2.7.4 Anticancer Peptides

Growing knowledge of the effect of diet on health offers new opportunities of cancer prevention through a change in eating habits. A variety of compounds from natural sources have been shown to be beneficial for cancer inhibition, such as fish [67], milk protein [106,107], and beef protein [51]. An increased consumption of milk or dairy products is associated with a significant reduction in cancer [10,108,109]. Cheeses and yogurt have been shown to decrease the risk of cancer by reducing the carcinogen itself, suppressing the enzyme activity that is responsible for carcinogenesis [110] and apoptosis induction [111–113]. Moreover, cysteine and cysteine-enriched proteins and peptides, or γ-glutamylcysteine dipeptides being efficient substrates for glutathione synthesis, can contribute to the suppression of tumorigenesis [108]. Many natural peptides show anticancer activity due to their capability to destroy target cells quickly, the broad spectrum of activity, and the specificity for cancer cells [114].

Animal models for colon and mammary tumorigenesis studies proposed that peptides derived from whey protein are more efficient in inhibiting tumor growth compared to other dietary proteins. High levels of γ-glutamylcyst(e)ine and cystine/cysteine dipeptides support this fact. These peptides are proficient substrates for the synthesis of glutathione, which is a ubiquitous cellular antioxidant that demolish reactive oxygen species and reduce the toxic effect of the carcinogens. Few infrequent studies on whey protein fractions, α-lactalbumin, β-lactoglobulin, and serum albumin advocate these components as potential anticancer moieties; moreover, these components are helpful in reducing the toxic effect of cancer [108]. A smaller fraction of lactoferrin showed significant results against intestinal tumors, as well as tumors at other sites. Mode of action attributed to lactoferrin is that it stimulates apoptosis, inhibits angiogenesis, modulates carcinogen metabolizing enzymes, and acts as an iron scavenger. Supplementation of cow feed with selenium results in elevated levels of selenoproteins in cow milk, which afterward is helpful in inhibiting the growth of colon cancer in rats [115].

Peptides, which are derived from casein hydrolysis, have verified antimutagenic properties [4]. Whole casein showed significant potential to reduce mutagenicity comparable with various other proteins [116]. Casein and peptides derived from digestion showed strong inhibitory effects [117]. However, the mechanism involved is not well established yet. It might be either due to physical connection by entanglement of mutagen with casein micelle or due to adsorption of mutagen on protein molecules and, in this way, preventing its reaction within the target cell. There are also chances of quenching reactions between proteolysis derived peptides and mutagens, or a chemical binding by a scavenging method.

Intact whey proteins have a nominal antimutagenic potential compared to derived peptides. Bosselaers et al. [117] proposed that low antimutagenic activity of whole whey protein molecules are due to their tight structure making them unapproachable to the mutagen. Caseins, on other hand, have a loose micellar structure because of which mutagen accesses them easily. Specific amino acid composition and the number of nucleophilic groups concerned to the reaction could be responsible for the binding of mutagen within the protein. Casein deprivation might raise the vulnerability of binding sites to mutagens.

10.2.7.5 Anti-inflammatory Peptides

Many age-related and degenerative disorders, such as atherosclerosis, arthritis, cancer, diabetes, osteoporosis, dementia, obesity, and metabolic syndrome, are caused by chronic inflammation [118]. In this context, different cytokines play a role in the development of inflammation. However, acute inflammation is associated with immune response of vascularized living tissue against infections, chemical and/or physical irritants, that functions to enclose injury, destroy invading microorganisms, inactivate toxins, and to recover the tissue or organ [119]. The process itself is not considered a disease, but failure to successfully resolve it may result in exacerbation of tissue damage and the modulation of signaling pathways [120].

Inflammation is an essential, normal immune response against microbial infections, lesions, and chemical and/or physical irritants. During defensive reactions, the activated macrophages secrete different bioactive inflammatory mediators, including nitric oxide (NO), necrosis factor-a, and interleukin-6 [121]. NO is an ubiquitous cellular mediator of physiological and pathological processes, being largely released at inflammatory sites for neurotransmission, vasodilation, and immune defense [122]. However, the uncontrolled production of NO by macrophages stimulation has been implicated in various inflammatory, arthritis, atherosclerosis, and cancer ailments [123]. Epidemiological investigations have exposed that chronic inflammation is caused by the expansion of 15%–20% malignancies, globally [124]. Many cancers arise from sites of infection and continuous irritation; for instance, ulcerative colitis is linked with the increased risk of colon adenocarcinoma [125] and chronic pancreatitis causes pancreatic cancer. Chemoprevention is considered an important strategy to suppress the inflammatory mediators. In this context, the inhibition of NO release is an attractive approach for remedial intervention in inflammation disorders.

10.2.7.6 Antimicrobial Peptides

Peptides having antimicrobial activities have been purified from several bovine milk protein hydrolysates, edible plants, fish, and eggs [126,127]. Antimicrobial peptides are an essential part of newborn immunity, mainly at mucosal surfaces like the small intestine and lungs, which are vulnerable to a broad spectrum of potent pathogenic microorganisms. A positive charge and an amphiphilic nature are known to be main structural motifs that determine contact mechanism with bacterial membranes and this has been acknowledged as a major target in their mode of action. It has also been proved through studies that a few milk-derived antimicrobial protein fragments can reach intracellular targets. Peptide with the strongest antimicrobial potential defined so far resembles a fraction from whey protein lactoferrin, called lactoferricin [128]. Afterward, other whey proteins, like α-LA and β-LG, were also investigated for their potential against various microorganisms, resulting in positive effects.

Lactoferrin derived peptides are antimicrobial in nature. Enzymatic hydrolysates of lactoferrin showed more antimicrobial potential compared to the parent protein molecule. Afterward, antibacterial peptides from bovine f(17–41) and human lactoferrin f(1–47) (Table 10.4) were discovered, purified, and named bovine and human lactoferricin [128]. A strong antibacterial potential against an extensive array of Gram +ve and Gram –ve bacteria was observed with these peptides [131].

Considering caprine and ovine species, a chemically-synthesized peptide fragment f (17–41) of goat milk lactoferrin showed antibacterial activity, though less compared to the corresponding bovine fraction. Antimicrobial peptides obtained by proteolysis of sheep and goat milk lactoferrin, homologous to lactoferricin, and corresponding to fraction f(14–42) were identified in caprine lactoferrin hydrolysates. Activity observed against *Escherichia coli* was lower, while analogous against *Micrococcus flavus* as shown by caprine lactoferricin when compared with bovine counterpart [72,132,133].

Antimicrobial peptides have a well-documented activity against a wide spectrum of pathogenic organisms, such as *Listeria, Salmonella, Escherichia, Staphylococcus, Helicobacter*, filamentous fungi, and yeasts [134]. Minimum concentration needed for inhibition depends upon the nature of that specific microorganism and it may differ from one to other bacteria. The antibacterial peptide αS$_2$-casein (f164–179) and (f183–207) demonstrated inhibitory activity against Gram +ve and Gram –ve bacteria at a minimum concentration of 8–95 μmol/L [133].

It is obvious (Table 10.4) that casein-like whey proteins is a rich source of antibacterial peptides [134]. At the primary stage of a study, fragments obtained by enzymatic hydrolysis (with pepsin, trypsin, and chymotrypsin) of ovine β-casein exhibited antibacterial activity against *Escherichia coli* (JM103), but exact peptides responsible for functionality were not identified [135]. Likewise, antimicrobial peptides have also been identified in αS$_1$-, αS$_2$-, and κ-CN [136].

TABLE 10.4
Antimicrobial Peptides Derived from Milk Proteins

Precursor Protein	Fragment	Released By
Lactoferrin	Bovine LF f(17–41/42), human LF f(1–11)S-S(12–47), caprine LF f(14–42)	Digestion with pepsin or chymotrypsin
α-Lactalbumin	α-La f(1–5), α-La f(17–31)S-S(109–114)	Digestion with trypsin
α Lactalbumin	α-La f(61–68)S-S(75–80)	Digestion with chymotrypsin
β-Lactoglobulin	β-Lg f(15–20), f(25–40), f(78–83), f(92–100)	Digestion with trypsin
α S1-Casein	α S1-Casein f(99–109)	Digestion with pepsin
α S2-Casein	α S2-Casein f(150–188)	Heated and acidified milk
α S2-Casein	α S2-Casein f(164–179)	Digestion with pepsin
α S2-Casein	α S2-Casein f(183–207), f(164–207), f(175–207), f(181–207)	Digestion with chymosin
κ-Casein	κ-Casein f(106–169)	Digestion with chymosin
κ-Casein	κ-Casein f(18–24), f(30–32), f(139–146)	Digestion with peptic enzyme
κ-Casein	Human κ-casein f(43–97)	Digestion with pepsin
β-Casein	β-Casein f(184–210)	Digestion with proteinase of *Lactobacillus helveticus* PR4

Source: Minervini, F. et al., *Appl. Environ. Microbiol.*, 69, 5297–5305, 2003; Lee, J.E. et al., *Korean J. Obstet. Gynecol.*, 55, 278–284, 2012.

10.3 BIOACTIVE LIPIDS

10.3.1 CONJUGATED LINOLEIC ACID (CLA)

Conjugated linoleic acid (CLA) refers to a group of polyunsaturated fatty acids with 18 carbons and two conjugated double bonds (C18:2) in *cis* or *trans* position [137]. The most biologically active isomers of CLA are reported to be *cis*-9, *trans*-11, which can be found in milk and dairy products. *Cis*-9, *trans*-11 CLA is also referred to as rumenic acid. In milk fat, approximately 75%–90% of the total CLA is in the *cis*-9, *trans*-11 form [138].

Bovine milk fat is composed of more than 400 fatty acids, which are esterified to the glycerol molecule as triacylglycerols [139]. Milk fat is rich in CLA contents ranging from 2 to –53.7 mg/g fat. Multiple health benefits have been demonstrated for dietary CLA. These positive effects include antidiabetic, antiobesity, augmentation of immune system [138], lower body weight and fat mass, increases lean body mass, reduction of serum cholesterol and triglyceride levels, and protection against various types of cancer, such as breast, prostate, and colon cancer, colorectal cancer [140].

Another biologically interesting lipid group in milk fat is the polar lipids, which are mainly located in the milk fat globule membrane (MFGM). The membrane consists of triglycerides, cholesterol, phospholipids (phosphatidylethanolamine, phosphatidylcholine, phosphatidylinositol, and phosphatidylserine), and sphingolipids (sphingomyelin, ceramides, and gangliosides). The polar lipids are involved in transmembrane signal transduction and regulation, growth, proliferation, differentiation, and apoptosis of cells, blood coagulation, immunity, and inflammatory responses, anticancer, cholesterol-lowering, and antibacterial activities prevent bowel-related diseases [133,136].

10.4 BIOACTIVE CARBOHYDRATES

10.4.1 LACTOSE

The lactose contents of goat, cow, and human milk are 4.1, 4.7, and 6.9 g/100 mL, respectively. It can stimulate the development of *bifidus* flora, decrease in the luminal pH, and increase colonization resistance against pathogenic organisms in the human intestine; thus, stimulating the vitamin D-independent component of the intestinal calcium transport system in animal models, enhancing calcium absorption. It is suitable in the diet of diabetics and has less cariogenic properties. Lactose-derived products are lactulose, lactitol, lactobionic acid, and galacto-oligosaccharides. Lactulose is mainly used in infant milk formulae and medicinal products for the treatment of constipation and chronic hepatic ailments. It also increased calcium absorption in postmenopausal women [141,142].

10.4.2 OLIGOSACCHARIDES

Milk contains minor forms of carbohydrates including oligosaccharides that comprise of 2–10 monosaccharide units. These carbohydrates contain galactose, fucose, *N*-acetylglucosamine, and *N*-acetylneuraminic acid (NANA). These sugars make a substantial contribution to the carbohydrate content; for example, in human milk up to 1.4% of the entire carbohydrate content. Oligosaccharides contain 3–10 monosaccharide units that are linked through glycosidic bonds [53,143]. A great deal of the previous research on oligosaccharides are mostly focused on human milk since they are highly abundant in human milk. The number of oligosaccharides in milk from other animals is low compared to human milk is the reason for a lack of studies on milk from other species [144,145]. There is increasing evidence that the principal role of oligosaccharides seems to be to administer the protection against pathogens, promoting the growth of *Lactobacillus bifidus* in the intestinal tract, and anti-infective properties. By functioning as competitive inhibitors on the binding site of the intestinal epithelial surface may give physiological protection [146,147].

10.5   GROWTH FACTORS (GF)

The growth factors (GF) are polypeptides with molecular masses ranging between 6,000 and 30,000 Daltons and amino acid residues of 53 (EFG) to about 425 (TGF-2), respectively. These can withstand pasteurization and ultra-high temperature (UHT) heat treatment of milk. There are different growth factors recognized in bovine mammary secretions: BTC (β -cellulin), EGF (epidermal growth factor), FGF1 and FGF2 (fibroblast growth factor), IGF-I and IGF-II (insulin like growth factor), TGF-1 and TGF-2 (transforming growth factor), and PDGF (platelet-derived growth factor) [148,149].

EGF and BTC stimulate the proliferation of epidermal, epithelial, and embryonic cells, inhibit the secretion of gastric acid, and promote wound healing and bone resorption. The TGF-family plays an important role in the development of the embryo, tissue repair, formation of bone and cartilage, and regulation of the immune system. Both forms of TGF are known to stimulate proliferation of connective tissue cells and inhibit proliferation of lymphocytes and epithelial cells. Both forms of IGF stimulate proliferation of many cell types and regulate some metabolic functions, by glucose uptake and synthesis of glycogen [148].

10.6   BIOACTIVE MINERALS

Milk, as a nutritional supply of minerals, contributes a significant role in human physiology and metabolism. Calcium is an essential mineral and one of the most abundant minerals in the human body. It is a crucial nutrient required in numerous biological functions, such as skeletal mineralization. Therefore, the loss of calcium through nail, skin, hair, as well as urine and feces must be replaced from the daily diet. However, the calcium requirement is reliant on the state of the calcium metabolism, which is based on the individual. Most calcium in found in milk and is bound to casein, and to minor extent to other milk proteins, phosphorus, and citrate. There is also a small fraction of calcium that exists in an unbound form [141]. During the past 20 years, research has proven that calcium in dairy products has a beneficial role, and the level of milk and dairy product consumption is correlated to many of the twenty-first century diseases [150].

Calcium is important for the development, strength, and density of bones in children and prevention of osteoporosis, reducing cholesterol absorption, and in controlling body weight and blood pressure in elders, gastrointestinal and immunological improvement, and antibiotic and probiotic action [1]. The phosphorus present in milk participates in different metabolic functions in the body, including bone mineralization, energy metabolism, fat and carbohydrate metabolisms, body buffer system, and formation and transport of nucleic acids and phospholipids across cell membranes for body cell functioning.

Milk also contains good amount of copper, zinc, manganese, and iron. Iron deficiency causes anemia, impaired growth, and lipid metabolism. Zinc is the greatest among the trace minerals. Its deficiency results in skin lesions, disturbed immune function, growth retardation, and impaired wound healing. In a feeding trial with rats, animals fed a goat milk diet exhibited a greater bioavailability of zinc and selenium compared to those fed a cow milk diet. The level of iodine in milk is important for human nutrition, since iodine and thyroid hormones are closely related to the metabolic rate of physiological body functions. Goat and human milk contain higher concentrations of selenium than cow milk. Other trace minerals, including Mo, Cr, Co, Mn, F, As, Sn, perform different metabolic activities in body [151].

10.7   BIOACTIVE VITAMINS

Milk is comprised of bioactive vitamins, which perform several physiological, biochemical, and metabolical activities. Both types, water-soluble and fat-soluble vitamins are present in milk. The physiologically important vitamins are riboflavin (B-2), vitamin B-12, vitamin A, niacin, thiamin, and folic acid. The folate is necessary for the synthesis of hemoglobin. The deficiency of these vitamins may cause megaloblastic anemia in infants [152–156].

10.8 CONCLUSION

Bioactive components, especially proteins and peptides present in milk and milk products, perform several physiological functions, such as antihypertension, anti-inflammatory, antioxidant, antibacterial, antitumor, weight management, improve immunity; and reduce infections, cholesterol, osteoporosis, and diabetes.

REFERENCES

1. Gobbetti M, Minervini F, Rizzello CG (2007) Bioactive peptides in dairy products. In: Hui YH (Ed.) *Handbook of Food Products Manufacturing*, John Wiley & Sons, Hoboken, NJ.
2. Hartmann R, Wal JM, Bernard H, Pentzien AK (2007) Cytotoxic and allergenic potential of bioactive proteins and peptides. *Curr Pharm Des* 13:897–920.
3. Rafiq S, Huma N, Rakariyatham K, Hussain I, Gulzar N, Hayat I (2017) Anti-inflammatory and anti-cancer activities of water-soluble peptide extracts of buffalo and cow milk Cheddar cheeses. *Int J Dairy Technol* 70:1–7.
4. Rafiq S, Huma N, Gulzar N, Murtaza A, Hussain I (2018) Effect of Cheddar cheese peptides extracts on growth inhibition, cell cycle arrest and apoptosis induction in human lung cancer (H-1299) cell line. *Int J Dairy Technol* 70. doi:10.1111/1471-0307.12533.
5. Philanto A (2006) Antioxidative peptides derived from milk proteins. *Int Dairy J* 16:1306–1314.
6. Park YW, Haenlein GFW (2006) Goat milk, its products and nutrition. In: Hui YH (Ed.) *Handbook of Food Products Manufacturing*. John Wiley & Sons, New York.
7. Korhonen H, Pihlanto A (2006) Bioactive peptides: Production and functionality. *Int Dairy J* 16:945–960.
8. Lopez-fandino R, Otte J, Van Camp J (2006) Physiological, chemical and technological aspects of milk-protein-derived peptides with antihypertensive and ACE-inhibitory activity. *Int Dairy J* 16:1277–1293.
9. FitzGerald RJ, Murray BA, Walsh DJ (2004) Hypotensive peptides from milk proteins. *J Nutr* 134:980–988.
10. Gill HS, Doull F, Rutherfurd KJ, Cross ML (2000) Immunoregulatory peptides in bovine milk. *Br J Nutr* 84:111–117.
11. Korhonen H, Pihlanto A (2003) Bioactive peptides: New challenges and opportunities for the dairy industry. *Austr J Dairy Tech* 58:129–134.
12. Korhonen HJ (2009) Milk derived bioactive peptides. From science to applications. *J Funct Foods* 1:177–187.
13. Luhovyy BL, Akhavan T, Anderson GH (2007) Whey proteins in the regulation of food intake and satiety. *J Am Coll Nutr* 26:704–712.
14. Politis I, Chronopoulou R (2008) Milk peptides and immune response in the neonate. *Adv Exp Med Biol* 606:253–269.
15. Earnest CP, Jordan AN, Safir M, Weaver E, Church TS (2005) Cholesterol-lowering effects of bovine serum immunoglobulin in participants with mild hypercholesterolemia. *Am J Clin Nutri* 81(4):792–798.
16. Kivinen A, Salminen S, Homer D, Vapaatalo H (1992) Gastroprotective effect of milk phospholipids, butter serum lipids and butter serum on ethanol and acetylsalicylic acid induced ulcers inrats. *Milchwissenschaft* 47(9):573–575.
17. Markus CR, Olivier B, Panhuysen GE, Van der Gugten J, Alles MS, Tuiten A, Westenberg HG, Fekkes D, Koppeschaar HF, de Haan EE (2000) The bovine protein α-lactalbumin increases the plasma ratio of tryptophan to the other large neutral amino acids, and in vulnerable subjects raises brain serotonin activity, reduces cortisol concentration, and improves mood under stress. *Am J Clin Nutri* 71(6):1536–1544.
18. Matsumoto H, Shimokawa Y, Ushida Y, Toida T, Hayasawa H (2001) New biological function of bovine α-Lactalbumin: Protective effect against ethanol- and stress-induced gastric mucosal injury in rats. *Biosci Biotechnol Biochem* 65(5):1104–1111.
19. Chatterton DEW, Rasmussen JT, Heegaard CW, Sørensen ES, Petersen TE (2004) In vitro digestion of novel milk protein ingredients for use in infant formulas: Research on biological functions. *Trends Food Sci Technol* 15(8):373–383.
20. Embleton ND, Berrington JE, McGuire W, Stewart CJ, Cummings SP (2013) Lactoferrin: Antimicrobial activity and therapeutic potential. *Semin Fetal Neonat Med* 18:143–149.
21. Legrand D, Mazurier JA (2010) Critical review of the roles of host lactoferrin in immunity. *Biometals* 23:365–376.

22. Actor JK, Hwang SA, Kruzel ML (2009) Lactoferrin as a natural immune modulator. *Curr Pharm Des* 15:1956–1973.
23. Turin CG, Zea-Vera A, Pezo A, Cruz K, Zegarra J, Bellomo S, Cam L, Llanos R, Castañeda A, Tucto L (2014) Lactoferrin for prevention of neonatal sepsis. *Biometals* 27:1007–1016.
24. Hernández-Ledesma B, Recio I, Amigo L (2008) β-lactoglobulin as source of bioactive peptides. *Amino Acids* 35:257–265.
25. Barras D, Widmann C (2011) Promises of apoptosis-inducing peptides in cancer therapeutics. *Curr Pharm Biotechnol* 12:1153–1165.
26. Vanessa H, Frederic S, Jean-Marie P, Stephanie B (2009) Goat whey fermentation by *Kluyveromyces marxianus* and *Lactobacillus rhamnosus* release tryptophan and tryptophan-lactokinin from a cryptic zone of alpha-lactalbumin. *J Dairy Res* 76:379–383.
27. Kussendrager KD, van Hooijdonk AC (2000) Lactoperoxidase: Physico-chemical properties, occurrence, mechanism of action and applications. *Br J Nutr* 84:19–25.
28. Seifu E, Buys EM, Donkin EF (2005) Significance of the lactoperoxidase system in the dairy industry and its potential applications: A review. *Trends Food Sci Technol* 16:137–154.
29. Manso MA, Lopez-Fandino R (2003) Angiotensin I converting enzyme-inhibitory activity of bovine; ovine; and caprine kappa-casein macropeptides and their tryptic hydrolysates. *J Food Protect* 66:1686–1692.
30. Jamie S, Salsman MJ, Conrad DM, Hoskin DW (2005) Bovine lactoferricin selectively induces apoptosis in human leukemia and carcinoma cell lines. *Mol Cancer Ther* 4:612–624.
31. Wang Y, Zhu F, Chen J, Han F, Wang H (2009) Effects of Pro-Arg, a novel dipeptide derived from protamine hydrolysate on H_2O_2 induced oxidative stress in human diploid fibroblasts. *Biol Pharm Bull* 32:389–393.
32. FitzGerald RJ, Murray BA (2006) Bioactive peptides and lactic fermentations. *Int J Dairy Technol* 59:118–125.
33. Ong L, Shah NP (2008) Release and identification of angiotensin-converting enzyme-inhibitory peptides as influenced by ripening temperatures and probiotic adjuncts in Cheddar cheeses. *LWT – Food Sci Technol* 41:1555–1566.
34. Mellander O (1950) The physiological importance of the casein phosphopeptide calcium salts II. Peroral calcium dosage of infants. *Acta Society Med Uppsala* 55:247–255.
35. Korhonen H, Pihlanto A (2006) Bioactive peptides: Production and functionality. *Int Dairy J* 16:945–960.
36. Gobbetti M, Stepaniak L, De-Angelis M, Corsetti A, Di-Cagno R (2002) Latent bioactive peptides in milk proteins: Proteolytic activation and significance in dairy processing. *Crit Rev Food Sci Nutr* 42:223–239.
37. Ardo Y, Lilbaek H, Kristiansen KR, Zakora M, Otte J (2007) Identification of large phosphopeptides from β-casein that characteristically accumulate during ripening of the semi hard cheese Herrgard. *Int Dairy J* 17:513–524.
38. Chockalingam A (2008) World hypertension day and global awareness. *Can J Cardiol* 24:441–444.
39. National Health Survey of Pakistan (2014) Pakistan Demographic and health survey, preliminary report. National Institute of Population Studies, Islamabad, Pakistan.
40. FitzGerald RJ, Meisel H (2000) Milk protein-derived peptide inhibitors of angiotensin-I-converting enzyme. *Br J Nutr* 84:33–37.
41. Amir OY, Hassan A, Sarriff A, Awaisu AN, Ismail O (2009) Incidence of risk factors for developing hyperkalemia when using ACE inhibitors in cardiovascular diseases. *Pharm World Sci* 31:387–393.
42. Ashar MN, Chand R (2004) Fermented milk containing ACE inhibitory peptides reduces blood pressure in middle aged hypertensive subjects. *Milchwissenschaft* 59:363–366.
43. Otte J, Shalaby SMA, Zakora M, Nielsen MS (2007) Fractionation and identification of ACE-inhibitory peptides from α-lactalbumin and β-casein produced by thermolysin-catalysed hydrolysis. *Int Dairy J* 17:1460–1472.
44. Chen GW, Tsai JS, Pan BS (2007) Purification of angiotensin I-converting enzyme inhibitory peptides and antihypertensive effect of milk produced by protease-facilitated lactic fermentation. *Int Dairy J* 17:641–647.
45. Ryhanen EL, Pihlanto-Leppala A, Pahkala E (2001) A new type of ripened, low fat cheese with bioactive properties. *Int Dairy J* 11:441–447.
46. Saito K, Jin DH, Ogawa T, Muramoto K, Hatakeyama E, Yasuhara T (2003) Antioxidative properties of tripeptide libraries prepared by the combinatorial chemistry. *J Agric Food Chem* 51:3668–3674.
47. Tonouchi H, Suzuki M, Uchida M, Oda M (2008) Antihypertensive effect of an angiotensin converting enzyme inhibitory peptide from enzyme modified cheese. *J Dairy Res* 75:284–290.

48. Wu J, Ding X (2002) Characterization of inhibition and stability of soy-protein derived angiotensin I-converting enzyme inhibitory peptides. *Food Res Int* 35:367–375.

49. Miquel E, Gomez JA, Alegria A, Barbera R, Farre R, Recio I (2005) Identification of casein phosphopeptides released after simulated digestion of milk-based infant formulas. *J Agri Food Chem* 53:3426–3433.

50. Fox PF, McSweeney PLH (1996) Proteolysis in cheese during ripening. *Food Rev Int* 12:457–509.

51. Jang A, Jo C, Kang KS, Lee M (2008) Antimicrobial and human cancer cell cytotoxic effect of synthetic angiotensin-converting enzyme (ACE) inhibitory peptides. *Food Chem* 107:327–336.

52. Kawasaki T, Seki E, Osajima K, Yoshida M, Asada K, Matsui T (2000) Antihypertensive effect of Valyl-tyrosine, a short chain peptide derived from sardine muscle hydrolyzate, on mild hypertensive subjects. *J Hum Hypertens* 14:519–523.

53. Ong L, Henriksson A, Shah NP (2006). Development of probiotic Cheddar cheese containing *Lb. acidophilus, Lb. paracasei, Lb. casei* and *Bifidobacterium spp.* and the influence of these bacteria on proteolytic patterns and production of organic acid. *Int Dairy J* 16:446–456.

54. Ong L, Henriksson A, Shah NP (2007) Angiotensin converting enzyme-inhibitory activity in cheddar cheeses made with the addition of probiotic *Lactobacillus casei* sp. *Le Lait* 87:149–165.

55. Meisel H, Walsh DJ, Murray BA, Fitzgerald RJ (2006) *ACE Inhibitory Peptides in Nutraceutical Proteins and Peptides in Health and Diseases.* CRC Press/Taylor & Francis Group, New York.

56. Lopez-Exposito I, Minervini F, Amigo L, Recio I (2006) Identification of antibacterial peptides from bovine k-casein. *J Food Protect* 69:2992–2997.

57. Costabel LM, Bergamini CV, Pozza L, Cuffia F, Candioti MC, Hynes E (2015) Influence of chymosin type and curd scalding temperature on proteolysis of hard cooked cheeses. *J Dairy Res* 16:1–10.

58. Seppo L, Jauhiainen T, Poussa T, Korpela R (2003) A fermented milk high in bioactive peptides has a blood pressure-lowering effect in hypertensive subjects. *Am J Clin Nutr* 77:326–330.

59. Gobbetti M, Minervini F, Rizzello CG (2004) Angiotensin I-converting-enzyme-inhibitory and antimicrobial bioactive peptides. *Int J Dairy Technol* 57:172–188.

60. Gobbetti M, Ferranti P, Smacchi E, Goffredi F, Addeo F (2000) Production of angiotensin-I-converting-enzyme-inhibitory peptides in fermented milks started by *Lactobacillus delbrueckii* subsp. *Bulgaricus* SS1 and *Lactococcus lactis* subsp. *cremoris* FT4. *Appl Environ Microbiol* 66:3898–3904.

61. Hernández-Ledesma B, Amigo L, Recio I, Bartolome B (2007). ACE-inhibitory and radical-scavenging activity of peptides derived from beta-lactoglobulin f(19–25). Interactions with ascorbic acid. *J Agric Food Chem* 55:3392–3397.

62. Gomez-Ruiz JA, Taborda G, Amigo L, Recio I, Ramos M (2006) Identification of ACE inhibitorypeptides in different Spanish cheeses by tandem mass spectrometry. *Eur Food Res Technol* 223:595–601.

63. Gobbetti M, Ferranti P, Smacchi E, Goffredi F, Addeo F (2000) Production of angiotensin-I-converting-enzyme-inhibitory peptides in fermented milks started by *Lactobacillus delbrueckii* subsp. *Bulgaricus* SS1 and *Lactococcus lactis* subsp. *Cremoris* FT4. *Appl Environ Microbiol* 66:3898–3904.

64. Donkor ON, Henriksson A, Singh TK, Vasiljevic T, Shah NP (2007) ACE-inhibitory activity of probiotic yoghurt. *Int Dairy J* 17:1321–1331.

65. Vermeirssen V, Augustijns P, Van CJ, Opsomer A, Verstraete W (2005) *In vitro* intestinal transport and antihypertensive activity of ACE inhibitory pea and whey digests. *Int J Food Sci Nutr* 56:415–430.

66. Chen S, Khan ZA, Cukiernik M, Chakrabarti S (2003) Differential activation of NF-kappa B and AP-1 in increased fibronectin synthesis in target organs of diabetic complications. *Am J Physiol Endocrinol Metab* 284:1089–1097.

67. Hernandez-Ledesma B, Hsieh CC, de Lumen BO (2014) Chemopreventive properties of peptide lunasin: A review. *Protein Pept Lett* 20:424–432.

68. Ren NQ, Guo WQ, Wang XJ, Xiang WS, Liu BF, Wang XZ (2008) Effects of different pre treatment methods on fermentation types and dominant bacteria for hydrogen production. *Int J Hydrogen Energy* 33:4318–4324.

69. Gulçin I (2010) Antioxidant properties of resveratrol: A structure activity insight. *Innov Food Sci Emerg Technol* 11:210–218.

70. Dimitrios B (2006) Sources of natural phenolic antioxidants. *Trends Food Sci Technol* 17:505–512.

71. Urso ML, Clarkson PM (2003) Oxidative stress, exercise, and antioxidant supplementation. *Toxicology* 189:41–54.

72. Igoshi K, Kondo Y, Kobayashi H, Kabata K, Kawakami H (2008) Antioxidative activity of cheese. *Milchwissenschaft* 63:424–426.

73. Davalos A, Miguel M, Bartolome B, Lopez-Fandino R (2004) Antioxidant activity of peptides derived from egg white proteins by enzymatic hydrolysis. *J Food Protect* 67:1939–1944.

74. Suja KP, Jayalekshmy A, Arumughan C (2004) Free radical scavenging behavior of antioxidant compounds of sesame (*Sesamumindicum L.*) in DPPH system. *J Agri Food Chem* 52:912–915.

75. Antolovich M, Prenzler P, Patsalides E (2002) Methods for testing antioxidant activity. *Analyst* 127:183–198.

76. Butterfield DA (2002) Amyloid beta-peptide (1–42)-induced oxidative stress and neurotoxicity: Implications for neurodegeneration in Alzheimer's disease brain. *Free Rad Res* 36:1307–1313.

77. Pownall TL, Udenigwe CC, Aluko RE (2010) Amino acid composition and antioxidant properties of pea seed (*Pisum sativum* L.) enzymatic protein hydrolysate fractions. *J Agric Food Chem* 58:4712–4718.

78. Ndiaye F, Vuong T, Duarte J, Aluko RE, Matar C (2012) Anti-oxidant, anti-inflammatory and immunomodulating properties of an enzymatic protein hydrolysate from yellow field pea seeds. *Eur J Nutr* 51:29–37.

79. Hernández D, Cardell E, Zárate V (2005) Antimicrobial activity of lactic acid bacteria isolated from Tenerife cheese: Initial characterisation of plantaricin TF711, a bacteriocin like substance produced by Lactobacillus plantarum TF711. *J Appl Microbiol* 99:77–84.

80. Lahart N, Callaghan YO, Aherne SA, Sullivan DO, FitzGerald RJ, O'Brien NM (2011) Extent of hydrolysis effects on casein hydrolysate bioactivity: Evaluation using the human Jurkat T cell line. *Int Dairy J* 21:777–782.

81. Phelan MA, Aherne RJ, FitzGerald M, O'Brien NM (2009) Casein derived bioactive peptides: Biological effects, industrial uses, safety aspects and regulatory status. *Int Dairy J* 19:643–654.

82. Anusha GP, Samaranayaka CY, Eunice D, Li C (2011) Food derived peptide antioxidants: A review of their production, assessment, and potential applications. *J Funct Foods* 3:229–254.

83. Hernández-Ledesma B, Amigo L, Ramos M, Recio I (2004) Angiotensin converting enzyme inhibitory activity in commercial fermented products. Formation of peptides under simulated gastrointestinal digestion. *J Agric Food Chem* 52:1504–1510.

84. Xie Z, Huang J, Xu X, Jin Z (2008) Antioxidant activity of peptides isolated from alfalfa leaf protein hydrolysate. *Food Chem* 111:370–376.

85. Suetsuna K, Ukeda H, Ochi H (2000) Isolation and characterization of free radical scavenging activities peptides derived from casein. *J Nutr Biochem* 11:128–131.

86. Rival SG, Boeriu CG, Wichers HJ (2001) Caseins and caseinhydrolysates. 2. Antioxidative properties and relevance to lipoxygenase inhibition. *J Agri Food Chem* 49:295–302

87. Kudoh Y, Matsuda S, Igoshi K, Oki T (2001) Antioxidative peptide from milk fermented with *Lactobacillus delbrueckii* subsp. *Bulgaricus*. IFO13953. *J Jap Soc Food Sci* 48:44–50.

88. Kullisaar T, Songisepp E, Mikelsaar M, Zilmer K, Vihalemm T, Zilmer M (2003) Antioxidative probiotic fermented goats' milk decreases oxidative stress mediated atherogenicity in human subjects. *British J Nutr* 90:449–456.

89. Hernandez-Ledesma B, Contreras MM, Recio I (2011) Antihypertensive peptides: Production, bioavailability and incorporation into foods. *Adv Colloid Interface Sci* 165:23–35.

90. Power O, Jakeman P, FitzGerald RJ (2013) Antioxidative peptides: Enzymatic production, in vitro and *in vivo* antioxidant activity and potential applications of milk-derived antioxidative peptides. *Amino Acids* 44:797–820.

91. Pena-Ramos EA, Xiong YL (2002) Antioxidant activity of soy protein hydrolyzates in a liposomial system. *J Food Sci* 67:2952–2956.

92. Gibbs BF, Zougman A, Masse R, Mulligan C (2004) Production and characterization of bioactive peptides from soy hydrolysate and soy-fermented food. *Food Res Int* 37:123–131.

93. Huma N, Rafiq S, Sameen A, Pasha I, Khan MI (2018) Antioxidant potential of buffalo and cow milk Cheddar cheeses to tackle human colon adenocarcinoma (Caco-2) cells. *Asian-Aust J Animal Sci* 31:287–292.

94. Sah BNP, Vasiljevic T, McKechnie S, Donkor ON (2015) Identification of anticancer peptides from bovine milk proteins and their potential roles in management of cancer: A critical review. *Compr Rev Food Sci Food Saf* 14:123–138.

95. Gupta A, Mann B, Kumar R, Sangwan RB (2009) Antioxidant activity of Cheddar cheeses at different stages of ripening. *Int J Dairy Technol* 62:339–347.

96. Suetsuna K, Ukeda H, Ochi H (2000) Isolation and characterization of free radical scavenging activities peptides derived from casein. *J Nutr Biochem* 11:128–131.

97. Rafiq S, Huma N, Pasha I, Shahid M, Xiao H (2016) Angiotensin-converting enzyme-inhibitory and anti-thrombotic activities of soluble peptide extracts from buffalo and cow milk Cheddar cheeses. *Int J Dairy Technol* 69:1–9.

98. Fan HY, Fu FH, Yan M, Xu HY, Zhang AH, Liu K (2010) Antiplatelet and antithrombotic activities of salvianolic acid A. *Thromb Res* 126:17–22.

99. Almoosa K (2002) Is thrombolytic therapy effective for pulmonary embolism. *Am Fam Physician* 65:1097–1102.

100. Silvia SV, Malcata FX (2005) Caseins as source of bioactive peptides. *Int Dairy J* 15:1–15.
101. Gomez-Ruiz JA, Recio I, Pihlanto A (2005) Antibacterial activity of ovine casein hydrolysates: A preliminary study. *Milchwissenschaft* 60:41–44.
102. Jolles P, Levy-Toledano S, Fiat A, Soria M, Gillessen C, Thomaidis D, Dunn A, Caen JP (1986) Analogy between fibrinogen and case in: Effect of an undecapeptide isolated from κ-casein on platelet function. *Eur J Biochem* 158:379–384.
103. Raha S, Dosquet C, Abgrall JF, Jollès P, Fiat AM, Caen JP (1988) KRDS a tetrapeptide derived from lactotransferrin inhibits binding of monoclonal antibody against glycoprotein IIb-IIIa on ADP-stimulated platelets and megakaryocytes. *Blood* 72:172–178.
104. Qian Y, Melikian HE, Rye DB, Levey AI, Blakely RD (1995) Identification and characterization of antidepressant sensitive serotonin transporter proteins using site specific antibodies. *J Neurosci* 15:1261–1274.
105. Nagaoka I, Hirota S, Niyonsaba FO, Hirata M, Adachi Y, Tamura H, Heumann D (2001) Cathelicidin family of antibacterial peptides CAP18 and CAP11 Inhibit the expression of TNF-OE± by blocking the binding of LPS to CD14+ Cells. *J Immunol* 167:3329–3338.
106. Murray BA, FitzGerald RJ (2007) Angiotensin converting enzyme inhibitory peptides derived from food proteins: Biochemistry, bioactivity and production. *Curr Pharm Des* 13:773–791.
107. Fiat AM, Migliore-Samour D, Jolles P, Drouet L, Sollier CB, Caen J (1993) Biologically active peptides from milk with emphasis on two examples concerning antithrombotic and immunomodulating activities. *J Dairy Sci* 76:301–310.
108. Perdigon G, Moreno D, LeBlanc A, Valdez J, Rachid M (2002) Role of yoghurt in the prevention of colon cancer. *Eur J Clin Nutr* 56:65–68.
109. Kandaswami C, Lee LT, Lee PP, Hwang JJ, Ke FC, Huang YT, Lee MT (2005) The antitumor activities of flavonoids. *In Vivo* 19:895–909.
110. Wakabayashi H, Yamauchi K, Takase M (2006) Lactoferrin research, technology and applications. *Int Dairy J* 16:1241–1251.
111. Roy MK, Kuwabara Y, Hara K, Watanabe Y, Tamai Y (2002) Peptides from the N-Terminal End of Bovine Lactoferrin Induce Apoptosis in Human Leukemic (HL-60) Cells. *J Dairy Sci* 85:2065–2074.
112. Moreno DE, de LeBlanc A, Matar C, LeBlanc N, Perdigon G (2005) Effects of milk fermented by *Lactobacillus helveticus* R389 on a murine breast cancer model. *Breast Cancer Res* 7:477–486.
113. Mader JS, Salsman J, Conrad DM, Hoskin DW (2005) Bovine lactoferricin selectively induces apoptosis in human leukemia and carcinoma cell lines. *Mol Cancer Ther* 4:612–624.
114. Jaiswal M, LaRusso NF, Burgart LJ, Gores GJ (2000) Inflammatory cytokines induce DNA damage and inhibit DNA repair in cholangiocarcinoma cells by a nitric oxide-dependent mechanism. *Cancer Res* 60:184–190.
115. Pepe G, Tenore GC, Mastrocinque R, Stusio P, Campiglia P (2013) Potential anti-carcinogenic peptides from bovine milk. *J Amino Acids* 9:39–41.
116. Hosono A, Shashikanth KN, Otani H (1988) Antimutagenic activity of whole casein on pepper-induced mutagenicity to streptomycin-dependent strain SD 510 of *Salmonella typhimurium* TA 98. *J Dairy Res* 55:435–442.
117. Bosselaers IM, Caessens PR, Van Boekel MS, Alink GM (1994) Differential effects of milk proteins, BSA and soy protein on 4NQO- or MNNG-induced SCEs in V79 cells. *Food Chem Toxicol* 32:905–911.
118. Troncon Rosa F, Zulet MA, Marchini JS, Martinez JA (2012) Bioactive compounds with effects on inflammation markers in humans. *Int J Food Sci Nutr* 63:749–765.
119. Bernstein CN, Fried M, Krabshuis JH, Cohen H, Eliakim R, Fedail S (2009) World gastroenterology organisation practice guidelines for the diagnosis and management of IBD in 2010. *Inflamm Bowel Dis* 16:112–124.
120. Chung HY, Cesari M, Anton S, Marzetti E, Giovannini S, Seo AY (2009) Molecular inflammation: Underpinnings of aging and age related diseases. *Ageing Res Rev* 8:18–30.
121. Lee C, Beuchat LR (1991) Changes in chemical composition and sensory qualities of peanut milk fermented with lactic acid bacteria. *Int J Food Microb* 13(4):273–83.
122. Pacher P, Beckman JS, Liaudet L (2007) Nitric oxide and peroxynitrite in health and disease. *Physiol Rev* 87:315–424.
123. Ritchlin CT, Haas-Smith SA, Li P (2003) Mechanisms of TNF-alpha-and RANKL-mediated osteoclastogenesis and bone resorption in psoriatic arthritis. *J Clin Invest* 111:821–831.
124. Kuper H, Adami HO, Trichopoulos D (2000) Infections as a major preventable cause of human cancer. *J Int Med* 248:171–183.

125. Nair J, Strand S, Frank N, Knauft J, Wesch H, Galle PR, Bartsch H (2005) Apoptosis and age-dependant induction of nuclear and mitochondrial etheno-DNA adducts in Long–Evans cinnamon (LEC) rats: Enhanced DNA damage by dietary curcumin upon copper accumulation. *Carcinogenesis* 26:1307–1315.

126. Pellegrini A, Dettling C, Thomas U, Hunziker P (2001) Isolation and characterization of four domains in the bovine β-lacto-globulin. *Biochim Biophys Acta* 1526:131–140.

127. Chandan CR (2007) Milk composition, physical and processing characteristics. In: Hui YH (Ed.) *Handbook of food products manufacturing*. John Wiley & Sons, Hoboken, NJ.

128. Bellamy W, Takase M, Wakabayashi H, Kawase K, Tomita M (1992) Antibacterial spectrum of lactoferricin B, a potent bactericidal peptide derived from the N-terminal region of bovine lactoferrin. *J Appl Bacteriol* 73:472–479.

129. Minervini F, Algaron F, Rizzello CG, Fox PF, Monnet V, Gobbetti M (2003) Angiotensin I-converting-enzyme-inhibitory and antibacterial peptides from *Lactobacillus helveticus* PR4 proteinase hydrolyzed caseins of milk from six species. *Appl Environ Microbiol* 69:5297–5305.

130. Lee JE, Kim M, Choi H, Ko JK, Lee C, Cho Y, Kim B, Yang K, Kwon JE (2012) A case of adhesive small bowel obstruction with pelvic inflammatory disease due to Chlamydia trachomatis. *Korean J Obstet Gynecol* 55:278–284.

131. Lòpez-Expòsito I, Recio I (2006) Antibacterial activity of peptides folding variants from milk proteins. *Int Dairy J* 16:1294–1305.

132. Tomita M, Bellamy W, Takase M, Yamanchi K, Wakabayashi H, Kawase K (1991) Antibacterial peptides generated by pepsin digestion of bovine lactoferrin. *J Dairy Sci* 74:4137–4144.

133. Recio I, Visser S (2000) Antibacterial and binding characteristics of bovine, ovine and caprine lactoferrins: A comparative study. *Int Dairy J* 10:597–605.

134. Haque E, Chand R (2008) Antihypertensive and antimicrobial bioactive peptides from milk proteins. *Eur Food Res Technol* 227:7–15.

135. Gomez-Ruiz JA, Ramos M, Recio I (2002) Angiotensin-I-converting enzyme inhibitory peptides in Manchego cheeses manufactured with different starter cultures. *Int Dairy J* 12:697–706.

136. Parodi PW (2007) A role of milk proteins and their peptides in cancer prevention. *Curr Pharm Des* 13:813–828.

137. Aro A, Männistö S, Salminen I, Ovaskainen ML, Kataja V, Uusitupa M (2000) Inverse association between dietary and serum conjugated linoleic acid and risk of breast cancer in postmenopausal women. *Nutr Cancer* 38(2):151–157.

138. Collomb M, Schmid A, Sieber R, Wechsler D, Ryhänen EL (2006) Conjugated linoleic acids in milk fat: Variation and physiological effects. *Int Dairy J* 16:1347–1361.

139. Jensen RG (2002) The composition of bovine milk lipids: January 1995 to December 2000. *J Dairy Sci* 85:295–350.

140. Larsson SC, Bergkvist L, Wolk A (2005) High-fat dairy food and conjugated linoleic acid intakes in relation to colorectal cancer incidence in the Swedish Mammography Cohort. *Am J Clin Nutr* 82:894–900.

141. Park Y, Leitzmann MF, Subar AF, Hollenbeck A, Schatzkin A (2008) Dairy food, calcium, and risk of cancer in the NIH-AARP diet and health study. *Arch Intern Med* 169:391–401.

142. Varnam AH, Sutherland JP (1994) *Milk and Milk Products*. Chapman & Hall, New York.

143. Mehra R, Kelly P (2006) Milk oligosaccharides: Structural and technological aspects. *Int Dairy J* 16:1334–1340.

144. Kunz C, Rudloff S, Baier W, Klein N, Strobel S (2000) Oligosaccharides in human milk. Structural, functional and metabolic aspects. *Ann Rev Nutr* 20:699–722.

145. Kunz C, Rudloff S (2002) Health benefits of milk-derived carbohydrates. *Bull Int Dairy Fed* 375:72–79.

146. Martinez-Ferez A, Rudloff S, Guadix A, Henkelm CA, Pohlentz G, Boza JJ (2006) Goat's milk as a natural source of lactose- derived oligosaccharides: Isolation by membrane technology. *Int Dairy J* 16:173–181.

147. Gopal PK, Gill HS (2000) Oligosaccharides and glycoconjugates in bovine milk and colostrum. *Brit J Nutr* 84:69–74.

148. Gauthier SF, Pouliot Y, Maubois JL (2006) Growth factors from bovine milk and colostrum: Composition, extraction and biological activities. *Le Lait* 86:99–125.

149. Dunbar AJ, Priebe IK, Belford DA, Goddard C (1999) Identification of betacellulin as a major peptide growth factor in milk: Purification, characterization and molecular cloning of bovine betacellulin. *Biochem J* 44:713–721.

150. Gaucheron F (2011) Milk and dairy products: A unique micronutrient combination. *J Am Coll Nutr* 30:400–409.

151. Little EM, Holt C (2004) An equilibrium thermodynamic model of the sequestration of calcium phosphate by casein phosphopeptides. *Eur Biophys J* 33:435–447.
152. Miller BDD, Welch RM (2013) Food system strategies for preventing micronutrient malnutrition. *Food Policy* 42:115–128.
153. Krishnan AV, Feldman D (2011) Mechanisms of the anti-cancer and anti-inflammatory actions of vitamin D. *Annu Rev Pharmacol Toxicol* 51:311–336.
154. Mamede AC, Tavares SD, Abrantes AM, Trindade J, Maia JM, Botelho MF (2011) The role of vitamins in cancer: A review. *Nutr Cancer* 63:479–494.
155. Patel A, Zhan Y (2012) Vitamin D in cardiovascular disease. *Int J Prev Med* 3:664.
156. Chun RF, Adams JS, Hewison M (2011) Immunomodulation by vitamin D: Implications for TB. *Expert Rev Clin Pharmacol* 4:583–591.

11 Safety and Quality Aspects of Animal Origin Foods

Tahir Zahoor, Atif Liaqat, and Nehdia Azhar

CONTENTS

11.1 INTRODUCTION

The search for food has influenced human economic, social, and political development throughout history, which also played a role in the organization of history and society. Foods from animal origins constitute human diet inducing a broad range of multifaceted scientific, economic, environmental, and political issues. These are viewed to be the most expensive component of diets; however, foods from animal origins provide high quantities of essential nutrients [1]. Livestock, such as cows, buffalos, goats, sheep, chickens, pigs, and lesser-known species, can be useful for human in various ways. Foods from these sources provide complete, easily digestible, high quality protein along with numerous essential micronutrients, such as calcium, zinc, iron, vitamins A, and B_{12}. On the contrary, overconsumption of some foods, especially those containing high amounts of cholesterol, saturated fat, salt (sodium), and total energy are associated with obesity, overweight, and followed by other lifestyle related disorders [2]. Moreover, foods of animal origin contain high quality nutrients being more readily absorbed [1].

Worldwide, quantity and quality are the main nutritional challenges to overcome diet deficiencies, predominantly in developing world. Accessibility and consumption of total energy in terms of kilo calories is the main concern of diet quantity, while diet quality is its ability to provide high biologic value protein (all essential amino acids) and adequate amounts of micronutrients (vitamins and minerals). Both quality and quantity of diet are equally important [3]. Food from animal origins contain readily digestible protein and a dense amount of energy. Protein from these sources contain all essential amino acids and highly similar to the protein of human body with respect to amino acids composition [4].

11.1.1 MEAT AND MEAT PRODUCTS

Meat and meat products are important in human diet, which can be seen by making their comparison with diet including maize and beans. In a child, consumption of 1.7–2.0 kg per day of maize and beans can meet the average daily requirements for energy, zinc, and iron, which is far beyond the amount a child, can tolerate. While consumption of 60 g (2 oz) of meat per day can fulfill the same requirement. Moreover, micronutrients in these foods are more readily available. Although iron, zinc, and calcium are present in relatively higher amounts in some plant foods, such as spinach and legumes; however, micronutrients from these foods are poorly absorbed. High amounts of oxalate in leafy plants form insoluble compounds, which reduce intestinal absorption of minerals. Similarly, high amount of phytates and fiber, chiefly found in unfermented or uncooked seeds, nuts, and cereals grains can also make insoluble complexes with calcium, zinc, and iron, reducing their availability. Similarly, high amounts of tannins are found in coffee, tea leaves, and spinach that also inhibit absorption of calcium, zinc, and iron. However, in meat, iron and zinc are associated with heme protein, which is readily incorporated into blood cells [5–7].

11.1.2 MILK AND MILK PRODUCTS

Milk and milk products have a significant role in nourishing, both urban and rural populations, because of its high nutritional value. Milk is the single most perfectly balanced food in nature and contains almost all nutrients in the right proportion and easily digestible form. Along with its products, it is nutritious, economical, potable, refreshing, and a convenient food for human beings. Produced on daily basis, milk is either sold for cash or processed into products [8–10]. Moreover, milk and its products are good sources of calcium [4].

11.1.3 FISH AND FISH PRODUCTS

Fish is an outstanding source of high quality animal protein. Also, it contains micronutrients and essential fatty acids, particularly long-chain polyunsaturated ones [11]. Worldwide, average annual per capita consumption of seafood was up to 16 kg around 2005, which ranged from less than 1 kg to over 90 kg depending on the country [12]. Fish and fish products can be classified as a functional food. Polyunsaturated fatty acids in fish especially those belonging to omega-3 family have a number of benefits such as improvement of body functions, reduction in cancer susceptibility and cardiovascular diseases [13]. Meat and fish also provide riboflavin, selenium, taurine, and pentaenoic and hexaenoic acids abundantly [4].

11.1.4 EGGS AND EGG PRODUCTS

Egg is a nutrient dense food, playing an important part in diet both alone or as a component with other foods [13]. These are economical sources of food and contain a complete protein. The World Health Organization (WHO) considers eggs to be the reference protein all around the world; that is, all other proteins are compared with it. The biological value of its protein is hundred and it contains all essential amino acids in a well-balanced proportion. Eggs also contain vitamins; A, D, E, and other water-soluble ones, and minerals—iron, zinc, phosphorous, potassium, iodine, and sulfur [14].

11.2 ISSUES AND HAZARDS ASSOCIATED WITH FOODS OF ANIMAL ORIGIN

Food safety, starting from the farm, acts as prerequisite for a food producer to survive in the market [12]. Improper handling of foods from animal origin can pose potential threats to human health. These foods may get contaminated with physical, chemical, or biological hazards at various steps of the supply chain. Pathogens and chemical residues can contaminate these foods during production at the farm or during transportation, storage, delivery, and preparation for consumption. Contamination may also occur from unhygienic handling and from diseased animals [15]. According to estimation, hundreds of millions of people are affected by foodborne diseases of animal origin annually, especially in developing countries. Moreover, globalization has also made food safety an international issue as import of contaminated foods from producing countries may result in disease outbreaks in importing countries [16–18].

11.2.1 PHYSICAL HAZARDS

Physical hazards are foreign materials, such as glass, wood, metal, pest, insulation, plastic, dirt, and others, which can cause illness or injury to the user. These may be present in milk because of contamination [19]. In poultry, these include bone, glass, metal, and plastics [20]. On farms, the probability of contamination of physical hazards to the final products is supposed to be minimal. However, their contamination on the farm must be removed at this step. In the case of milk, physical contaminants are removed by filtration used by most dairy farms. In the past, introduction of these hazards during processing has occasionally happened [19,21,22].

11.2.2 CHEMICAL HAZARDS

Chemical hazards include antibiotics and other animal drugs; agricultural chemicals, such as fertilizer, herbicides, insecticides, pesticides, and rodenticides; allergens; naturally occurring toxins or toxic chemicals from industrial processes; food additives; and cleaning residues. These can contaminate food indirectly through plants and animals or directly during processing [23]. Table 11.1 summarizes the association of various chemical hazards with food products of animal origin and diseases due to those hazards.

11.2.2.1 Antibiotic Residues

Antibiotic residues can enter into animal products through various ways, such as their use for disease prevention, as growth promoters, or illegal uses [24]. Animals grown in high stock and closed confinement experience high stress, which favor incidence and spread of infectious diseases. Therefore,

TABLE 11.1
Association of Different Hazards with Food of Animal Origin

Hazard Type	Chemical Nature	Examples	Foods Associated with	Diseases
Physical Hazards		Glass, plastic, metal, bone, pests, dirt, dust	Poultry meat	Injuries or other illnesses
Chemical Hazards	Antibiotic residues	Chlortetracycline, erythromycin, gentamycin, penicillin, sulphaquinoxaline etc.	Meat, milk, fish and their products	Allergy, antibiotic resistance in bacteria, disturb intestinal microflora, cancer
	Biogenic amines	Histamine, cadaverine, putrescine, tryptamine, Tyramine, etc.	Meat, milk, fish and their products	Headaches, migraines, intestinal and gastric problems, pseudo-allergic reactions
	Heavy metals and radioactive elements	Lead, mercury, Iodine 89, Strontium 90, Barium140	Poultry meat, milk	
	Hormones	Steroid, bovine growth hormones	Milk	Endocrine disruption
	Insecticide and pesticide residues	DDT, dieldrin	Poultry meat, milk and milk products	
	Microbial toxins	Ochratoxin A, aflatoxin	Poultry meat, milk	Carcinogenic, mutagenic, hepatotoxic, tetratogenic
Biological Hazards	*Mycobacterium*		Meat, milk, and milk products	Tuberculosis
	Brucella		Milk, infected animal products	Brucellosis
	Bacillus		Milk	Gastroenteritis
	Campylobacter spp.		Undercooked meat, milk	Campylobacteriosis
	Clostridium		Poultry meat, fish	
	Escherichia		Meat, milk	Haemorrhagic colitis, haemolytic ureamic syndrome
	Helicobacter		Milk	Stomach cancer
	Listeria		Meat, milk	Listeriosis
	Staphylococcus		Meat, milk	Pyogenic infections, boils, pustules, skin lesions
	Streptococci		Milk	Sore throat, scarlet fever
	Salmonella		Meat, milk, eggs	Gastroenteritis, typhoid fever
	Shigella		Milk	Dysentery
	Viruses		Milk and ready-to-eat foods	Hepatitis
	Parasites		Undercooked meat	Cysticercosis, hydatidosis

Source: Karshima, N.S., *Rev. J. Anim. Prod. Adv.*, 3, 57–68, 2013; Mead, G.C., *Poultry Meat Processing and Quality*, Elsevier, Oxford, UK, 2004; Girma, K. et al., *World J. Dairy Food Sci.*, 9, 166–183, 2014; Adams, M.R., and Moss, M.O., *Food Microbiology*, RSC Publishing, Cambridge, UK, 2008.

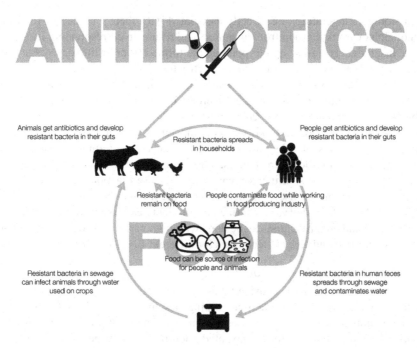

FIGURE 11.1 Bacterial resistance and transfer in humans, animals and foodstuffs. (From Kirbis, A., and Krizmana, M., *Proc. Food Sci.*, 5, 148–151, 2015.)

antibiotics are regularly administered to animals through feed, water, or injection for the treatment of diseases or their prevention. A part of this administered medicine is metabolized in animal's body, while the rest is eliminated through feces or urine. Pollution of soil, surface, as well as ground water also occurs through these excreted drugs and their metabolites [25]. Figure 11.1 shows the occurrence of bacterial resistance and transfer of bacteria in humans, animals, and food stuffs. Chlortetracycline and sulphaquinoxaline are the antimicrobial residues that may be present in poultry meat [20]. Treatment of dairy animals frequently involves intramammary infusion of antibiotics for mastitis control. Some drugs are also used to control ecto- and endo-parasites, as well as to increase milk production [26]. There are five major classes of commonly used antibiotics in dairy animals, including the tetracyclines (e.g. oxytetracycline, tetracycline, and chlortetracycline), beta-lactams (e.g. penicillins and cephalosporins), amino glycosides (e.g. streptomycine, neomycin, and gentamycin), macrolides (e.g. erythromycin), and sulfanomides (e.g. sulfamethazines). After treatment, quantifiable levels of antibiotic are usually detected in milk for some days [22,27]. Besides cattle and poultry, antibiotics are also used extensively in aquaculture to treat bacterial diseases, usually for prevention of disease occurrence. Unlike terrestrial animals, these drugs are directly or indirectly administered to culture water. Consequently, these chemicals or their metabolites also affect the non-target organisms, such as bacteria and algae. These antibiotics become risks to consumers when they exceed the thresholds levels [25] and can result in numerous potential health problems, like allergies. Their use can also develop resistance in bacteria and can make it difficult or impossible to make products from milk [15]. While the overuse of amino glycosides, sulfonamides, and tetracyclines in cattle production and their residues in food products cause allergic reactions, their therapeutic or sub-therapeutic levels may disturb the microflora in the human gut. Moreover, dimetridazole and nitrofurans can lead to carcinogenicity problems [22].

11.2.2.2 Biogenic Amines (BAs)

These low-molecular weight substances are primarily produced by amino acid decarboxylase enzymes from some microorganisms. These are tested in foods due to their toxicity and as food quality indicators [28]. Different factors, such as spoilage or starter bacteria, amino acid composition packing, and storage temperature, are directly associated with their presence in food items [29]. Elimination of alpha-carboxyl group from an amino acid results in corresponding Biogenic Amines (BAs); that is, histamine, tyramine, and tryptamine are formed from histidine, tyrosine, and tryptophan, respectively [30,31]. Based on the chemical structure, number of amine groups, biosynthesis, or physiological functions, these bioactive amines can be classified into various groups [32]. Therefore, these can be aliphatic, aromatic, or heterocyclic; monoamines, diamines or polyamines; natural or biogenic; polyamines and biogenic amines [32–35].

Besides spoiled foods, fermented foods also contain significant amounts of BAs [30,36]. Eating foods containing high levels of BAs can result in headaches, migraines, intestinal and gastric problems, as well as pseudo-allergic responses. These foodborne diseases chiefly result from the toxic action of tyramine and histamine, known as the "cheese reaction" and "histamine poisoning," respectively. Symptoms of disease appear after some minutes or a few hours of food ingestion [30,33,34,37]. Meat, fish, dairy, and fermented products are likely to contain high levels of BAs. Their detection and quantification can be done with high performance liquid chromatography, which is a highly sensitive and reliable technique for different BAs [33,37].

11.2.2.2.1 BAs in Meat and Meat Products

The presence of BAs in meat can be considered as a marker of freshness or bad conservation [38]. Fermented foods made from high protein-containing raw material, such as fermented sausages, show elevated amounts of BAs [39]. Their presence in meat and meat products can also be used as a quality index tool and as an indicator of unwanted microbial activity. Numerous factors affect the concentration of these amines, such as type and degree of contamination of raw material, manufacturing practices, and the use of starter culture [35]. Bioactive amines have been found in various chicken-based products, like frankfurters, mortadella, meatballs, and nuggets. However, these products have usually lower levels of biogenic amines [40].

11.2.2.2.2 BAs in Milk and Milk Products

Milk and milk products indicate elevated level of histamine due to improper processing. Fresh milk generally contains a very small amount of histamine, while commercially available Pasteurized or UHT milk demonstrates a little higher histamine content. Upon fermentation of milk, often a significant rise in histamine contents occurs and a drastic increase is seen in cheese production [31]. Spermine and spermidine have been found as the major amines in the raw milk from goats. Similarly, tyramine is the major amine in cheese produced from raw milk, while putrescine and cadaverine are mainly present in cheese made from pasteurized milk. Polyamines are most abundantly found in milk [32,41].

11.2.2.2.3 BAs in Fish and Fish Products

Among amines, histamine is the most frequent foodborne intoxication, also known as scombroid poisoning. Scombroid (bonito, tuna, mackerel, and saury) and non-scombroid fish species (amberjack, salmon, mahi-mahi, herring, sardines, marlin, bluefish, etc.) contain elevated histidine levels in their flesh. Histamine at high concentrations is a risk factor for food intoxication, while at moderate levels may result in food intolerance [30,32,36,42]. A significant amount of BAs has been found in fish products, principally those produced in all Southeast Asian countries. Sauces, canned, smoked-dried, and packed seafood are usually designated as a potential risk for BAs intoxication [32,43].

11.2.2.3 Hormone Residue

11.2.2.3.1 Steroid Hormones

Milk may contain sufficient amounts of steroid hormones. Fat content of dairy products affects the quantities of lipophilic hormones as estrogen and progesterone rise with fat. Processing operations, like churning and heating, do not affect their amounts in dairy products. In fresh and ripened cheese, testosterone has been found up to 0.1–0.5 mg kg^{-1} [22,44].

11.2.2.3.2 Bovine Growth Hormones

Bovine Growth Hormone (BGH), or Bovine Somatotropin (BST), is a protein product of genetic engineering that is similar to the natural bovine pituitary hormone. Its main function is to raise milk production in milk-producing animals, so BST administered cows eat enough feed quantities to fulfill their energy needs for extra milk synthesis. The United States (US) Food and Drug Administration (FDA) stated this hormone as safe in 1993, but it can rise the occurrence of mastitis in some animals, such as cows and ewes. Consequently, higher use of antibiotics for mastitis treatment may result in increased drug residues in milk. Therefore, BGH is not a risk for human health, instead it is the presence of antibiotic residues used for treatment of udder infections that pose the risk [22,45].

11.2.2.4 Pesticides and Insecticides Residue

Pesticides include a broad range of chemicals like fungicides, herbicides, insecticides, rodenticides, and plant growth regulators. Carbamates, organochlorines, organophosphates, and pyrethroids are some examples of pesticides [46]. Animals can ingest pesticide residues through contaminated feed. Consumption of such animals as food can make their way into the human body [15].

Dieldrin and DDT might be present in poultry meat as pesticide residues [20]. Pesticide treatment in fields results in contamination of feeds. Chlorinated pesticides, Dioxins, DDT, and Polychlorinated biphenyls (PCBs) can enter into milk and milk products. Chlorinated hydrocarbons are highly strong, persistent, endocrine disrupting, bioaccumulating, and widely distributed toxic compounds. While controlling environmental or animal pests, these chemicals make their way in to the food chain [47].

Around 20% of administered chlorinated hydrocarbon is released in milk. These chlorinated hydrocarbons adhere to milk fat; thus, higher proportions are found in butter. DDT may accumulate in fatty tissues and released into milk [48].

11.2.2.5 Mycotoxins Residue

Several poisonous metabolites are produced by some molds under appropriate temperatures and moisture conditions. These toxic metabolites are harmful to human health and called mycotoxins [49]. Cattle feed, with growth of fungi, can transfer aflatoxins to milk, and they are known as M1, M2, M4, and so on. These toxins may appear in milk within 48 hours of eating contaminated feed. Some of these toxins are carcinogenic so their control is highly advisable. Aflatoxin M1 (AFM1) is found in milk of animals when they are given feed contaminated with Aflatoxin B1 (AFB1). Mycotoxins are described to be carcinogenic, mutagenic, hepatotoxic, and tetratogenic in most animals and humans [22].

11.2.2.6 Heavy Metals Residue

Lead and mercury are the heavy metals that may be present in poultry meat [20]. Similarly, lead, arsenic, mercury, cadmium, and others are the heavy metals reported in milk. These heavy metals enter into the human body primarily by ingestion and inhalation routes. Children are more sensitive to these metals than adults. While copper and zinc are the essential micronutrients, which take part in different biochemical functions in all living organisms, they can be toxic in excess amount [50]. Radioactive substances are rarely found in milk. Major radioactive substances include Iodine 89, Strontium 90, Barium 140 [20].

11.3 MICROBIAL HAZARDS

Foodborne bacteria are diverse groups present everywhere in food production areas, including soil, freshwater, marine ecosystems, and so forth. They are also present in the food processing areas, such as the food industry or restaurants [51]. Their presence can be seen in red meat, poultry, seafood processing, and storage areas. Fresh meat and most of its products provide a favorable medium for growth of microorganisms. Therefore, the microbiological safety is important throughout the food chain, starting from slaughter of the animals to the finished product [12]. Table 11.1 summarizes the association of various microbiological hazards with food products of animal origin and diseases due to those hazards.

Milk is virtually a sterile fluid at the time of secretion into the udder's alveoli. Beyond this stage, microbial contamination occurs usually from three major sources—interior of udder, exterior of udder, and milk handling and storage equipment. Other possible sources may include feed, soil, surrounding air, feces, and grass. Contamination may also occur at other stages like procurement, processing, and distribution. Diseased animals, environment and unhygienic workers milking the animal can also cause contamination. Milk in raw or processed form is a good growth medium, supporting the growth of numerous microorganisms. Therefore, microbial safety of dairy products with respect to foodborne diseases is considered important all around the globe, particularly in developing countries. Several bacteria such as *Lactobacillus, Streptococcus, Enterobacter, Salmonella, coliforms, Klebsiella, Listeria, Corynebacterium, Pseudomonas, Acinetobacter, Flavibacterium, B. subtilis, S. aureus* can be isolated from raw milk [10]. Eggs also require careful handling, like any other perishable commodities. Contamination of eggs with *S. typhimurium, S. enteriditis, E. coli,* and similar pathogens can result in serious human health problems [12].

11.3.1 MYCOBACTERIUM

The Mycobacterium genus mainly consists of harmless environmental organisms; however, it can sometimes be foodborne and cause tuberculosis (TB) and leprosy. The species are generally Gram-positive, non-spore forming. *Mycobacterium bovis* is mesophilic bacterium [52] and a member of *Mycobacterium tuberculosis* complex, which is responsible for bovine tuberculosis [53,54]. It is a contagious and chronic infectious bacterial zoonosis of domesticated animals, wildlife species, and humans [55]. The disease forms granulomas in tissues particularly in, lymph nodes, lungs, liver, intestines and kidney [56] *Mycobacterium bovis* shows resistance against drugs that are used against *Mycobacterium tuberculosis* [57]. Tuberculosis has been eradicated in most developed countries; however, it still persists in developing countries [58].

Mycobacterium bovis is shed in milk, feces, respiratory secretions, and sometimes in urine, semen, or vaginal secretions of cattle. Transmission among cattle mostly occurs with aerosols during close contact. Raw or undercooked meat can also be source of this organism, but ingestion of unpasteurized dairy products is the primary route of infection in humans. This organism can also infect through breaks in the skin. Pasteurization can destroy this organism [22]. Human tuberculosis continues to be reported from poorly controlled bovine disease areas. The incidence is higher in workers working with animals. Humans can also get infection from other species, such as goats, seals, and rhinoceros. The symptoms of respiratory infection in humans may include cough, fever, chest pain, and so on [22,59,60].

11.3.2 BRUCELLA

Bacteria from the genus Brucella cause infectious disease known as brucellosis, a widespread and globally distributed disease [61]. Brucellosis has been reported in humans, domestic animals, and in many wildlife species across Africa with more than 500,000 reported cases annually around the globe. It is one of the examples of milk-borne zoonosis. In various parts of world, three major species of Brucella; *Brucella melitensis, Brucella suis,* and *Brucella abortus,* have been isolated from milk of dairy animals, all of which can infect humans. *Brucella melitensis* causes severe infection in humans [15,62].

Contact with infected animals or consumption of their products can result in human infections [63]. Symptoms of disease may include headache, sweats, physical weakness, fatigue, back, and joint pain. Heart lining or central nervous systems may also be severely infected. Common sources of human infection include goats, sheep, and buffalos [64,65]. These organisms can be destroyed by pasteurization [62].

11.3.3 Bacillus

Contamination of bacillus spores in raw milk often occurs at the farm. However, incidence of *Bacillus cereus* in raw milk can be reduced by following sanitation of the teats prior to milking. Processed dairy product may contain this bacterium because of the survival of spores to pasteurization. It may colonize in tanks, pipes, and filling machines [66].

11.3.4 Campylobacter

Campylobacters are characterized by non-spore forming, Gram-negative, and oxidase-positive rods [53]. These are responsible for campylobacteriosis. The disease causes zoonotic diarrhea in both developed and developing countries. Human infection is caused by domestic animals, particularly poultry. *Campylobacter coli* and *Campylobacter jejuni* are the main causes of acute bacterial food-borne gastroenteritis. Transmission of these bacteria from animals has been recognized with the highest risk in children. Species of campylobacter can live in the intestinal tract of domestic ruminants and swine [15]. As commensals, these can exist in domestic poultry and livestock. However, in humans these can show clinical signs like low fever, headache, myalgia, and enteritis. Acute campylobacteriosis frequently starts with abdominal cramps followed by a high fever and diarrhea during the initial days of disease [15,67].

Campylobacter either can live as a normal commensal organism or can cause subclinical infections in animals including rodents, cattle, and wild birds. Some insects can also carry this organism on their exoskeleton. Outbreaks have been reported due to milk, and pasteurization generally eliminates the organism. Several reports have been published on the detection of *Campylobacter* in farm bulk tanks [68].

Consumption of undercooked meat, undercooked infected poultry, unpasteurized milk and water contaminated with faeces of infected animals can result in human infection. Several workers have reported campylobacteriosis in humans, animals and milk [15]. In UK, *Campylobacter jejuni* has resulted in severe outbreaks of enteritis in the recent years due to consumption of unpasteurized milk. Symptoms of the disease are profuse diarrhea (sometimes bloody), fever, nausea, dizziness and stomach cramps. Pasteurization can destroy this organism [22,69].

11.3.5 Escherichia

Escherichia belong to the family Entero bacteriaceae. The member, *Escherichia coli* is catalase-positive, oxidase-negative, Gram-negative, non-spore forming rod and very closely related to the genus Shigella [52]. *Escherichia coli* is a normal resident of warm-blooded animals. They also reside in human intestines. These can contaminate food products during animal slaughtering and evisceration or during food manipulation [51]. Naturally, it is found in environments like in water, soil, faeces, or the digestive tract of humans and animals. The presence of this organism indicates poor hygiene practices or improper processing. Infection symptoms include fever, vomiting, stomach cramps, and diarrhea. Pasteurization can destroy this organism [70]. *E. coli* O157:H7 is a newly recognized strain, which causes haemorrhagic colitis and haemolytic ureamic syndrome in humans. Haemolytic ureamic syndrome can result in acute renal failure. This organism is found in fecal material and the gut of infected humans and cows. Contamination of milk may result from cow feces or unhygienic handling. Shiga toxin-producing *E. coli*, especially, O157:H7 harbor in cattle; however, it has also been isolated from other animals, such as goat, sheep, horse, dog, pig, and flies [22,71].

11.3.6 Helicobacter

The transmission of *Helicobacter pylori* may occur through contaminated milk. If infection occurs, it can be a strong factor in the development of stomach cancer. Clinical cases require expensive treatment and gastric biopsy is needed for accurate diagnosis in humans. The organism can be destroyed by pasteurization [72].

11.3.7 Listeria

Among different species of Listeria, *Listeria monocytogenes* is an important human pathogen; however, *Listeria ivanovii*, *Listeria seeligeri* and *Listeria welshimeri* have also been associated with human illness, just occasionally [52]. Listeria is divided into eight species. *Listeria monocytogenes* was first detected in rabbits in 1924. It is Gram-positive, catalase positive, oxidase-negative, haemolytic, motile at 20°C–28°C with one to five peritrichous flagella. *L. monocytogenes*, associated with processed meat, results in 2–10 cases per million people in Europe. In 2006, it was found to be the fifth most common zoonotic infection. It is also the most common foodborne pathogen causing deaths in the US [73].

Listeria monocytogenes often contaminates raw poultry. It is rarely found on live birds but makes its way to meat as a result of contamination, especially during processing. Raw meat products containing listeria can cross contaminate other foods in the kitchen, particularly ready-to-eat ones [20]. *Listeria monocytogenes* has gained the highest attention in dairy industry operations. The ability of the organism to grow at low temperatures makes it necessary to obey strict temperature control for its growth restriction. Many studies have been conducted for the detection or surveillance of *Listeria monocytogenes* in bulk tank milk, representing more than 66,000 samples from 24 countries. A little portion of the samples examined showed the absence of the organism that is 641 samples across five countries [74].

This bacterium is naturally found in environment. Consumption of raw milk can lead to interaction with this organism. Infection with this bacterium can result in symptoms such as flu-like illnesses to meningitis. It can also lead to abortion in pregnant women. Infected persons have mortality rate of 30%. Pasteurization can destroy this organism [75].

11.3.8 Staphylococcus

Sir Alexander Ogston, a Scottish surgeon, first stated the Staphylococci as the causing agent of numerous pyogenic (pus producing) infections in humans. In 1882, he named them as 'staphylococcus' (from Greek: *staphyle* meaning a bunch of grapes and *coccus*, a berry or grain), after looking at them under a microscope. *Staphylococcus aureus*, a member of this genus, is a Gram-positive coccus producing spherical to ovoid cells. Cells divides in multiple planes resulting in irregular clumps, which most resemble the grape bunches [52].

Staphylococcus aureus, associated with dairy products, most likely comes from raw milk. Human infections with pathogenic staphylococci commonly lead to boils, pustules, skin lesions, and are often detected in farm workers. Staphylococcus is also frequently detected in older cows from small ulcers on teats or sub-clinical mastitis. Pasteurization can destroy this bacterium; however, its toxin is not destroyed [22,76].

11.3.9 Streptococcus

Group A streptococci, originated from human carriers, can affect udder of animal. The organism causes sore throat, scarlet fever, and mastitis. The organism can rapidly multiply in unpasteurized or inefficiently cooled milk. However, pasteurization can destroy this organism [22,73].

11.3.10 SALMONELLA

Salmonella belongs to the family Enterobacteriaceae, which are Gram-negative, oxidase-negative, catalase-positive, facultative anaerobes, non-spore forming rods, and are generally motile with peritrichous flagella [52]. Bacteria of genus *Salmonella* causes Salmonellosis, a foodborne bacterial zoonosis. Species of *Salmonella enterica* and *Salmonella bongori* belong to this genus and more than 2,400 serotypes have been identified. Zoonotic serotypes of *Salmonella* infect both humans and animals resulting in non-typhoidal salmonellosis. Globally, it is the most common foodborne bacterial disease [77]. Animals may or may not get disease from *Salmonella*. However, these produce diseases in specific species that they are adapted to like *Salmonella abortus ovis* (sheep), *Salmonella gallinarum* (poultry), *Salmonella abortus equi* (horse), *Salmonella cholerae suis* (pigs), and *Salmonella dublin* (cattle). These are also thought to be less pathogenic to humans, but can lead to severe septicemia in immunocompromised people [22,78].

Various studies of *Salmonella* incidence in meat are reported around the world and many go unreported [74]. Numerous serotypes are capable of causing infection in poultry. Usually, these relatively poorly colonize alimentary tract and flourish best in young birds. Invasive strains that can reach internal organs, such as spleen, liver, and reproductive tract, are the most challenging strains for poultry industry [20]. *Salmonella* are not the natural pathogens of milking animals. However, these are transmitted by milk in regions where pasteurization of milk is not compulsory [22,79]. Infection transmits from animals to humans with consumption of undercooked or raw meat, egg, and its products, as well as unpasteurized milk and dairy products. Trade of live animals, contaminated feed, and non-heat-treated animal products can result in the spread of organisms from one region to another [15]. Generally, freshly laid eggs are sterile from the inside, but *Salmonella enteritidis* has been detected in some eggs [14]. Symptoms associated with the infection of this organism include vomiting, nausea, headache, abdominal pain, chills, and diarrhea. Pasteurization can destroy this organism [22,79].

11.3.11 SHIGELLA

Kiyoshi Shiga, a Japanese microbiologist, identified genus Shigella in 1898 as a causing agent of bacillary dysentery. This genus includes four species: *Shigella dysenteriae*, *Shigella boydii*, *Shigella flexneri*, and *Shigella sonnei*. All of these are considered human pathogens, though differ in severity of disease. Shigella belong to family Enterobacteriaceae. These are Gram-negative, oxidase-negative, non-motile, non-spore forming, and facultative anaerobic rods. These produce acid but generally no gas from glucose and are unable to ferment lactose except some strains of *Shigella sonnei*, a characteristic these share with most *Salmonellas* [52].

In humans, shigella infections are often linked with the consumption of raw milk. Its occurrence is worldwide, but common in people living under poor conditions like crowding, malnutrition, and poor sanitation. Milk handlers, flies, and water act as sources of these bacteria. Pasteurization can destroy this organism [22,72].

11.3.12 VIRUSES

These are the smallest microorganisms, which can result in foodborne illnesses. By just looking at a food, one cannot judge their presence. Viruses can contaminate milk through unhealthy animals, hands, milking utensils, or water. These are different from bacteria in the way that these cannot grow in food and simply use the food as a transfer vehicle from one person to another. Mostly, sources of viral foodborne illnesses are water, iced drinks, shellfish, salads, and other ready-to-eat foods. Some of the viruses that contaminate milk and other food stuffs are infectious hepatitis virus, Entero viruses, foot-and-mouth disease virus, and tick-borne Encephalitis virus [22].

11.4 PARASITIC DISEASES

11.4.1 CYSTICERCOSIS

Tapeworms of the genus Taenia at larval stages are responsible for cysticercosis, a foodborne parasitic zoonosis. Serious human cysticercosis is caused by larvae of the beef tapeworm (*Taenia sagina*) and pork tapeworm (*Taenia solium*). Human infection is caused by the consumption of undercooked or raw beef or pork [15].

11.4.2 ECHINOCOCCOSIS (HYDATIDOSIS)

Tapeworms of the genus Echinococcus at larval stages (hydatid cyst) cause hydatidosis, a widespread foodborne parasitic disease [80]. Larvae infect humans, domesticated animals, and a wide range of wildlife species. There are four species from this genus that are a public health concern; *Echinococcus multicularis* causing alveolar echinococcosis, *Echinococcus granulosus* causing cystic echinococcosis, *Echinococcus Oligarthus*, and *Echinococcus vogeli* both have been responsible for polycystic echinococcosis [81]. The disease has a worldwide distribution and poses serious public health concerns, veterinary concerns, and economic reduction to pervasive countries [15].

11.5 SAFETY ASPECTS IN FOODS OF ANIMAL ORIGIN

To guard the consumer from foodborne diseases, integration of all steps in the food supply chain, such as animal feed production, farm practices, transportation and slaughtering of animals, processing, storage, delivery, sale, cooking, and hygienic service, is needed. It links the whole food chain from animal breeding to the time the food is put on the consumer's table. This can simply be adapted in all types of food including meat, fish, milk, eggs, and their products [15].

The risk of physical contamination can be greatly reduced by preventive maintenance of equipment as equipment breakage can make a way for physical hazards to get entry in to foods, generally, during the processing stage. In this regard, routine inspection and maintenance of the equipment is good practice. Moreover, regular inspection of screens or filters can reduce the contamination of objects from equipment, such as broken machine parts or rubber seals. The risk of chemical hazards can be reduced by implementing a management system that identifies sampling points and sampling levels. During processing and storage of milk and milk products, control points for chemical hazards must be identified. Hazard analysis technique can be useful in this regard [22].

Moreover, livestock farmers should be provided training related to food related hazards. Veterinarians must ensure clean handling of animals on farm. Hygienic collection and processing of animal products at farm and their safe transportation are also mandatory. Inspection of live animals and carcasses in slaughterhouse plays a vital role in a surveillance system for animal diseases and their transfer to humans. These also guarantee the safety of meat and its products. Animals can be immunized with vaccines against anthrax and other diseases that ultimately reduces risk for transfer of these diseases to humans. Correct prescription and administration of veterinary drugs are necessary for food safety. Monitoring the usage of these drugs is important for withdrawal periods to control antibiotics in animal products [15].

Cross-contamination must be managed to produce safe food. Production equipment, and processing and storage sites must be sanitized, cleaned, and disinfected regularly. Packing and distribution of products must also be looked after to avoid contamination by any hazard. Moreover, information to consumers about correct storage and heat treatment of the product can further decrease the food safety risks [22].

Several processing and preservation methods can maintain the safety and quality of foods of animal origin. For example, freezing stops increase of microorganisms while thermal processing kills them [22]. There is also rising interest in non-thermal processes, such as pulsed electric fields, oscillating magnetic fields, high-intensity ultrasound, high hydrostatic pressure, and ultraviolet light.

Hurdle technology uses a combination of two or more preservation methods with synergistic or combined antimicrobial effects. Natural antimicrobial compounds, such as bacteriocins or organic acids, have recently been proposed to control foodborne microorganisms. Furthermore, these biological hazards can be controlled by packaging methods and types. Various novel methods, such as filling inert gases (N_2, CO_2 etc) in packaging, active packaging, modified atmosphere packaging, bacteriostatic films, intelligent (indicator) packaging, can also improve stability, safety, and quality of food products including those from animal origin [12]. Several thermal and chemical methods have been developed to control or eradicate *Salmonella enteritidis* in eggs. Use of organic acids, quaternary ammonium compounds, high pH, microwaves, gamma irradiation, ozone are other methods of decontamination that can also be employed separately or in combination [12]. Control of viruses can be best achieved by preventing their entry into food. Once they have entered, cooking might not destroy them [22].

11.5.1 Control/Quality

Safety and quality of foods can be achieved in a good manner by making an integrated, multi-disciplinary approach and applying it to the whole food supply chain. Control or elimination of foodborne hazards at the source point—a preventive approach—can more effectively eliminate or reduce the risk than its control in final product. Traditional control systems involved good practices, such as Good Agricultural Practices and Good Hygienic Practices. From these old systems, current food safety approaches have advanced through more targeted systems based on hazard analysis and critical control points (HACCP) and food safety risk analysis [15]. Use of HACCP is one of the useful methods to control hazards (physical, chemical, biological/microbiological) in foods [22].

Quality refers to the expectations of the clients about a certain product or service. Quality can be achieved through Total Quality Management (TQM), International Standardization Organization systems (ISO), Good manufacturing practices (GMPs), and HACCP. ISO is a laborious, costly, and very non-specific to make it workable for a dairy farmer. However, HACCP is the best choice for a quality control program of dairy farms as it is highly farm specific, cost effective, process and product oriented, requiring less labor, and easy to link with operational management. HACCP involves various procedures to be adopted, such as hazard and risk identification, process breakdown, designation of critical control points, monitoring system, documentation, and verification of the program. TQM can be thought as a merger of HACCP and GMP concepts [82]. HACCP is a written food safety management plan and procedures. It is an internationally recognized system of food safety management and recommended to adopt [73].

Also, there are authorities and administrations concerned with safety and quality. In the US, the United States Department of Agriculture (USDA) controls veterinary drugs, the Food and Drug Administration (FDA) controls additives and chemical resides in processed foods, and the Environmental Protection Agency (EPA) controls chemicals applied at the farm [23].

11.6 SUMMARY

Foods of animal origin are the part of human diets that are excellent sources of energy, nutrients, vitamins, and minerals. These contain good quality protein and fats (fatty acids), providing essential amino acids and fatty acids, respectively. Foods of animal origin include meat, milk, fish, eggs, and their products. These foods can get contaminated at any step in their production to the time they reach the table—at the farm, during handling, transportation, processing, storage, and so on. Various hazards associated with these foods can be grouped into physical, chemical, and biological.

Physical hazards include wood, paper, metal, broken equipment parts, and others that may become part of the food during various steps of food chain. Similarly, chemical hazards include antibiotic residues, pesticides, hormones, toxins, biogenic amines, and heavy metals added to these foods at any step of supply chain. Biological hazards include bacteria, viruses, molds, and parasites (such as *listeria, salmonella, shigella, staphylococcus* spp.). Similar to other hazards, these can also be incorporated into these foods from farm to fork. Several workers necessitating their control or eradication have reported negative health effects of various hazards.

To provide safe foods to the consumers, control of these hazards has become essential and can be achieved by applying control measures, particularly at the step of origin for these hazards. Various systems and approaches have been introduced for this purpose like HACCP, Good Agricultural Practices, Good Manufacturing Practices, and Good Hygiene Practices for production of safe food. ISO systems of quality management and total quality management can further be adopted to bring about quality. Furthermore, a functional epidemiological surveillance system is necessary to ensure the risk assessment of animal originated foods to prevent their future hazards.

11.7 CONCLUSION

Animal-sourced foods are a healthy part of human diet. However, these can pose risks to the consumer if contaminated at any stage from production to consumption. The application of various control and quality systems are essential to ensure their safe production and good quality.

REFERENCES

1. Schönfeldt HC, Pretorius B, Hall N (2013) The impact of animal source food products on human nutrition and health. *S Afr J of Anim Sci* 41: 394–412.
2. WHO (2007) Protein and Amino Acid Requirements in Human Nutrition. Report of a Joint WHO/FAO/UNU Expert Consultation, Rome, Italy. World Health Organisation Technical Report Series no 935.
3. Scrimshaw N (1994) The consequences of hidden hunger for individuals and societies. *Food Nutr* 15: 3–23.
4. Neumann C, Harris DM, Rogers LM (2002) Contribution of animal source foods in improving diet quality and function in children in the developing world. *Nutr Res* 22: 193–220.
5. Murphy SP, Beaton GH, Calloway DH (1992) Estimated mineral intakes of toddlers: Predicted prevalence of inadequacy in village populations in Egypt, Kenya, and Mexico. *Am J Clin Nutr* 56: 565–572.
6. Sanders TAB (1995) Vegetarian diets and children. *Pediatr Clin North Am* 42: 955–965.
7. Gibson RS (1994) Content and bioavailability of trace elements in vegetarian diets. *Am J Clin Nutr* 59: 1223–1232.
8. Kashifa K, Ashfaque M, Iftikhar H, Masood A (2001) Bacteriological studies on raw milk supplied to Faisalabad city during summer months. *Pak Vet J* 21: 77–80.
9. Abebe B, Zelalem Y, Ajebu N (2012) Hygienic and microbial quality of raw whole cow's milk produced in Ezha district of the Gurage zone, Southern Ethiopia. *WJAR* 1: 459–465.
10. Abate M, Wolde T, Nigussie A (2015) Bacteriological quality and safety of raw cow's milk in and around Jigjiga City of Somali region, Eastern Ethiopia. *Int J Res Stud Biosci* 3: 48–55.
11. Beveridge MCM, Thilsted SH, Phillips MJ, Metian M, Troell M, Hall SJ (2013) Meeting the food and nutrition needs of the poor: The role of fish and the opportunities and challenges emerging from the rise of aquaculturea. *J Fish Biol* 83: 1067–1084.
12. Konieczny P, Kijowski J (2005) Animal origin food preservation and its safety issues. *Pol J Food Nutri Sci* 14: 21–29.
13. Usydus Z, Szlinder-Richert J (2012) Functional properties of fish and fish products: A review. *Int J Food Prop* 15: 823–846.
14. Vaclavik VA, Christian EW (2008) *Essentials of Food Science*. Springer, New York, pp. 205–230.
15. Karshima NS (2013) The roles of veterinarians in the safety of foods of animal origin in nigeria. *Rev J Anim Prod Adv* 3: 57–68.
16. Abdou EA (2002) Application of food safety in developing countries. Epidemiology of meatborne and milkborne infections in the Mediterranean region. *Inf Circ WHO/Mediter Zoon Control Centre* 54: 6–9.
17. Slorach SA, Maijala R, Belveze IT (2002) Examples of comprehensive and integrated approach to risk analysis in the food chain: Experiences and lessons learned. Conference paper.
18. Hathaway SC (1999) Management of food safety in international trade. *Food Control* 10: 247–253.
19. Olsen AR (1998) Regulatory action criteria for filth and other extraneous criteria for filth and other extraneous materials. I. Review of hard or sharp foreign objects as physical hazards in foreign objects as physical hazards in food. *Reg Food Tox Pharm* 28: 181.

20. Mead GC (2004) *Poultry Meat Processing and Quality.* Elsevier, London, UK.

21. Gorham RJ (1999) Hard foreign objects in food as a cause of injury and disease: A review. In *Foodborne Disease Handbook*, Vol. 3, Hui YH, Gorham JR, Murrell KD, Cliver DO (Eds.). Marcel Dekker. New York.

22. Girma K, Tilahun Z, Haimanot D (2014) Review on milk safety with emphasis on its public health. *World J Dairy Food Sci* 9: 166–183.

23. Roberts CA (2001) *The Food Safety Information Handbook.* Greenwood Publishing Group, Westport, CT.

24. Gaudin V, Fontaine J, Maris P (2001) Screening of penicillin residues in milk by a surface plasmon resonancebased biosensor assay: Comparison of chemical and enzymatic sample pre-treatment. *Anal Chim Acta* 436: 191–198.

25. Hu Y, Cheng H (2016) Health risk from veterinary antimicrobial use in China's food animal production and its reduction. *Environ Pollut.* doi:10.1016/j.envpol.2016.04.099.

26. Korsrud GO, Boison JO, Nouws JFM, MacNeil JD (1998) Bacterial inhibition tests used to screen for antimicrobial veterinary drug residues in slaughtered animals. *J AOAC Int* 81: 21–24.

27. Mitchell JM, Griffiths MW, McEwen SA, McNab WB, Yee AE (1998) Antimicrobial drug residues in milk and meat: Causes, concerns, prevalence, regulations, tests and test performance: A review. *J Food Prot* 61: 742–756.

28. Önal A (2007) A review: Current analytical methods for the determination of biogenic amines in foods. *Food Chem* 103: 1475–1486.

29. Halász A, Baráth Á, Simon-Sarkadi L, Holzapfel W (1994) Biogenic amines and their production by microorganisms in food. *Trends in Food Sci Technol* 5: 42–49.

30. Bodmer S, Imark C, Kneubühl M (1999) Biogenic amines in foods: Histamine and food processing. *Inflamm Res* 48: 296–300.

31. Gloria MBA, Hui YH (2005) *Handbook of Food Science, Technology and Engineering.* Boca Raton, FL: Taylor & Francis Group, p. 38.

32. De la Torre CAL, Conte-Júnior CA (2013) Chromatographic methods for biogenic amines determination in foods of animal origin. *Braz J Vet Res Anim Sci* 50(6): 430–446.

33. Shalaby AR (1996) Significance of biogenic amines to food safety and human health. *Food Res Int* 7: 675–690.

34. Silla Santos MH (1996) Biogenic amines: Their importance in foods. *Int J Food Microbiol* 29: 213–231.

35. Ruiz-Capillas C, Jiménez-Colmenero F (2004) Biogenic amines in meat and meat products. *Crit Rev Food Sci Nutri* 44: 489–499.

36. Hungerford JM (2010) Scombroid poisoning: A review. *Toxicon* 56: 231–243.

37. Efsa (2011) Scientific opinion on risk based control of biogenic amine formation in fermented foods. *EFSA J* 9: 2393.

38. Vinci G, Antonelli ML (2002) Biogenic amines: Quality index of freshness in red and white meat. *Food Control* 13: 519–524.

39. Suzzi G, Gardini F (2003) Biogenic amines in dry fermented sausages: A review. *Int J Food Microbiol* 88: 41–54.

40. Soriano-Santos J, Guerrero-Legarreta I, Hui YH (2010) Dietary products for special populations. In *Handbook of Poultry Science and Technology*, Hoboken, New Jersey: John Wiley & Sons. Vol. 2, pp. 275–289.

41. Novella-Rodríguez S, Veciana-Nogués MT, Roig-Sagués AX, Trujillo-Mesa AJ, Vidal-Carou MC (2004) Evaluation of biogenic amines and microbial counts throughout the ripening of goat cheeses from pasteurized and raw milk. *J Dairy Res* 71: 245–252.

42. Richard N, Pivarnik L, Ellis PC, Lee C (2008) Effect of matrix on recovery of biogenic amines in fish. *J AOAC Int* 91: 768–776.

43. Prester L (2011) Biogenic amines in fish, fish products and shellfish: Part A chemistry, analysis, control, exposure and risk assessment. *Rev Food Addit Contam* 11: 1547–1560.

44. Hartmann S, Lacorn M, Steinhart H (1998) Natural occurrence of steroid hormones in food. *Food Chem* 62: 7–20.

45. Layman P (1998) Murky to ruling on hormone treated beef. *Chem Eng News* 76: 12–12.

46. Aktar W, Sengupta D, Chowdhury A (2009). Impact of pesticides use in agriculture: Their benefits and hazards. *Interdiscip Toxicol* 2: 1–12.

47. Mukerjee D (1998) Health risk of endocrine disrupting ortho substituted PCBs emitted from incinerators. *Environ Eng Sci* 15: 157–169.

48. Wong SK, Lee WO (1997) Survey of organochlorine pesticide residues in milk in Hong Kong. *J AOAC Int* 80: 1332–1335.

49. Chen J, Gao J (1993) The Chinese total diet study in 1990. Part I: Chemical contaminants. *J AOAC Int* 76: 1193.

50. Raghunath R, Tripathi RM, Khandekar RN, Nambi KSV (1997) Retention times of Pb, Cd, Cu and Zn in children's blood. *Environ Sci* 207: 133–139.

51. Kirbis A, Krizmana M (2015) Spread of antibiotic resistant bacteria from food of animal origin to humans and vice versa. *Proc Food Sci* 5: 148–151.

52. Adams MR, Moss MO (2008) Food microbiology. RSC Publishing, Cambridge, UK.

53. Collins CH, Grange JM (1983) A review of bovine tuberculosis. *J Appl Bacteriol* 55: 13–29.

54. Pfeiffer DU (2003) Tuberculosis in animals. In: *Clinical Tuberculosis*, 3rd ed., Davies PD (Ed.). Arnold, London, UK.

55. Radostits OM, Blood DC, Hinchcliff KW, Gay CC (2007) Veterinary medicine: A textbook of the diseases of cattle, sheep, pigs, goats and horses. Bailliere-Tindall, London, UK, p. 1763.

56. Shitaye JE, Tsegaye W, Pavlik I (2007) Bovine tuberculosis infection in animals and human populations. *Vet Med* 52: 317–332.

57. Davies PDO (2006) Tuberculosis in humans and animals: Are we a threat to each other? *J R Soc Med* 10: 539540.

58. Amanfu W (2006) The situation of tuberculosis and tuberculosis control in animals of economic interest. *TB* 86: 330–335.

59. Cassidy JP (2006) The pathogenesis and pathology of bovine tuberculosis with insights from studies of tuberculosis in humans and laboratory animal models. *Vet Microbiol* 112: 151–161.

60. O'Reilly LM, Daborn CJ (1995) The epidemiology of Mycobacterium bovis infections in animals and man: A review. *Tuber Lung Dis* 76: 1–46.

61. Pappas G, Papadimitriou P, Akritidis N, Christou L, Tsianos EV (2006) The new global map of human brucellosis. *Lancet Infect Dis* 6: 91–99.

62. Githui WA, Hawken ES, Juma ES, Godfrey Faussett P, Swai DK, Kibuga JDH, Porter SM, Wilson, Drobniewski FA (2000) Surveillance of drugresistant tuberculosis and molecular evaluation of transmission of resistant strains in refugee and non refugee populations in North Eastern Kenya. *Int J Tuber Lung Dis* 4: 947–955.

63. Godfroid J, Scholz H, Barbier T, Nicolas C, Wattiau P (2011) Brucellosis at the animal/ecosystem/human interface at the beginning of the 21st century. *Prev Vet Med* 102: 118–131.

64. Applebaum GD, Mathsen G (1997) Spinal brucellosis in a Southern California resident. *West J Med* 166: 61–65.

65. Arimi SM, Koroti E, Kang'ethe EK, Omore AO, McDermott JJ (2005) Risk of infection with Brucella abortus and Escherichia coli O157:H7 associated with marketing of unpasteurized milk in Kenya. *Acta Tropica* 96: 1–8.

66. Christiansson A, Bertilsson J, Svensson B (1999) Bacillus cereus spores in raw milk: Factors affecting the contamination of milk during the grazing period. *J Dairy Sci* 82: 305–314.

67. Blaser MJ (1997) Epidemiologic and clinical features of Campylobacter jejuni infections. *J Infect Dis* 2: 103–105.

68. Savolainen S, Schildt M, Hänninen ML (2006) Long-lasting Campylobacter jejuni contamination of milk associated with gastrointestinal illness in a farming family. *Epidemiol Infect* 134: 401–405.

69. Orr KE, Lightfoot NF, Sisson PR, Harkis BA, Tweddle JL, Boyd P, Carroll A, Jackson CJ, Wareing DRA, Freeman R (1995) Direct milk excretion of Campylobacter jejuni in a dairy cow causing cases of human enteritis. *Epidemiol Infect* 1: 15–24.

70. Cobbold R, Desmarchelier P (2000) A longitudinal study of Shiga-toxigenic Escherichia coli (STEC) prevalence in three Australian dairy herds. *Vet Microbiol* 71: 125–137.

71. Hussein HS, Sakuma T (2005) Invited review: Prevalence of shiga toxin producing Escherichia coli in dairy cattle and their products. *J Dairy Sci* 88: 450–465.

72. Jayarao BM, Henning DR (2001) Prevalence of food borne pathogens in bulk tank milk. *J Dairy Sci* 84: 2157.

73. Kerry JP, Kerry JF (2011) *Processed Meats: Improving Safety, Nutrition and Quality.* Elsevier, Oxford, UK.

74. Jensen NE, Aarestrup FM, Jensen J, Wegener HC (1996) Listeria monocytogenes in bovine mastitis. Possible implication for human health. *Int J Food Microbiol* 32: 209.

75. Ryser ET, Marth EH (1999) *Listeria, Listeriosis and Food. Safety*, 2nd ed. Marcel Dekker, New York.

76. Mossel DAA, Van Neten P (1990) Staphylococcus aureus and related staphylococci in foods: Ecology, proliferation, toxinogenesis, control and monitoring. *J Appl Bacteriol Symp Suppl* 69: 123.

77. Forshell LP, Wierup M (2006) *Salmonella* contamination: A significant challenge to the global marketing of animal food products. *Rev Sci Tech Off Int Epiz* 25: 541–554.

78. Acha PN, Szyfres B (1987) *Salmonella.* In *Zoonoses and Communicable Diseases Common to Man and Animals.* Pan American Health Organization (PAHO), Washington, DC, pp. 147–155.

79. Murinda SE, Nguyen LT, Ivey SJ, Gillespie BE, Almeida RA, Draughon FA, Oliver SP (2002) Molecular characterization of *Salmonella* spp. Isolated from bulk tank milk and cull dairy cow fecal samples. *J Food Prot* 65: 1100–1105.

80. Magaji AA, Oboegbulem SI, Daneji AI, Garba HS, Salihu MD, Junaidu AU, Mohammed AA et al. (2011) Incidence of hydatid cyst disease in food animals slaughtered at Sokoto central abattoir, Sokoto state, Nigeria. *Vet World* 5: 197–200.

81. Bouree P (2001) Hydatidosis: Dynamics of transmission. *World J Surg* 25: 4–9.

82. Noordhuizen JPTM, Metz JHM (2005) Quality control on dairy farms with emphasis on public health, food safety, animal health and welfare. *Livest Prod Sci* 1: 51–59.

12 Strategies for Improving the Quality of Animal Origin Foods

Sana Mehmood, Muhammad Issa Khan, and Hira Shakoor

CONTENTS

12.1 INTRODUCTION

Anthropology has previously recognized the importance of food and diet variations among time periods. It is possible to sum up the profile of meat consumption during human evolution in four periods: the first could be characterized by opportunist hunting; while in the second, hunting had grown to a bigger scale and lasted 2–3 million years; in the third period, men started to domesticate animals and plants, which began 10,000 years ago; during the fourth and last period studies determined that meat contained compounds that could increase disease risk [1]. It has been stated that human genes had not changed since the Paleolithic period. Human beings are animals, submitted to the same environmental pressures as other animals and living species [2]. With this, scientists have proposed several possible influences on diet in human evolution in which some can be highlighted: cranial-dental and bowel morphologic changes and increased energy needs leading to an elevated quotient between brain and body size [3]. Anthropological data have also suggested an important influence of meat consumption in human erect posture. Bipedalism is probably the first and most important characteristic that distinguished humans from their ancestors as it allowed a more efficient locomotion and load carrying, which are important advantages in hunting [4]. Cranial–dental changes are quite visible when analyzing hominids fossils. Molar teeth size has decreased, and the jaws and front teeth have become stronger. Shearing crests have also been grown to manipulate the feeding needs. These changes could be explained through the urgent need of tearing and chewing meat rather than grinding leaves, fruits, seeds, and cereals [1,3].

In European legislation, the term meat refers to the edible parts removed from the carcass of domestic ungulates including bovine, porcine, ovine, and caprine animals as well as domestic solipeds; poultry; lagomorphs; wild game; farmed game; and small and large wild game [5]. Generally, meat is an important source of several nutrients. It is particularly rich in high biological value protein, as well as micronutrients like iron, selenium, zinc, and vitamin B12. Likewise, organ meats especially liver are rich source of heme iron, Vitamin A and folic acid to reduce the burden of anemia [6].

12.2 NUTRITIONAL IMPORTANCE OF FOODS OF ANIMAL ORIGIN

Animal-sourced foods are energy dense and excellent sources of protein, minerals, vitamins and essential fatty acids [7]. The protein in foods of animal origin contains essential amino acids that the human body cannot produce, some of which resembles that in the human body in terms of amino acid composition. Iron, zinc, and vitamin A are the main micronutrients available in meat, while vitamin B12, riboflavin, calcium, and conjugated linoleic acid are available from milk.

The bioavailability of these nutrients is high, compared to those in plants, because of the presence of the heme protein and the absence of fiber and phytates in foods of animal origin. Iron serves many roles in the human body, as a component of haemoglobin (the protein that carries oxygen), myoglobin (a protein found in muscle), and of some enzymes. Thus, iron deficiency reduces capacity for physical work, diminishes cognitive function in children, and has been associated with anorexia. Zinc plays a significant role in gene expression, cell division and differentiation, and in DNA and RNA synthesis as it is a constituent of several enzymes involved in these processes. Zinc deficiency is of particular importance in maternal, foetal, infant, and child health and survival [8].

Vitamin B12 is involved in the formation of normal blood and of neurological development and function [9]. It plays an essential role in the synthesis of DNA and RNA components (purines and pyrimidines), transfer of methyl groups, synthesis of proteins from amino acids and carbohydrates and fat metabolism. Vitamin B12 deficiency results in reduced cognitive functions and is associated with anaemia. Vitamin A is a fat-soluble vitamin that promotes good vision, growth, and strengthens the immune system. Vitamin A deficiency results in stunted growth, impaired vision and blindness, compromises the immune system and, in severe cases, may result in mortality. Conjugated linoleic acid (CLA) is a generic term for a mixture of geometric and positional isomers of C18:2 that contain a conjugated double bond [10]. These compounds have shown to have anticarcinogenic effects. They also have antidiabetogenic, anti-atherogenic, and anti-obesity effects, as well as supporting immunomodulation and modulation of bone growth [6,11].

Milk, meat, and eggs currently provide around 13% of the energy and 28% of the protein consumed globally; in developed countries, this rises to 20% and 48% for energy and protein, respectively [12]. The world's 17 billion livestock occur in three main types of production systems: confined intensive, mixed crop–livestock, and open grazing systems [13]. Estimates, based on data for 2001–2003, suggest that grazing systems supply 9% of the world's meat and 12% of milk; mixed crop–livestock systems contribute 46% of meat, 88% of milk, and 50% of cereals; while intensive systems provide 45% of meat. By consuming feedstuffs that people could consume directly, such as grains and legumes, animals reduce the total amount of food available. Today, about half the world's production of grain is fed to animals, especially monogastrics [14], and 77 million tons of plant protein are fed to livestock to produce 58 million tons of animal protein contributing 13% of the energy to the world's diet.

Feed crops occupy an estimated a half a billion hectares of land; including grazing land, and livestock accounts for four-fifths of all agricultural land [15].

12.3 HEALTH IMPACT OF OUTBREAKS OF FOODBORNE ILLNESS FROM ANIMAL FOODS

Potential negative effects of foods of animal origin on human nutrition and health are also an important matter to be discussed. The sections above have highlighted the positive effects of consuming foods of animal origin on human and nutrition outcomes. However, there are also potential risks that need to be considered, indicating the need to devise strategies for their mitigation.

12.3.1 FOODBORNE DISEASES

Because of their rich nutrient content, foods of animal origin tend to be susceptible to microbial contamination which can lead to foodborne diseases. Microbial contaminants include bacteria, fungi, viruses, or parasites that result in more than 3 million premature deaths worldwide each year. Improved access to foods of animal origin also requires parallel access to food safety education aimed at reducing incidences of foodborne diseases. Studies that have combined increased animal production with nutrition education have generally resulted in improved nutritional status of households [10,16].

12.3.2 ZOONOTIC DISEASES

In recent years, there has been an increase in zoonotic diseases (i.e. diseases that are transmittable from animals to humans), such as Rift Valley fever, avian influenza, bovine tuberculosis, and foot-and-mouth disease. Keeping livestock may increase the risks of such outbreaks yet improving access to foods of animal origin by vulnerable households requires increasing the number of animals or increasing production [11]. This means that better methods of detection and control of zoonoses are required, including the participation of communities who own the animals together with veterinary and health professionals [5].

12.3.3 CHRONIC DISEASE

Foods of animal origin present a risk of chronic disease because of the purported association between consumption of the saturated fat present in foods of animal origin and the occurrence of cardiovascular disease and development of type 2 diabetes. This association is based on studies of diets with over consumption of foods of animal origin [8]. However, in developing communities, consumption of foods of animal origin is low and broad generalizations relating to fat consumption and its links to chronic diseases are inappropriate given recent findings about fat quality [9].

The polyunsaturated fatty acids in animal origin food consist of CLAs and sphingolipds which have phenomenal effects on brain development. Humans and plants are unable to synthesize these polyunsaturated fatty acids and they need to be supplied in the diet by the consumption of foods of animal origin. Consequently, there have been several efforts to increase the content of these polyunsaturated in meat and milk. It has been reported on strategies to increase milk fatty acids that are beneficial to human health through nutritional management of dairy cows [17].

In a similar vein, it is reported that amounts of CLA in both meat and milk can be enhanced through nutrition. Dietary manipulations aimed at increasing CLA content in beef and concluded that fresh forage diets offered the best option. In most developing communities, ruminants are fed on fresh forage, at least during the wet season, and thus could have beneficial fatty acids profiles [2]. Recent evidence suggests that the relationship between foods of animal origin and cancer is very tenuous at best. Thus, the risk of chronic diseases because of consuming low to moderate levels of food from animal origins in the diets of developing communities is extremely limited [7,10].

12.3.4　Water Contamination

While the risk of contamination of water resources by livestock waste is outside the scope of this chapter, suffice to say that this risk can be mitigated through appropriate management of livestock waste, such as using biogas digesters and recycling manure on crops.

12.3.5　Global Warming

Increasing livestock numbers has the potential to impact greenhouse gases (GHGs), such as carbon dioxide, methane and nitrous oxide. Already, livestock have been estimated to contribute about 18% of the global emission of GHG [18]. However, in terms of livestock owned by the poor, the contribution would be small given the smaller number in poor areas, compared to developed areas, and the limited transportation of livestock over long distances in these areas. The evidence above indicates that the risks to human health and the environment posed by ownership of livestock and consumption of foods of animal origin by poor communities are negligible compared to the individual and societal benefits that accrue as a result of combating nutritional deficiencies. Therefore, it is desirable to increase access to and consumption of foods of animal origin [3] (Figure 12.1).

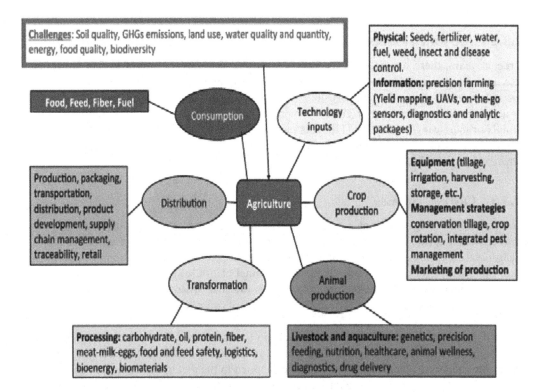

FIGURE 12.1 Current agricultural and livestock challenges. (Adapted from Pearson, A.M., and Gillett, T.A., *Processed Meats*, Springer, Dordrecht, the Netherlands, 2012; Koldovsky, O., *J. Nutr.*, 119, 1543–1551, 1989.)

12.4 PROCESSING OF ANIMAL ORIGIN FOODS

12.4.1 MEAT PROCESSING

Meat is the fleshy edible portion removed from the carcass of domestic animals, including goat, camel, buffalos, and poultry [10].

Meat processing techniques, such as salting and smoking, have been performed for decades before the invention of refrigeration. Both smoking and salting protect the meat from harmful physiological changes, including organoleptic characteristics like color, taste, and appearance, and preserve them to keep them safe and healthy to eat for longer periods of time.

There are many other ways to process meat for improving consumption in both the developed and industrialized world. The major purpose of processing is to develop healthy and nutritious products adding good mouth feel and texture to food. The processed meat products, such as sausages, salami, beef, and mutton, are traditionally important in many parts of world. The potential hazards associated with consumption of meat products make them unfit for consumption as meat products are perishable commodities and contaminated through bacterial growth, autolysis, and destruction by endotoxic enzymes.

The process of canning has been used since the nineteenth century for handling of meat to prevent against contamination and sterilized method. Freezing is a modern processing technique for meat with a storage temperature of 4°C for few days. Under hygienic conditions and suitable handling practices, these techniques can prolong the storage life to about 1 month. Chilling for meat products is also advantageous for inactivating bacterial pathogens and enzyme activity at a temperature range of −15°C, while growth of many harmful microorganisms stops at −10°C [4,16].

12.4.2 MILK PROCESSING

From a nutritional point of view, milk is nature's most perfect and wholesome food. Milk is full of all essential nutrients that are required to fulfill the basic needs for growth and development. It is the chief source of important macronutrients, such as calcium, vitamin D, phosphorous, and are necessary for the healthy teeth and bones development [3].

There has been extensive research on milk and dairy products used worldwide as a source of a balance diet. As a valuable food commodity milk requires careful processing and handling. In addition to its use as complete food, milk is a food product that has less storage time and can be easily exposed to microbial growth leading to damage and various fatal diseases in human. The processing of milk requires the maintenance of milk properties for hours, days, weeks, or months and prevents many illnesses caused by harmful pathogenic microorganisms [19]. Milk processing is beneficial in terms of providing healthy nutrition, more profits rather than selling raw milk, means of income, and overall improvement in safety and quality of milk products consumed by human.

The techniques that are important from a processing point of view for improving the shelf life of dairy products include refrigeration for enhancing the raw milk attributes, fermentation, and pasteurization. Pasteurization and ultra-high temperature (UHT) techniques prolong the shelf life of milk and other dairy products by lowering the risk of contamination from life threatening microorganisms. Furthermore, for high quality and easily manageable products with longer shelf life, milk can be further processed to products like cheese, butter, and ghee. Seasonal changes are better managed due to availability of processed milk products in local and urban market. The modification of fresh milk into various products is also beneficial for the whole society by providing the opportunities in collection of milk from various sources as well as marketing the products [14].

12.5 ANIMAL PRODUCTS CONSUMPTION PATTERN

For the majority of people who are residents of developing countries, the consumption of milk and other dairy products is estimated at more than 6 billion people. Since the early 1960s, per capita milk consumption in developing countries has increased almost twofold. However, the consumption of milk has grown more slowly than that of other livestock products; meat consumption has more than tripled and egg consumption has increased fivefold. Over the last two decades, per capita milk consumption decreased in sub-Saharan Africa. In India, about 50% of milk is consumed on-farm. Milk provides 3% of dietary energy supply in Asia and Africa, compared with 8% and 9% in Europe and Oceania; 6% and 7% of dietary protein supply in Asia and Africa, compared with 19% in Europe; and 6%–8% of dietary fat supply in Asia and Africa, compared with 11%–14% in Europe, Oceania and the Americas [10,20].

Among the animal derived foods, which are major source of healthy and wholesome diet, the milk and dairy products are most important and wide group of animal foods. Milk or dairy products are defined as the liquid foods derived from animal milk, such as goat, buffaloes, camels, and cows. Milk is consumed in many parts of world as a nutritious commodity that is required for the health and growth of children and adults. There are many modified forms of dairy products available for people globally. The total nutrient content of milk is basically determined by the energy density and is considered a complete food group.

On the basis of the fat content, milk is divided into low fat or skim milk and whole milk containing about 90–120 kcal of calories per cup. The consumption of dairy products is more than 150 kg/capita/year in Pakistan and many other Asian countries. In India and south African regions, the per capita consumption is moderate, while there is a low (less than 30 kg) intake of milk products in central Africa and east Asia [21]. It is expected that by 2030 the global intake of milk and milk products will be enhanced in south Asia by 125%. Some important and consumer friendly dairy products, which are considered as safe and healthy are yogurt, cheese, butter, and ghee. These products have rich sources of all macronutrients and micronutrients needed by the human body.

12.5.1 GHEE

Ghee is commonly called vegetable ghee manufactured by butter extracted from cream or curd. Ghee is a solid form of fat residue that remained as the supernatant obtained from whey processing. Its organolaptic characteristics depend upon the type of milk which is used for processing, butter quality, and time of exposure to production techniques [20].

12.5.2 SKIM MILK

It is the type of milk from which the solid cream portion has been removed and generally categorized as low fat or no fat milk. It contains reduced amount of most of the worthwhile fat-soluble vitamins required for healthy growth and development of brain [3].

12.5.3 STANDARDIZED MILK

Nowadays, a commonly used milk product is standardized milk, which is obtained by the partial adjustment of fat or cream from milk to make the milk medium fat. It can also be prepared by mixing the whole milk with skim milk to get the desired concentration. Being mostly used for individuals, it is aimed to promote bone and teeth health without excessive weight gain [10].

12.5.4 FORTIFIED MILK

Food fortification is the addition of nutrients in food, which are either deficient or absent in specific food to meet the nutritional requirement of larger population. The milk also acts as a common vehicle for food fortification through the addition of different micronutrients such as Ca, vitamin D, and iron [21]. Fortified milk is nutritionally stable and plays an important role to ameliorate the detrimental disorders and improves the overall health of people.

12.5.5 CONDENSED MILK

Condensed milk is the type of milk from which the liquid or watery portion has been removed to increase the concentration of nutrients especially sugar content. Most often, condensed milk is regarded as milk with added sugar or sweetened milk. Its consistency and density are quite high, which make it concentrated source of energy. The shelf life of this type of milk is almost up to years if stored at refrigerated temperature. It is used to make different dessert dishes across the region [17].

12.5.6 POULTRY

Among the animal sources that are part of our daily diet, poultry meat is one of them. Basically poultry or chicken meat is categorized as lean meat or white meat, which offers protein for body development. Almost 70%–80% of daily meal dishes comprises of poultry chicken/meat including homemade and fast food restaurants [22].

12.5.7 EGGS

Another common animal product used in everyone's daily diet is eggs. Eggs are obtained from birds like hens and pigeons that are used for preparation of many recopies and can be consumed as a whole either in boiled or fried form. Egg protein offers high-quality protein, which means if you consume an egg then bioavailability will be 100% and will become the part of body [1,2].

12.5.8 BEEF/MUTTON

Both of these animal sourced foods are derived from milk-giving animals like buffalo, cow, goat, and camel. Beef or mutton often called as red meat could be used as whole or minced form in different foods [6]. The consumption pattern of these foods varies according to region-to-region and socio-cultural acceptance regarding meat [4, 23]. Due to their high-quality protein content, Iron and B complex vitamins, mutton and beef are recommended for the population to prevent malnutrition especially for children and pregnant females.

12.5.9 FISH

It is the only animal derived food product which is enriched or packed with all essential nutrients needed for health promotion and disease prevention. Fish and its various types are widely used in every community, along seaside, Mediterranean regions, and western society as an important source of nutrition. Among the key nutrients are essential fatty acids such as omega-3 fatty acid and omega-6 fatty acids, which are worthy to describe. Fish due to its high nutritional quality is recommended for hypertension and CVD (cardiovascular diseases) patients [17].

12.6 ANIMAL FEED PRODUCTION CODE OF ETHICS

According to expert health bodies and quality assurance firms, it has been recommended that the safety and quality of animal feed depends upon the species being fed and type of fodder. To define the quality of the feedstuffs to be accepted, ingredient combinations and qualities are chief factors to be considered by quality assurance processor whenever the new materials are established for feed processing. For the final feed formulation, which includes any added chemical, should meet the governmental regulatory standards and must satisfy the key objectives of the animal production by customer. Among the other quality assurance factors are the manufacturing and distribution of the feed products. For the effective and satisfactory feed production, facility quality assurance forms need to confirm the sampling techniques, microscopy and laboratory testing, quality control in-plant, proper control of drugs, sanitation of plant and integrated pest management, cleanliness of plant, storage, and transportation [14]. There must be proper monitoring systems for future quality assurance procedures documentation and records maintenance.

Clear guidance regarding required features of feed quality assurance programs to industries and manufactures must be provided as a single preventive approach to safe feed for animals. Codes of practice for the animal feed and livestock sectors are playing their role for the provision of such guidance to industries by occupying all the major strategies of feed production, and their handling and storage for ultimate consumption by animals [8]. It has been well elaborated that handlers and producers who are the key actors in animal feed production must ensure that their processing practices and documentation describe the close relationship with the principles of hazard analysis critical control point (HACCP).

Inspection and labeling meat and poultry products are inspected by US Department of Agriculture's Food Safety and Inspection Service (FSIS) every day. Inspectors monitor plant sanitation, proper processing, and cooking, when applicable. As part of their duties, inspectors also check to be sure that labels accurately reflect product ingredients. Any ingredient used in a processed meat or poultry product must be declared on the product label. Processed meat and poultry products have an excellent safety record. Some processed meats, like a marinated chicken breast, require additional cooking [24]. Consumers should follow instructions on packages carefully and use an instant read thermometer to ensure that the product has reached the proper internal temperature.

12.7 OVERCONSUMPTION OF ANIMAL-SOURCED FOODS

Overconsumption of animal-sourced foods can harm human health and well-being, impacting whole societies as well as individual households. Overconsumption of fatty red meats and hard cheeses, which have increased concentrations of saturated fats, can lead to cardiovascular disease, while overconsumption of processed meats, such as bacon and ham, has been associated with some cancers [25]. Increased consumption of energy-dense meat, milk, and eggs also contributes to the global obesity epidemic. This is not an issue confined to developed countries, and it is multi-faceted, with differences within a single household, and a diversity of views on "how much is too much" and how to influence.

Due shifts in dietary patterns of the world and rapid urbanization, meat and meat products are the main food for people. Quality of meat products is mandatory for safe and adequate consumption. The major cause of deterioration in meat is the oxidation process that occurs due to elevated levels of heme-pigments, monounsaturated fatty acids, metallic catalyst, and a variety of oxidizing compounds. Oxidative stress is responsible for production of free radical damage by reactive oxygen species (ROS) and reactive nitrogen species (RNS) that leads to the destruction of macromolecules, such as proteins and lipids. Synthetic antioxidants have been used for decades for the prevention of health-related maladies related to stress and to enhance the physiological integrity of oxidized meat, but it still remained a challenge for large scale meat industry [22].

Basically, the chief cause of oxidative stress is the continuous progression of modulators that disturb the homeostasis of animal before slaughter. At present, amongst the most important issues in meat industry is protein and lipid oxidation. The major alterations in meat are limited shelf life, reduced the nutritional quality, decreases the market value, and increases toxicity of meat and meat products. Natural antioxidants are more preferable for sustaining the nutritional quality and shelf life of meat. The most important role of bioactive components found in medicinal plants is main phyto-pharmaceutical strategy against lipid–protein oxidation [13,18]. The application of natural antioxidants, such as thyme leaves, rosemary extract olive, and grape seed extract, can be delivered through the technological and dietary strategies to ameliorate and prevent oxidative damage in muscles portion. Prevention and reduction of oxidative damage in meat, antimicrobial activities, and improvement in functional qualities is the key role of these natural antioxidants.

Despite its nutritional value, meat consumption has been considered a disease-promoting food. Recently, research has started to demystify this negative health image and has helped to point out the crucial role of meat in human evolution, especially red meat. Meat consumption has contributed to human gastrointestinal tract development, as well as crucial cranio-dental features and posture, helping distinguish man from other hominids. Meat continues to supply nutrients and play a vital role in human life because of its high biological value protein, iron, zinc, selenium, and vitamin B_{12} contents being a crucial component of a well-balanced diet [14]. Fat content, a matter of concern regarding meat consumption, is highly variable depending on species, origin, feeding system, and the cut. Leaner cuts like pork or beef loin do not differ significantly from skinless turkey or chicken breast and the nutritional richness justifies their inclusion in a well-balanced diet.

12.8 MAJOR MILESTONES OF STRATEGIES

12.8.1 FORUM ESTABLISHMENT FOR ANIMALS

The objective of this forum must be to create the harmony among different members of the animal welfare research community working either at local or international animal welfare firms and animal-sourced food sector to discuss the major issue regarding animal welfare issues, policies, and practices for the improvement of food quality of animal origin foods at both national and global level. It can also be promoted through awareness campaigns, outreach activities, communities support groups, and educational advertisements to preserve the animal welfare for better consumption patterns [17].

12.8.2 SCIENCE BASED ANIMAL WELFARE STANDARDS ESTABLISHMENT AND PRACTICING

By taking into account regional perspectives and related ethical considerations, best scientific and practical expertise on animal welfare has resulted in better quality of animal origin foods production.

12.8.3 ENCOURAGEMENT OF REGIONAL ANIMAL WELFARE STRATEGIES (RAWS)

The key approach for the improvement of food quality and sustainability for prolonged period of time it has been suggested to reserve the in-practice feed quality and safety strategies. To achieve this, there is dire need to encourage and support the current evolution, development, and implementation of regional animal welfare strategies (RAWS). Professionals in this field must provide the detailed procedures for development of animal welfare legislation, policies, and region-specific activities. It is also important to consider ensuring that in every part of a region there is implementation of upgraded scientific knowledge and developmental techniques in animal welfare [13].

12.8.4 LOCAL VETERINARY SERVICES STRENGTHENING

Locally available facilities must be utilized for increasing the total output and improved quality of animal-sourced foods without any harmful risk and impact on the end consumer. Among the most common veterinary services are the application of better quality drugs, fodder, equipments, and hormonal therapies, which are used for increasing the overall yield of animal welfare. This all can be achieved through capacity building activities by giving worth to national animal welfare bodies. It is an important issue to provide training and awareness on animal welfare preservation.

12.8.5 DEVELOPING RELATIONSHIPS WITH OTHER SCIENCE AREAS

For better and long-term improvement of animal-sourced food quality, the association with other key areas of science will be supportive. Experts suggest strengthening and expansion of relationships between animal welfare science and other areas of sciences. These science areas include environmental, soil, pharmaceutical, social and economic science with the help of close collaboration and participation in developing policies, research, and seminars at local and international level across the globe [6,19].

12.9 CONCLUSION

It has been well recommended by expert health bodies that there must be proper legislations and monitoring systems for ensuring quality and safety of animal origin foods which provides the basis for adequate control and prevention of animal feed hazards associated with life threatening risks to general community and public health. For the improvement of the quality of foods of animal sources, certain biological agents and chemical substances are injected into feed at any stage of synthesis. The local and international strategies, which are currently in practice, need further strengthening for the production of quality foods, and there must be close collaboration among the researchers for smooth provision of facilities and to determine the possible hazard and risk level.

REFERENCES

1. Pereira, P.M.D.C.C., and Vicente, A.F.D.R.B. 2013. Meat nutritional composition and nutritive role in the human diet. *Meat Sci* 93:586–592.
2. Larsen, C.S. 2003. Animal source foods to improve micronutrient nutrition and human function in developing countries animal source foods and human health during evolution. *Health (San Francisco)* 1(2):3893–3897.
3. Bradbear, N. 2009. *Bees and Their Role in Forest Livelihoods: A Guide to the Services Provided by Bees and the Sustainable Harvesting, Processing and Marketing of Their Products.* Non-wood Forest Products. Food and Agriculture Organization of the United Nations, Rome, Italy.
4. Speedy, A.W. 2011. *FAO and Pre-Harvest Food Safety in the Livestock and Animal Feed Industry.* Animal Production and Health Division. FAO, Rome, Italy.
5. Pearson, A.M., and Gillett, T.A. 2012. *Processed Meats.* Springer, Dordrecht, the Netherlands.
6. Smith, J., Sones, K., Grace, D., Macmillan, S., Tarawali, S., and Herrero, M. 2013. Beyond milk, meat, and eggs: Role of livestock in food and nutrition security. *Anim Front* 3:6–13.
7. Koldovsky, O. 1989. Search for role of milk-borne biologically active peptides for the suckling. *J Nutr* 119:1543–51.
8. Eaton, S.B., and Konner, M.J. (1997). Review paleolithic nutrition revisited: A twelve-year retrospective on its nature and implications. *Eur J Clin Nutr* 51(4):207–216.
9. Zucoloto, F. (2011). Evolution of the human feeding behavior. *Psychol Neurosci* 4(1):131–141.
10. Larsson, S.C., and Wolk, A. 2012. Red and processed meat consumption and risk of pancreatic cancer: Meta-analysis of prospective studies. *Br J Cancer* 106:603–607.
11. European Comission REG (EC) No835/2004. 2002 Regulation (2004). EUOJ L139/55.
12. Venes, D. 2017. *Taber's Cyclopedic Medical Dictionary.* F.A. Davis Company, Philadelphia, PA, p. 2557.
13. U.S. Food and Drug Administration, Federal Food, Drug, and Cosmetic Act, Chapter II, Sec. 201.
14. Herrero, M., Thornton, P.K., Notenbaert, A.M., Wood, S., Msangi, S., Freeman, H.A. et al. 2010. Smart investments in sustainable food production: Revisiting mixed crop–livestock systems. *Science* 327:822–825.
15. Fairweather-tait, S.J., Collings, R., and Hurst, R. (2010). Selenium bioavailability: Current knowledge and future research. *Am J Clin Nutr* 91(2). doi:10.3945/ajcn.2010.28674.
16. Bender, A.E. 2012. *Meat and Meat Products in Human Nutrition in Developing Countries.* FAO, Rome, Italy.
17. FAO. 2011. *World Livestock 2011—Livestock in Food Security.* FAO, Rome, Italy.
18. O'Mara, F.P. 2011. The significance of livestock as a contributor to global greenhouse gas emissions today and in the near future. *Anim Feed Sci Technol* 166–167:7–15.
19. IAASTD. 2009. *International Assessment of Agricultural Knowledge, Science, and Technology for Development Global Report.* Island Press, Washington, DC.
20. D'Evoli, L., Salvatore, P., Lucarini, M., Nicoli, S., Aguzzi, A., Gabrielli, P. et al. 2009. Nutritional value of traditional Italian meat-based dishes: Influence of cooking methods and recipe formulation. *Int J Food Sci Nutr* 60(Suppl. 5):38–49.
21. Thornton, P.K., and Herrero, M. 2009. *The Inter-linkages Between Rapid Growth in Livestock Production, Climate Change, and the Impacts on Water Resources, Land Use, and Deforestation.* World Bank Policy Research Working Paper, WPS 5178. World Bank, Washington, DC.

22. Ingram, J., Ericksen, P., and Liverman, D. (Eds.). 2010. *Food Security and Global Environmental Change*. Earthscan, London, UK.
23. Wijk, M.T. 2012. Conservation agriculture in mixed crop–livestock systems: Scoping crop residue trade-offs in sub-Saharan Africa and South Asia. *Field Crops Res* 132:175–184.
24. Sherraden, M. 1991. *Assets and the Poor: A New American Welfare Policy*. M. E. Sharpe, Armonk, NY.
25. Grace, D., Mutua, F., Ochungo, P., Kruska, R., Jones, K., Brierley, L. et al. 2012. *Mapping of Poverty and Likely Zoonoses Hotspots*. Report to the Department for International Development. International Livestock Research Institute, Nairobi, Kenya.

13 Issues and Policies to Promote Animal Origin Food Consumption

Muhammad Issa Khan, Hira Shakoor, and Sana Mehmood

CONTENTS

13.1   INTRODUCTION

There are pivotal linkages between health, nutrition, and animal-sourced food that are instrumental to attract the attention of scientific community to promote better health in a society. However, animal foods are rich in saturated fat but on other side, it provides essential nutrients that are necessary for the development of body. World is marching towards the progress, which not only changed the lifestyle of a man but also eating pattern. Although, there are large number of food industries but still, world is facing some problems, which needs to be address and measures should be taken accordingly. For instance, developed world has been focusing on the plant-based diet and nutraceutical foods; thereby, ignoring the animal food. While, on the other hand, underdeveloped countries are unable to purchase expensive animal origin food. So, in this chapter we highlighted some of the issues, due to which consumption of animal food like milk, cheese, poultry, fish, red meat, and eggs are affected and some strategies are suggested to promote the intake of safe and healthy animal food herewith.

13.1.1 GLOBAL SCENARIO OF ANIMAL ORIGIN FOOD CONSUMPTION AND ECONOMIC TRANSITION

Food and water are the fundamental resources needed to produce food. Population growth, economic development, and environmental changes pushed these resources into an extreme danger. In future, farmer should have to produce more food from limited resources, which is a strenuous task. Nowadays, world is progressing so fast, food production and meeting market or consumer demands are challenging, because it is deeply rooted with the reduction of poverty, malnutrition from society, and improve health, ecosystem and maintain biological diversity [1]. However, this is an era of nutritional transition: a radical shift in dietary patterns occurs especially calories saturation, thereby, traditional food is replaced by expensive food like meat, fruits, and vegetables [2]. It is observed that per capita demands of meat depend upon per capita income. Secondly, per capita income and meat consumption don't show a linear trend: poor population basically avoid meat consumption until their income reach lower threshold whereas, richer population remain satiated beyond an upper threshold. Thirdly, increasing meat demand raised the needs of more feed for animal production. Consequently, meat demand is increasing quite faster than crop production [3]. According to an estimate, with increasing world population, food demands is also rising at a rate of 1.1% per year between now and 2050 at an average [4]. The Food and Agriculture Organization (FAO) suggested that food security is determined through socioeconomic status and some local specific factors than by the food producing capacity of the world [4]. Whereas, in food insecure countries like Africa, more than 300 million people will remain undernourished by 2050. Currently in the developed world, overconsumption is also a big issue leading toward various detrimental health problems, and 50% UK adults will suffer from obesity by 2050 [5].

Certainly, economic transition and urbanization in the world, meat consumption dramatically rose from 23.1 kg per person per year in 1961 to 42.20 kg per head per year in 2011. In addition, similar trend shown by dairy products. Over a period of 50 years (1961–2011), animal-based protein (ABP) consumption raised from 61–80 g per person per day, eventually [6]. Therefore, animal products play a significant role in the growth of food in the world; can supply 17% of total energy and 35% of the protein to the body [7]. Moreover, raw milk demands are predicted to increase from the current scenario, which is 704 million tons, to 1077 million tons by 2050 [8]. The reason is that in developed world milk consumption is approximately stable and contrarily, 50% volume will increase in developing world [4,8]. A yearly consumption rate in Mexico is 355 eggs per individual; in China, it is 344 eggs and in Japan, it is 325 eggs. In 2009, the production of eggs was recorded 64 million tons; China had the highest level of production, which accounted for 36% of the production globally [9]. The aforementioned consumption pattern of animal food showed that trends have been changing with the passage of time.

13.2 MYTHS AND CONTROVERSIES REGARDING ANIMAL FOOD CONSUMPTION

Animal origin food consumption is ubiquitous, but level of intake and types of animal food varies. Increasing animal-sourced food consumption affect ecosystem and bio-diversity. In addition, intake of animal food and food products is more likely to increase modern species extinction rate, overfishing, pollution, climate change, deforestation, and loss of wild life as shown in Figure 13.1 [10]. Contrarily, animal foods are rich in nutrients like protein, calcium, minerals, iron, and some bioactive components, which are highly bioavailable; it is basic food for children, pregnant, lactating women, and the elderly. Evidence has proved that even small quantities of meat and dairy products help to improve the nutritional statuses [8].

Red meat refers to mammalian muscle meat including beef, veal, pork, lamb, mutton, horse, and goat and are supposed to be the reason of various health problems and increase mortality [11–13]. Similarly, long term consumption of red meat increases the risk of cardiovascular diseases, diabetes, and cancer [14–16]. However, there are several proposed mechanisms for the disease-promoting effects of red meat: formation of N-nitorso compounds (NOCs), synthesis of mutagens, and generation

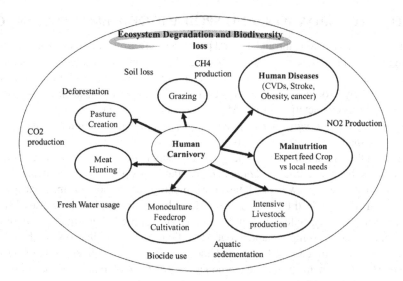

FIGURE 13.1 Effect of increased production and consumption of animal origin food (Machovina, B., Feeley, K.J., Ripple, W.J., *Sci. Total Environ.* 536, 419–431, 2015). [10]

of trimethylamine-Noxide (TMAO). All these compounds are formed during meat processing like grilling, baking, and frying [17]. Heterocyclic amines (HCAs) and Polycyclic aromatic hydrocarbons (PAHs) are also present in fish and chicken, which are processed at high temperature, grilled, or fried. But poultry and fish consumption are not associated with cancer despite of the fact that grilled or fried chicken contains much higher content of HCAs as compared with beef [18]. It is reasonable to say, according to the aforementioned factors, that still there is no authentic explanation available for the carcinogenic effect of meat either processed or non-processed [19,20]. Although, red meat may be contaminated with some inorganic toxins including arsenic, cadmium, mercury, lead, pesticides during cooking or industrial processing of meat. Nevertheless, these compounds are also present in some other food sources; so, again it is not proved that the presence of these compounds increased the risk of diseases, which are specifically supposed to be associated with red meat consumption [21]. Moreover, meat contains saturated fats and its oxidation lead to the production of oxysterols and aldehydes, which cause a proliferation of cells [22]. But carcinogenesis, obesity, and inflammation are not specifically associated with red meat, because other foods also contain certain proportion of saturated fats. Thereby, recent evidences demonstrated the inconsistent relationship between saturated fats intake and risk of cancer: breast and prostate [23,24]. Similar trends shown by high salt contents of meat and meat products, but meat is not the major culprit to cause cardiovascular diseases (CVDs), hypertension, and renal diseases; there might be some other factors involved [17].

Furthermore, the consumption of eggs provides extreme health benefits and is expected to provide several ranges of nutrients to the body. Several studies have tested the relationship between the intake of eggs and heart disease risks but no consistent findings occurred. Some studies provided negative relation while, some did not provide any relation at all. The controversy exists between cardiovascular disease risk and egg consumption [25]. For an individual to have a healthy life, an intake of 300 mg cholesterol in a day is recommended by American Heart Association. However, the consumption of egg is expected to contribute to 200 mg intake of cholesterol; hence, dietitians are recommending to reduce the consumption of eggs [26]. But, no limit has been put on the dietary cholesterol intake and egg consumption by British Heart Foundation and the Diabetes United Kingdom. However, a limit of 200 mg dietary cholesterol is placed by National Lipid Association (NLA) for dyslipidemic patients. The health benefits that eggs are expected to provide to the individuals forced world to increase in the production and consumption of eggs all over the world [27].

13.3 SHELF LIFE, OXIDATION, AND SPOILAGE OF ANIMAL ORIGIN FOOD

Foods of animal origin have gone through several processes before consumption. These include slaughtering, ageing, transformation, storage, and so forth, and they can impair the quality of final products. Admittedly, meat and meat products are good source of protein; structural and storage lipids, like phospholipids and triacylglycerols, respectively. However, for a long period of time lipid oxidation in meat is considered to impair its characteristics [28]. Meat in raw form is more prone to the attack of pathogens and spoilage. For instance, *Campylobacter jejuni* is a bacterium that contaminates raw or undercooked meat, poultry, and shellfish; *Clostridium* spoils meats and meat products; *Escherichia coli* O157:H7: is harmful bacteria that contaminates uncooked beef (especially ground beef); Listeria monocytogenes effects dry sausages, meat, and poultry; *Salmonella* contaminates poultry and meat, and *Vibrio vulnificus* contaminates uncooked or raw fish. All the above-mentioned microorganisms destroy food texture, taste, shorten shelf life, and lead to the number of food-borne illnesses in the world [28]. According to some authorities, like Food Safety and Inspection Service of the US, about 3000 people died every year due to spoiled meat consumption and about 48 million food borne illnesses are the reasons of this outbreaks. Likewise, according to the European Union, 5550 foodborne illness were responsible for 48 deaths in 2009. Thereby, fish, meat, and meat products cause 26.3% of total outbreaks; pork meat causes 7.8%; bovine accounted for 2.5%, and fish and fish product are the source of 5.4% outbreaks [29].

In muscle food, protein oxidation (PROTOX) involved in the progression of several diseases [30,35] may be induced in meat and meat products directly through reactive oxygen species (ROS), reactive nitrogen species (RNS), and indirectly through oxidative stress [31]. Moreover, some precursors of protein oxidation are described in Figure 13.2.

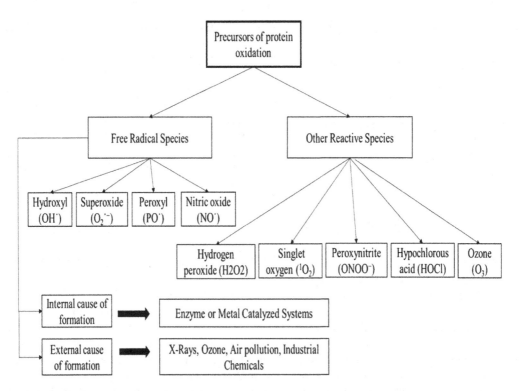

FIGURE 13.2 Factors that initiate PROTOX in meat system either by modifying the amino acid side chains or attacking the polypeptide backbone of the protein (From Lund, M.N. et al., *Meat Sci.* 76, 226–233, 2007; Lund, M.N. et al., *Mol Nutr. Food Res,* 55, 83–95, 2011; Xiong, Y.L. *Protein Oxidation and Implications for Muscle Food Quality. Antioxidant in Muscle Foods.* Wiley, Chichester, UK, pp. 85–111, 2000; Calkins C.R., and Hodgen J.M., *Meat Sci,* 77, 63–80, 2007). [30, 35, 36, 37]

Oxidative stress results in a modification of the amino acid side chain and causes fragmentation, aggregation, and polymerization of the protein. Hence, it eventually leads to both biochemical and structural disruption, which results in a change of sensory, technological, and nutritional properties of fleshy food [31,32]. Moreover, protein oxidation is also caused by a cleavage of protein bond. Fragmentation may occur when free radical reacts with the polypeptide backbone of protein and α-amidation or diamide pathways, results in cleavage of alkoxyl radicals and alkyl peroxide (derivatives of protein) [33]. Furthermore, N-pyruvyl derivatives are formed due to the oxidation of glutamyl and aspartyl residue, which causes destruction of peptide bond. In addition, modification in the structure of protein march towards protein oxidation and lose sulfhydryl group. A sulfur-containing amino acids, like cysteine and methionine, are quite sensitive to reactive oxygen species, and their loss in meat is an indication of oxidative stress to specific meat proteins [34].

In addition, lipids oxidation is also known as autoxidation, which mostly occurs in three simultaneous phases: initiation, propagation, and completion. The product from these reactions are unsaturated fatty acid, which depends upon substrates. The first two phases caused the formation of radicals that immediately transformed into non-radical compounds, like conjugated di-enes and hydroperoxides; they are prime products of lipid oxidation. Further decomposition of this compound give rise to secondary products including carbonyl compounds, ketones, alcohols, and aldehydes. Although, lipid oxidation effects the taste and odor of meat due to development of aromatic compounds [38–40]. Secondary lipid oxidative products (aldehydes) also effect organoleptic, nutritional properties and react with proteins. Moreover, fluctuation or decrease in the amount of polyunsaturated fatty acid, may leads to increase saturated fatty acid content in animal origin food [28]. Consequently, due to lipid and protein oxidation, unhealthy products are form within animal food and it also has impact on shelf life and flavor. Hence, acceptability and consumption of animal-sourced food is affected. Adequate cooking/processing, good packaging, proper transportation, and reducing oxidation process are the key factors to improve its intake.

13.4 ANTIMICROBIAL AGENT: DEVELOPMENT OF RESISTANCE IN HUMAN BODY

Modern animal production practices are basically linked with the excessive use of antimicrobial agents that results in sustainable livestock production [40]. Antimicrobial agents have been used in human and veterinary medicine for more than 60 years to prevent, control, treat infection, and improve growth [41]. Although, excessive and misuse of antibiotics give birth to the term "antibiotic resistance" [42]. According to the World Health Organization, antibiotic resistance refers to the resistance of bacteria or other microorganisms from so-called antimicrobial drugs and this leads to a decrease in the effectiveness of treatment [43]. Like everything, antimicrobial agents have some pros and cons, despite of some negative consequences of antimicrobial resistance in body, there are lack of quantitative measurement for use of antimicrobial agents in livestock [40]. But according to an estimate, average annual consumption of antimicrobials in animal origin food are about 45 mg per kg cattle, 148 mg per kg for chicken, and 172 mg per kg for pigs in the world. Antimicrobial consumption is ubiquitous, and it will increase up to 67% from 63,151 (±1,560) tons in 2010 to 105,596 (±3,605) tons in 2030. In countries like Brazil, Russia, India, China, and South Africa probably, antimicrobial consumption in livestock is predicted to increase by 99% [40]. Similar trends are shown in Table 13.1 in which the percentage of antimicrobial agents used in animal food in various countries is described.

Introduction of antimicrobial agent in veterinary medicine eventually improve animal health and productivity [45]. Moreover, it is indispensable tool for declining the morbidity and mortality rate that can cause by infection in host: animals and humans. But resistance to antimicrobial drugs now has become a global issue of both medicinal and agricultural field [46]. Thereby, intensive and inappropriate use may lead to loss in efficacy. Antimicrobial resistance pathogens not only possess harm in animal but also effect public heath because it is transmitted as food born contaminants. However, common antimicrobial drugs that are given to animals may belongs to these

TABLE 13.1

Comparison between Percentage of Antimicrobial Agent Consumption in 2010 and 2030

Countries	2010	2030
China	23%	30%
United States	13%	10%
Brazil	9%	8%
India	3%	4%
Germany	3%	–

Source: Angulo, F.J, et., *Semin Pediatr. Infect. Dis*, 15, 78–85, 2004; Griggs, D.J. et al., J. *Antimicrob. Chemother*. 33, 1173–1189, 1994). [40, 44]

classes: beta-lactams, tetracyclines, macrolides, aminogylcosides, and sulphonamides [47]. Animal and human bacterial pathogens are becoming resistant to several frontline bacteria: expanded-spectrum cephalosporins, aminoglycosides, and even fluoroquinolones [45,48]. Admittedly, when antimicrobial pressure is introduced in environment, which immediately develops resistance and starts spreading. It's like a chain reaction that can move one microbial species to the next. Plasmid: an extra-chromosomal DNA segment, is involved in transformational process. Therefore, DNA may possess various antimicrobial resistance genes and responsible to spread these gene among different bacterial species [49,50]. With the passage of time, in the presence of pressure, antimicrobial resistant bacteria might displace the antibiotic-susceptible population [51,52]. Recent studies have demonstrated that different resistance determinants have the potential to aggregate and form a cluster on one mobile element; likely different classes of antibiotics and non-antibiotic substances: heavy metals, disinfectant, probably chosen for antimicrobial resistant bacteria [53,54]. The ecology of antimicrobial resistance creates hurdles and makes it difficult to control infection. Whereas, in the population of bacteria, certain cells exist that may possess traits that enable them to survive even in the presence of some notorious stuff and components. Further, susceptible organism: lacking good traits, starts eliminating and leave only resistant population behind. Hence, resistant commensal bacteria immediately synthesize as a component of normal flora of various host species [49,55]. Emergence and dissemination of resistant antimicrobial genes have undergone some pathways in Figure 13.3 and

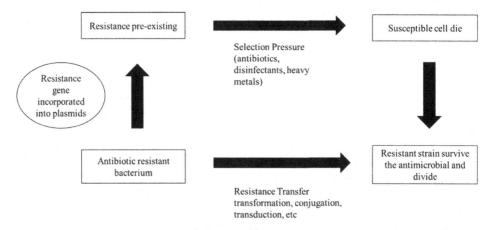

Emergence of Antimicrobial Resistance

FIGURE 13.3   Possible pathways of emergence and transfer of antimicrobial resistant strain and gene (Bush, K. et al., *Antimicrob. Agents Chemother*, 39, 1211–1233, 1995). [46]

created an ecology of resistance in the body. Consequently, resistance is an inevitable biological phenomenon; the challenge is to tackle disastrous consequences and prevent from chronic health problems [46].

13.5 ANIMAL ORIGIN FOOD INCREASE THE RISK OF CANCER

There is a strong epidemiological association between red meat and risk of carcinomas and mortality [13]. An increased intake of processed red meat is associated with cancer; for instance, 1 g of processed red meat increased the risk of cancer two to ten times [56]. It is estimated that 34,000 deaths from cancer every year occur due to diets high in processed meat [57]. Colorectal cancer is the third most frequently diagnosed cancer in the world and it effects more than 1 million people every year [58]. Prostate cancer is the second most common cancer in men worldwide; 1.1 million new cases appear every year [59]. Breast cancer effects more than 1.2 million people in the world [60]. Larsson and Wolk [61] illustrated that populations with the highest quartile of red meat consumption showed an increased risk of colorectal cancer about 1.35 fold, and processed meat raised 1.31 fold risk. Hence, foods of animal origins are associated with increased risk of cancer [62].

13.5.1 MILK AND CANCER

Hormones are chemical messengers, that helps to regulate physiological and behavior functions [63] Recombinant bovine growth hormone (rBGH): is a steroidal transgenic substance, which is injected in cattle in order to increase milk production. It can approximately enhance 8–10 pounds per day [64]. Synthetic hormones are like a two-edged sword that have both merits and demerits; however, the adverse effects outweigh its merits because it increases the risk of prostate, breast, and ovarian cancers [65,66]. DNA plays an important role in the production of bovine growth hormone in cattle, which is combined with the plasmid vector of *E. Coli* bacteria and reproduces latterly, enriching the quantity of rBGH hormone [64,67,68]. Insulin-like growth factor (IGF-1) is a hormone synthesized by the liver in response to somatotropin. IGF-1 promotes growth of tumor cells because of apoptosis, cell proliferation, and angiogenesis [69]. Correspondingly, IGF-1 acts as mitogen for the epithelial cells of the prostate [70]. To increase milk production in cattle, the Food and Drug Administration (FDA) approved the following hormones: Bovine somatotropin (bST) bovine growth hormone (bGH), recombinant bovine somatotropin (rbST), and recombinant bovine growth hormone (rbGH) [71]. But, the FDA also acknowledged that these hormones raised the IGF-1 level in milk [72,73]. The recombinant bovine growth hormone (rbGH) injection in cattle, consequently, causes various diseases in human beings due to the consumption of bovine milk, as shown in Figure 13.4. The human gut absorbs IGF-1, in turn effecting the endogenous IGF-1 in circulation. Consequently, this leads to the elevation of the circulating IGF-1 level. Bovine IGF-1 in milk is quite similar to the human IGF-1 [72]. Likewise, milk intake elevates the circulating IGF-1 level [74,75] and, eventually, increases the risk of cancer. On other hand, some studies showed a week association between milk and breast cancer [76]. While, evidence has proved that high levels of circulating IGF-1 increased the risk of breast cancer seven times and four-fold the risk of prostate cancer. Moreover, shortening the average girls age entering early puberty and menstruation [64]. Furthermore, the combination of IGF-1 in BST-milk and IGF-1 in the human gastrointestinal lumen may cause intraluminal concentrations of this hormone; raised the carcinogenic effects on gut tissues [77].

13.5.2 MEAT AND CANCER

Globally, about <5%–100% red meat is consumed, as a source of basic nutrient whereas, processed meat consumption is less than 2%–65% approximately. Average daily meat intake is 50–100 g per person and high consumption is more than 200 g per person per day. Red meat consumption either

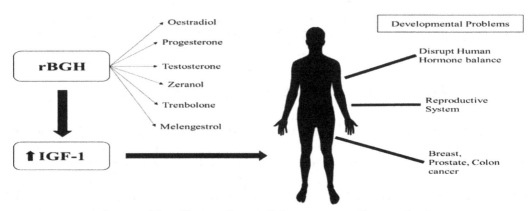

Adverse side effects of growth hormone on human body

FIGURE 13.4 Effect of injecting growth hormone in cattle, disrupt developmental problem in human body (Epstein, S.S. *Int. J. Health Serv*, 26, 173–185, 1996; Juskevich, J.C. Guyer, C.G. *Science*, 249, 875–884, 1990. Bouvard, V. et al., *Lancet Oncol*, 16, 1599–1600, 2015). [64, 71, 78]

processed or unprocessed may lead to pancreatic, prostate, stomach cancer [79]. According to World Cancer Research Foundation, red meat is considered among top ten factors that are linked with the incidence and progression of carcinomas in all population [80]. Although, carcinomas risk is enhanced in tissues, especially colonic epithelium, mostly adenomas can progress into carcinomas through molecular changes in oncogene and tumor suppressor genes [81]. A meta-analysis illustrated that 100 g of red meat daily increased the risk of colorectal cancer by 17% and 50 g of processed meat increased the risk by 18% [58].

The International Agency for Research on Cancer (IARC) represent different classification of carcinogens; in which processed meat is classify in group one and red meat in group 2 as shown in Figure 13.5. There is a mechanistic approach for the carcinogenesis of red meat: formation of mutagens by grilling, DNA damage due to N-nitroso compound, and free radical formation by heme iron [82]. Substantially, red and proceed meat consumption induce N-nitroso compounds (NOC) in the digestive tract. Moreover, high red meat consumption about 300–420 g/day increased DNA adducts due to NOC [83,84]. Heme iron also mediates the generation of NOC and leads to lipid oxidation products in the digestive tract [79]. Heterocyclic amine (HCA) are formed by reaction of amino acid and sugar; according to the type of meat, chemical environment, and temperature [85]. HCA is converted into genotoxic metabolites by Cytochrome P450, N-Acetyltransferases (NAT), Sulfotransferases (SULT), and results in formation of DNA reactive substances [85]. Red and processed meat intake increased colorectal cancer risk. However, meat consumption may impart cancer differently in various region of colorectum: proximal colon, distal colon, and rectum [86]. Moreover, high consumption of red and processed meat increased postmenopausal breast cancer [87].

To put all above in a nut shell, processed and red meat may cause cancer but still it needs a strong evidenced to prove. However, we cannot deny the beneficial effect of meat. Altering cooking methods and processing techniques prevent the formation of carcinogenic compound in meat. Therefore, for healthy milk production, limit the use of growth hormone in cattle. By taking simple steps, a new perspective can be presented to reduce the risk of cancers and to promote healthy animal food in a better way.

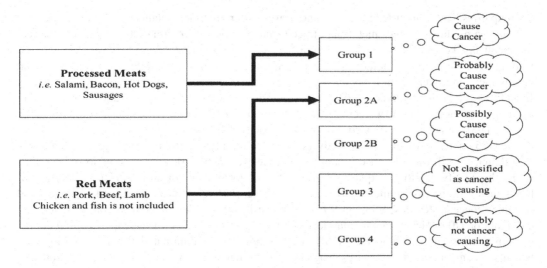

FIGURE 13.5 Carcinogenic classification of meat groups (Steinfeld, H. et al., Food & Agriculture Organization of the United Nations (FAO), Rome, Italy, pp. 79–125, 2006). [88]

13.6 LIVESTOCK AND ENVIRONMENTAL PROBLEM

Livestock disrupts the carbon balance of land that is used for the pasture and feed crops; hence, leads to indirect release of carbon in the atmosphere. Further, fossil fuels are used to produce feed and that releases gasses [89]. Livestock has been increasing considerably with the passage of time, but it may lead to global warming, loss of biodiversity, and water and air pollution [90]. Livestock production rise with the growth in population and with economic boost, results in increase in consumption of animal origin food [91]. For instance, one-third of the land is served for feed production and about a third of global cereal production is used to feed animals [91]. That is why, livestock production contributes toward global warming: anthropogenic methane about 35%–40% and 9% anthropogenic CO_2. Emissions from livestock manure and urine contribute approximately 64% of global anthropogenic ammonia emission [92]. Hence, emission from livestock leads to major environmental problems. Firstly, it causes air pollution because of emission of ammonia (NH3) and nitrogen oxides that contribute to the formation of secondary particulate matter and tropospheric ozone [93]. Secondly, livestock systems contribute about 14.5% greenhouse gases in the world [94]. Moreover, greenhouse gases: methane, nitrous oxide, carbon dioxide produce the use of fossil fuel and land [95]. Livestock production effect terrestrial biodiversity by use of land because of ammonia emission, deposition, and climate change [96]. Moreover, it also causes the deterioration of fresh water quality by increasing phosphorus and N loss from water system. According to an evidence, 25 mg L^{-1} nitrate (NO_3^-) in drinking water, basically increase the risk of colon cancer by about 3% [97]. Subsequently, livestock production and consumption of animal-sourced food is influenced.

13.6.1 ACCUMULATION OF METALS IN FISH

In aquatic food chain, fish acquire a remarkable place. Heavy metals can easily accumulate in fish body through food, water, and sediments [98,99]. Heavy metals: cadmium, copper, zinc, iron, considered as toxic substance for the body [100]. Heavy metals that pollute the aquatic environment are comes from atmospheric deposition, geologic weathering, through agriculture discharge, municipal/residential/industrial wastes, and waste water treatment plants [101]. Moreover, coal combustion produces various metals and trace elements [102]. There are certain factors that effect the metal uptake: gender, age, size, reproductive cycle, swimming patterns, water ecology, and feeding behavior [99,103]. Metals are mostly concentrated in the edible parts of fish muscles and organs including liver, kidney, heart, bone, digestive tract, brain, and reproductive system [104]. In addition, the gills and liver are the target organ for accumulation; concentrations in gills is an indication of concentration in water whereas, accumulation in liver reflects the storage of metals [100]. Accumulation of heavy metals accounts towards toxicity, which may counteract the positive effects of fish [105]. This may cause several adverse effects to the human body including kidney failure, liver damage, cardiovascular diseases, and sometime even death [106,107]. International programs assess the quality of fish for aquatic environment and for human consumption [108]. Presence of heavy metals in the environment disrupt aquatic and terrestrial organism. Metals like mercury and selenium concentrates in fish; about 90% of human health problem related to contaminated fish consumption [109]. Heavy metals may lead to production of reactive oxygen species by inducing oxidative stress and carcinogenesis [101]. That is how the contaminated fish instead of giving benefits become a reason of diseases progression in human body. Aquatic life should be protected from toxic wastes of industry. So, fish can be consumed as healthy food, which contains omega-3 fatty acid that reduce the risk of heart disease, inflammation, and cancer.

13.7 ORGANIC LIVESTOCK PRODUCTION

Organic farming and livestock are crucial to prevent human beings from the detrimental effects of fertilizers, antibiotics, steroids, and other chemical compounds. For the promotion of animal food, it is necessary to provide food that are free range and healthy for the body. For this purpose, drugs, and other chemical should be limited. Alternative ways should be used that reduce the risk of cancer, early menstruation, antibiotic resistance, and hormones problems. Disastrous consequences can be prevented through organic production of food.

13.7.1 REDUCE USE OF ANTIBIOTICS AND BANNING GROWTH PROMOTERS IN FEED

Long term use of antimicrobial agents disrupts the microbial ecology dramatically. So, ratio of resistant organisms will increase in a society. Five principles are proposed by Levy [110] through which we can understand and promote possible solution of this problem: (1) there should be sufficient time and proper use of antibiotics; (2) resistance to antibiotic is progressive that evolve from low level to intermediate and then to high level; (3) resistance to one antimicrobial may leads towards other; (4) once resistance is develop, it decrease slowly; (5) use of antimicrobial agent in one individual may affect others in their surrounding environment. The use of antimicrobials should be very concise and focused in order to treat and prevent animal from disease. Although, bacterial pathogens: *Escherchia coli*, *Salmonella*, *Enterococcus*, *Staphylococcus*, *Campylobacter* are acquiring various antibiotic resistance phenotypes, which results in limiting and diminishing of therapeutic choices (Table 13.2).

In order to considered alternatives for antimicrobials, the scope and benefits of antibiotics should acknowledge. Use of antibiotics can be limited by developing immunization program and introducing vaccinations at low cost [43]. Another way to reduce antibiotics and prevention from diseases, is the improvement of gut health: promote gut bacterial flora by introducing probiotics, prebiotics, and synbiotics [114,115]. However, good gut health is an indication of immune functionality, contribution of nutrients, and reduce pathogen colonization. For instance, *Salmonella* colonization is significantly reduced by the commensal anaerobic bacteria administration in poultry. Although, *Butyricicoccus pullicaecorum* isolated from broiler cecum is directly linked with inflammatory bowel disease, which can be reversed through oral administration of beneficial bacteria [116]. Yeasts possessing certain characteristics and genetically modified strains may also use as probiotics [117]. This provide a promising health benefits, but it is crucial to access the

TABLE 13.2

Antimicrobial Resistance Pathogens and Diseases

Micro Organisms	Diseases Caused	Resistances
Streptococcus pneumoniae	Meningitis, pneumonia	Aminoglycosides, chloramphenicol, penicillin, macrolides
Streptococcus aureus	Bacteremia, pneumonia	Chloramphenicol, macrolodes, trimethoprim, tetracycline, betalectams
Enterococcus	Bacteremia, wound infections, urinary tract infection	Aminoglycosides, beta-lectams, erythromycin, glycopeptides
Enterobacteriaceae	Bacteremia, pneumonia, diarrhea, urinary tract infection	Aminoglycosides, chloramphenicol, trimethoprim, FQs
Shigelladysenteriae	Severe diarrhea	Ampicillin, chloramphenicol, tetracycline
Plasmodium falciparum	Malaria	Chloroquine
Mycobacterium tuberculosis	Tuberculosis	Aminoglycosides, ethanbutol, isoniazid, rifampin

Source: Salyers, A.A., and Amiable-Cuevas, C.F., *Antimicrob Agents Chemother*, 41, 2321–2325, 1997; Hall, R.M. et al., *Ann NY Acad Sci.*, 870, 68–80, 1999; Gold, H.S., and Moellering, R.C., *N. Eng. J. Med.*, 335, 1445–1453, 1996; Piddock, L.J.V. *Drugs Suppl.*, 2, 29–35, 1995; Callaway, T.R., et al., *Anim. Health Res. Rev.*, 9, 217–225, 2008). [51, 52, 110, 111, 112, 113]

effectiveness and underlying mechanisms [116,118,119]. Interestingly, pathogens are neutralized during the lytic phase of their cycle by using phages. The use of phages is quite compatible with the use of antibiotics agents, but it is limited to the treatment of tropical infection in human, neutralization of food borne pathogens in animals and also control plant pathogens [120–122]. Moreover, they are more specific than antibiotics because they exhibit variable specificity, primarily influence through phage titer and effect of phage on microbiota is lesser than antibiotics [123,124]. In addition, another alternative are antimicrobial peptides: some has a toxic effect on mammalian cell, while some are supposed to lack toxicity; for example, bacteriocins that are ribosomally synthesized peptides can also be used as food preservatives [125]. They are generally recognized as a safe fermentate, act as starter culture, and reduce Listeria from food [126,127]. So, bacteriocins may be sufficient for pathogens destruction. One other alternative way to reduce antibiotics are the use of predatory bacteria: *Bdellovibrio bacteriovorus* and *Micavibrio aeruginosavorus* [124,128]. Evidence showed that these bacteria prey on multidrug-resistant pathogens including *A. baumannii*, *E. coli*, *Klebsiella pneumonia*, *Pseudomonas aeruginosa*, and *Pseudomonas putida* without the discrimination among antibiotic resistance and antibiotic susceptible strains [129]. Intriguingly, they act as an antibiotic as well as probiotic organism. Therefore, in this way antibiotic resistance from society will be diminished and everyone will have an easy approach to nutritious animal food. Furthermore, growth promotion and hormones in animals should be banned to enhance the quality and safety of meat and milk.

The global situation regarding antibiotic resistance is at alarming rate. World Health Organization in 2001, has set the foundation for the establishment of measure to control antibiotic resistance [44]. The control measures involved in reducing emergence and spreading of antibiotic resistant strain, develop better surveillance system, make proper use of antibiotics, enforce legislation, and motivate the development and production of new vaccines and other drugs [43]. However, in the Third World Healthcare Associated Infection Forum (WHAIF) in 2011, present antibiotic resistance action and awareness strategies. WHAIF involve 70 experts, who represent 33 countries, and, at the end of this forum, all of them agreed on the formation of 12 priority actions shown in Table 13.3.

TABLE 13.3

Third World Healthcare Association Infection Forum Accept Priority Actions

Stakeholders	Priority Actions and Steps
Policy makers and health authorities	• Stop the administration of antibiotics in human medicine and limit it to only therapeutic use • Ban use of antibiotic as growth promoter in animal feed • Regulate the sale and prohibit over the counter sale of antibiotic • International organization develop a good antibiotic stewardship, signed by all ministries and commit to respect it in the world
Human and veterinary health care communities	• There should be a standardized, universal surveillance of antibiotic use; resistance; monitor the emergence of new bacterial resistance • Establish job training programs according to cultural specificities of every country with special reference to training in bacterial resistance and use of bacteria for health care worker
General public	• Establish culturally sensitive awareness campaigns and explaining the importance of protecting antibiotics and use them only in absolute necessary • Educate regarding fundamental hygiene and prevent from infection spreading • Involve consumers in the implementation and development of action plan
Industry	• Develop diagnostic tests and point of care, to guide the prescription of antibiotics and avoid their prescription for viral infection • Stimulate research and development of novel antibiotics • Develop new economic models in order to reconcile public health interests with industry needs for profitability

Source: World Health Organization, 2001; Griggs, D.J. et al., Quinolone resistance in veterinary isolates of *Salmonella. J. Antimicrob. Chemother.*, 33, 1173–1189, 1994). [43, 44]

Note: Stakeholders: national and international health authorities and policy makers, the medical and veterinary communities, the general public, and industry.

13.8 TECHNIQUES TO INCREASE SHELF LIFE OF FOOD

Shelf life of animal-sourced food increases through natural material that scavenge free radicals and reduces lipid oxidation. For that purpose, honey is added and it contains phenolic acid, vitamins, and enzymes [130]. Besides honey, chitosan acts as an antioxidant for animal origin food because it delays lipid oxidation and hinders reactive oxygen species by donating a hydrogen atom and a lone pair of electrons [131]. In addition, freezing is the easiest and economical technique to preserve animal-sourced food, especially meat. It stops microbial activity by decreasing water activities and slows down the rate of chemical reaction. Furthermore, high pressure processing is an alternative to the heating process because it maintains organoleptic properties. This method ruptures the cell membrane of microorganisms. In this type of processing, food is exposed to high pressure to deactivate microorganisms with or without addition of heat. The additional benefit of this technique is that it maintains the freshness and quality of food without breaking covalent bond [132]. Moreover, meat packaging is very crucial for extending shelf life and enhancing the acceptability. Although, some packaging techniques is very effective to slow down the oxidation of meat (2015). Modified atmosphere packaging (MAP) has a potential to increase myosin cross links protein carbonyls and reduce thiol group in high oxygen 70%–80% MAP [31,133,134]. Notably, PROTOX can be induces by high oxygen MAP. However, 100% nitrogen or vacuum packaging prove to reduce PROTOX [31,134]. PROTOX in vivo studies cause life threatening disorder: Alzheimer's disease, chronic renal failure, and diabetes. So, oxygen should be replaced by nitrogen in MAP for better packaging and good quality meat and meat products [33]. Therefore, in this way animal food with greater shelf life will encouraged.

13.9 VALUE ADDITION AND PROMOTION OF FUNCTIONAL FOOD OF ANIMAL ORIGIN

Value addition of foods is a traditional method to increase the functional value by adding more nutritive value, making food attractive to the consumers. With the advancement in technology, the food industry is flourishing and is known as a sunrise industry because it adds value to the raw products and provides convenient food packages. Meat and meat products intake may lead to the development of obesity, cancer, and stroke because it has saturated fatty acid. Whereas this concept neglects the positive potential of meat on the human health. Nevertheless, meat contains essential nutrients naturally, but its value enhanced by adding bioactive compounds that have beneficial physiological effect on body. For instance, fish contains bioactive compound like omega-3 that helps to lower the risk of triglycerides, reduce the risk of heart attack, inflammatory disorders, and various other diseases. Adding omega-3 in eggs and meat enhance the quality and functionality of them. Similarly, polyphenolic components help in the formation of stable protein network in meat and meat products. In value addition, high fats contents in meat can be reduce and replace by good fats contents. Ideally, there should be optimal balance between omega-3 and omega-6 contents and ratio of omega-6 to omega-3 should be less. The World Health Organization (WHO) and FAO suggested a ratio of omega-3 and saturated fat should be between 0.4 and 1.0 respectively. Saturated fats elevate lipid oxidation and cause the development of fishy flavor. Adding Eicosapentaenoic (EPA), Docosahexaenoic (DHA), Alpha linolenic acid (ALA), and antioxidants in meat mince, sausages recipe, and other meat products enhance its value. Moreover, reduction of cholesterol content in meat can be achieved by adding conjugated linoleic acid (CLA) through supplementation in animal feed with linoleic acid. In dairy products, processing is beneficial; cooking that raise CLA content. CLA has positive potential includes: cholesterol lowering effect, anticarcinogenic, antidiabetic, antiatherogenic effect, bone metabolism, strengthening immune system, and body composition [135].

The main source of long-chain polyunsaturated fatty acids are plants oil, oil seed, marine algae, flaxseed, and canola. They are added into the feed of poultry to enhance the quality of poultry meat and eggs. However, beef's functional value is also enhanced by the addition of these substances in the feed [136]. The omega-3 fatty acids, Docosahexaenoic acid (DHA) and Alpha linolenic acid (ALA), which are present in the yolk of eggs increases with a diet enriched with flaxseeds. When the amount of flaxseed consumption is increased in the diet, a decline in the ratio of omega-6 to omega-3 in egg yolk is observed [137]. The major component of poultry diets are vegetable protein sources, which are available in comparatively greater quantity and can be efficiently incorporated in poultry diets. Among vegetable protein sources, the soybean meal is well known due to its best profile of certain essential amino acids [138]. Over the past 30 years, rapeseed meal has successfully produced high quality (canola) cultivator with low erucic acid (<2%) in the oil and low glucosinolates (<30 micro moles/gram) in the meal, increasing the use of the oil in the vegetable oil market and in the meal in animal feeds [139].

Lipids oxidation in meat decreases the shelf life of frozen, fermented meat like sausages. While in precooked meat, reheating leads to the development of off-flavor in meat. This problem can be tackled by the addition of an antioxidant that scavenges free radicals and thereby, terminates the chain reaction. For example, vitamin E, lycopene, and lutein not only reduce the lipid oxidation of meat but are also good for health. Natural antioxidants are proved to be more beneficial compared to synthetic, which are added in form of spices in meat [135]. Although milk has high content of calcium but calcium fortification in milk is done in order to enhance functional, nutritional, and technological properties [140]. In addition to calcium, probiotics are also supplemented having a protective effect on the intestine of goats, and, in return, they produce milk that is high in polyunsaturated fatty acid [141]. Considerably, through this valuable addition, the nutritional value of animal-sourced food is enhanced and, along with basic nutrients, it can also provide extra health benefits as a functional food.

13.10   MAINTAINING BIODIVERSITY AND PROMOTION OF ANIMAL-SOURCED FOOD

Certain strategies have been suggested to raise sustainability in livestock production including efficiency strategy: increase productivity by improving feeding, feed efficiency, improving digestibility; consistency strategy: in livestock ration reduce the use of food-competing feed components that has impact on availability of livestock products [90]. According to the FAO, 843 million people suffer from hunger in 2013 globally. In poor areas of the world, people are mostly suffering from protein and micronutrients (vitamin A, iron, folate, and zinc) deficiencies [142]. It is estimated that one billion people in the world are facing chronic inadequate protein intake or protein energy malnutrition [143]. Foods of animal origins are rich in protein; that is, eggs, meat, dairy products, poultry, sea food, beef, and mutton. More than 40% of protein on dry matter contributed by these foods is relatively high level. On the other hand, foods of plant origins, except legumes, contributed less than 15% protein only on a dry matter basis. Vitamins (B6, B12, and A) and minerals (iron and zinc) are essential for the human body and present in animal origin food. Moreover, animal protein is a complete protein whereas plant protein is considered as incomplete [144]. Animal origin food provides an adequate and balanced amount of amino acids that are necessary for optimal growth, development, and health. Food of animal origins should be promoted to build a healthy nation. Certain policies should be adopted for the promotion of food of animal origin. For instance, conserve and use agro-biodiversity for the production of inexpensive protein rich food and encourage diet diversification [145]. Promote animal-sourced food, particularly in those areas where protein and micronutrients intake are low. In addition, promote the use of mechanism-based means including optimizing the proportion of essential and non-essential amino acid to enhance the efficiency of livestock and poultry production; thus, stimulating protein synthesis and inhibiting protein degradation. Moreover, continue exploring radical innovation in the field of animal-sourced food. Production of healthy food with less strain to the environment is a bigger challenge. Valuable tools should be used for effective environmental management [143]. Livestock meat production can be replaced by laboratory meat production in order to lessen the environmental burden. Further, monitor fish biomarker that induce heavy metals in fish and cause alteration in fish quality [146]. Treatment of waste water, sewage and agriculture waste must be properly conducted before discharge into aquatic system. Laws and legislation are enforced for the protection of aquatic environment [144]. According to the aforementioned strategies, issues related to animal origin food consumption can be resolve. So, encourage animal food because it is healthy for human consumption due to several benefits. In addition, sources of micronutrients that are essential for growth and development of body are demonstrated in Table 13.4.

TABLE 13.4

Sources of Micronutrients in Animal Sourced Food

Micronutrients	Sources
Thiamin, Riboflavin, Niacin, Vitamin B6, B12 Pantothenic acid, Biotin, Vitamin K	Meat, liver, milk, eggs and other animal products
Vitamin D	Milk, eggs and liver is a good source of vitamin D3
Vitamin C, E and A	Liver, milk, eggs, butter, fats
Iron	Meat, liver, blood, milk and other animal products
Zinc, Copper, Selenium, Molybednum	Meat, liver, blood, eggs and animal product

Source: Wu, G. *Amino Acids: Biochemistry and Nutrition.* CRC Press, Boca Raton, FL, 2013. [143]

13.11 CONCLUSION AND FUTURE PERSPECTIVE

Human health depends upon dietary protein with adequate amounts of amino acids, which are present in animal food. However, production of meat increases pressure on the environment and causes health problems. Therefore, trends have been shifting towards lower meat consumption. But, we cannot deny the wonders of animal food and how important it is for the human body. At present, there is a concern to produce animal food at low costs and without strain on the environment and human health. A balance diet with adequate protein consumption are a radical step towards sustainability. Moreover, there is need to adopt some strategies for the promotion of animal food including increase the role of extrinsic cues in quality perception of meat; production and transport of good quality meat; encourage better packaging and storage systems; make meat/milk/eggs easily available to everyone; increase the intake of less processed meat and milk with limited use of preservatives, hormonal growth promotant, and antibiotics; last but not least increase purchasing power and promote diet diversification. Although, industries are now focusing on producing value-added animal origin products that not only raise the quality of food but also enhance its functionality. With the growth in food industries, meat production will also increase to fulfill the demand of the world's population. Thereby, the interaction of consumer lifestyles and food chains will exploit many possibilities of the biological variation in animal food that add part for the consumer welfare and well-being.

REFERENCES

1. Schneider UA, Havlík P, Schmid E, Valin H, Mosnier A, Obersteiner M, Fritz S (2011) Impacts of population growth, economic development, and technical change on global food production and consumption. *Agric Sys* 104:204–215.
2. Popkin BM (2006) Global nutrition dynamics: The world is shifting rapidly toward a diet linked with noncommunicable diseases. *Am J Clin Nutr* 84:289–298.
3. Keyzer MA, Merbis MD, Pavel IFPW, Van Wesenbeeck CFA (2005) Diet shifts towards meat and the effects on cereal use: Can we feed the animals in 2030? *Ecol Econ* 55:187–202.
4. Alexandratos N, Bruinsma J (2012) *World Agriculture Towards 2030/2050: The 2012 Revision*, Vol. 12, No. 3. FAO, Rome, Italy, ESA Working paper.
5. Butland B, Jebb S, Kopelman P, McPherson K, Thomas S, Mardell J, Parry V (2007) Foresight. Tackling obesities: Future choices. Project report. *Foresight. Tackling Obesities: Future Choices. Project Report.* 2nd ed.
6. Sans P, Combris P (2015) World meat consumption patterns: An overview of the last fifty years (1961–2011). *Meat Sci* 109:106–111.

7. Council for Agriculture Science and Technology (1999) *Animal Agriculture and Global Food Supply*. Task Force Report no. 135. Ames, IA.

8. Van Hooijdonk T, Hettinga K (2015) Dairy in a sustainable diet: A question of balance. *Nutr Rev* 73:48–54.

9. Miranda JM, Anton X, Redondo-Valbuena C, Roca-Saavedra P, Rodriguez JA, Lamas A, Cepeda A (2015) Egg and egg-derived foods: Effects on human health and use as functional foods. *Nutrients* 7:706–729.

10. Machovina B, Feeley KJ, Ripple WJ (2015) Biodiversity conservation: The key is reducing meat consumption. *Sci Total Environ* 536:419–431.

11. Larsson SC, Orsini N (2013) Red meat and processed meat consumption and all-cause mortality: A meta-analysis. *Am J Epidemiol* 179:282–289.

12. Pan A, Sun Q, Bernstein AM et al. (2012) Red meat consumption and mortality: results from 2 prospective cohort studies. *Arch Intern Med* 172:555–563.

13. Sinha R, Cross AJ, Graubard BI, Leitzmann MF, Schatzkin A (2009) Meat intake and mortality: A prospective study of over half a million people. *Arch Intern Med* 169:562–571.

14. Aune D, Ursin G, Veierod MB (2009) Meat consumption and the risk of type 2 diabetes: A systematic review and meta-analysis of cohort studies. *Diabetologia* 52:2277–2287.

15. Aune D, Chan DS, Vieira AR et al. (2013) Red and processed meat intake and risk of colorectal adenomas: A systematic review and meta-analysis of epidemiological studies. *Cancer Causes Control* 24:611–627.

16. Micha R, Wallace SK, Mozaffarian D (2010) Red and processed meat consumption and risk of incident coronary heart disease, stroke, and diabetes mellitus: A systematic review and meta-analysis. *Circulation* 121:2271–2283.

17. Alisson-Silva F, Kawanishi K, Varki A (2016) Human risk of diseases associated with red meat intake: Analysis of current theories and proposed role for metabolic incorporation of a non-human sialic acid. *Mol Aspects Med* 51:16–30.

18. Heddle JA, Knize MG, Dawod D, Zhang XB (2001) A test of the mutagenicity of cooked meats in vivo. *Mutagenesis* 16:103–107.

19. Cross AJ, Leitzmann MF, Gail MH, Hollenbeck AR, Schatzkin A, Sinha R (2007) A prospective study of red and processed meat intake in relation to cancer risk. *PLoS Med* 4:325–331.

20. Huxley RR, Ansary-Moghaddam A, Clifton P, Czernichow S, Parr CL, Woodward M (2009) The impact of dietary and lifestyle risk factors on risk of colorectal cancer: A quantitative overview of the epidemiological evidence. *Int J Cancer* 125:171–180.

21. Domingo JL, Nadal M (2016) Carcinogenicity of consumption of red and processed meat: What about environmental contaminants? *Environ Res* 145:109–115.

22. Biasi F, Mascia C, Poli G (2008) The contribution of animal fat oxidation products to colon carcinogenesis, through modulation of TGF-beta1 signaling. *Carcinogenesis* 29:890–894.

23. Pelser C, Mondul AM, Hollenbeck AR, Park Y (2013) Dietary fat, fatty acids, and risk of prostate cancer in the NIH-AARP diet and health study. *Cancer Epidemiol Biomarkers Prev* 22:697–707.

24. Xia H, Ma S, Wang S, Sun G (2015) Meta-analysis of saturated fatty acid intake and breast cancer risk. *Medicine* (*Baltimore*) 94:1–10.

25. Ballesteros MN, Valenzuela F, Robles AE, Artalejo E, Aguilar D, Andersen CJ, Fernandez ML (2015) One egg per day improves inflammation when compared to an oatmeal-based breakfast without increasing other cardiometabolic risk factors in diabetic patients. *Nutrients* 7:3449–3463.

26. Rong Y, Chen L, Zhu T, Song Y, Yu M, Shan Z, Liu L (2013) Egg consumption and risk of coronary heart disease and stroke: Dose-response meta-analysis of prospective cohort studies. *British Med J* 346:1–13.

27. Miranda JM, Anton X, Redondo-Valbuena C, Roca-Saavedra P, Rodriguez JA, Lamas A Cepeda A (2015) Egg and egg-derived foods: Effects on human health and use as functional foods. *Nutr.* 7:706–729

28. Guyon C, Meynier A, De Lamballerie M (2016) Protein and lipid oxidation in meat: A review with emphasis on high-pressure treatments. *Trends Food Sci Technol* 50:131–143.

29. European Food Safety Authority (EFSA) (2013) The European union summary report on trends and sources of zoonoses, zoonotic agents and food-borne outbreaks in 2011. Available at http://www.eurosurveillance.org/content/10.2807/ese.18.15.20449-en. Accessed March 17, 2018.

30. Stadtman ER (1993) Oxidation of free amino acids and amino acid residues in proteins by radiolysis and by metal-catalyzed reactions. *Annual Rev Biochem* 62:797–821.

31. Lund MN, Hviid MS, Skibsted LH (2007) The combined effect of antioxidants and modified atmosphere packaging on protein and lipid oxidation in beef patties during chill storage. *Meat Sci* 76:226–233.

32. Estevez M, Ventanas S, Heinonen M (2011) Formation of Strecker aldehydes between protein carbonyls—α-aminoadipic and γ-glutamic semialdehydes—and leucine and isoleucine. *Food Chem* 128:1051–1057.

33. Soladoye OP, Juarez ML, Aalhus JL, Shand P, Estevez M (2015) Protein oxidation in processed meat: Mechanisms and potential implications on human health. *Compr Rev Food Sci Food Saf* 14:106–122.

34. Hawkins CL, Morgan PE, Davies MJ (2009) Quantification of protein modification by oxidants. *Free Radic Biol Med* 46:965–988.

35. Shacter E (2000) Quantification and significance of protein oxidation in biological samples. *Drug Metabol Rev* 32:307–326.

36. Lund MN, Heinonen M, Baron CP, Estevez M (2011) Protein oxidation in muscle foods: A review. *Mol Nutr Food Res* 55:83–95.

37. Xiong YL (2000) *Protein Oxidation and Implications for Muscle Food Quality. Antioxidant in Muscle Foods*. Wiley, Chichester, UK, pp. 85–111.

38. Calkins CR, Hodgen JM (2007) A fresh look at meat flavor. *Meat Sci* 77:63–80.

39. Maarse H (1991) *Volatile Compounds in Foods and Beverages*, 44th ed. Marcel Dekker, New York, pp. 107–178.

40. Boeckel V, Brower TP, Gilbert C et al. (2015) Global trends in antimicrobial use in food animals. *Proc Natl Acad Sci* 112:5649–5654.

41. Angulo FJ, Baker NL, Olsen SJ, Anderson A, Barrett TJ (2004) Antimicrobial use in agriculture: Controlling the transfer of antimicrobial resistance to humans. *Semin Pediatr Infect Dis* 15:78–85.

42. Davies J, Davies D (2010) Origins and evolution of antibiotic resistance. *Microbiol Mol Biol Rev* 74:417–433.

43. Economou V, Gousia P (2015) Agriculture and food animals as a source of antimicrobial-resistant bacteria. *Infect Drug Resist* 8:49–61.

44. World Health Organization (2001) WHO global strategy for containment of antimicrobial resistance. Available at http://www.who.int/drugresistance/WHO_Global_Strategy_English.pdf. Accessed February 22, 2018.

45. Griggs DJ, Hall MC, Jin YF, Piddock LJV (1994) Quinolone resistance in veterinary isolates of *Salmonella. J Antimicrob Chemother* 33:1173–1189.

46. McDermott PF, Zhao S, Wagner DD, Simjee S, Walker RD, White DG (2002) The food safety perspective of antibiotic resistance. *Animal Biotechnol* 13:71–84.

47. Bush K, Jacoby GA, Medeiros AAA (1995) Functional classification scheme for b-Lactamases and its correlation with its molecular structure. *Antimicrob Agents Chemother* 39:1211–1233.

48. Singh M, Chaudhry MA, Yadava JN, Sanyal SC (1992) The spectrum of antibiotic resistance in human and veterinary isolates of Escherichia coli from 1984–1986 in Northern India. *J Antimicrob Chemother* 29:159–168.

49. Davies JE (1997) *Origins, Acquisition and Dissemination of Antibiotic Resistance Determinants. In Antibiotic Resistance: Origins, Evolution, Selection and Spread*. John Wiley and Sons, Chichester, UK, pp. 15–35.

50. Kruse H, Sorum H (1994) Transfer of multiple drug resistance plasmids between bacteria of diverse origins in natural environments. *Appl Environ Microbiol* 60:4015–4021.

51. Levy SB (1994) Balancing the drug-resistance equation. *Trends Microbiol* 10:341–342.

52. Salyers AA, Amiable-Cuevas CF (1997) Why are antibiotic resistance genes so resistant to elimination? *Antimicrob Agents Chemother* 41:2321–2325.

53. Hall RM, Collis CM, Kim MJ, Partridge SR, Recchia GD, Stokes HW (1999) Mobile gene cassettes and integrons in evolution. *Ann NY Acad Sci* 870:68–80.

54. Recchia GD, Hall RM (1997) Origins of the mobile gene cassettes found in integrons. *Trends Microbiol* 10:389–394.

55. Marshall B, Petrowski D, Levy SB (1990) Inter- and intraspecies spread of *Escherichia coli* in a farm environment in the absence of antibiotic usage. *Proc Natl Acad Sci USA* 87:6609–6613.

56. Hammerling U, Laurila JB, Grafstrom R, Iiback NG (2015) Consumption of red processed meat and colorectal carcinoma: Possible Mechanisms underlying the significant association. *Food Sci Nutr* 56:614–634.

57. World Health Organization (2015) Links between processed meat and colorectal cancer. Available at http://www.who.int/mediacentre/news/statements/2015/processed-meat-cancer/en/. Accessed March 26, 2018.

58. Chan DS, Lau R, Aune D, Vieira RV, Greenwood DC, Kampman E (2011) Red and processed meat and colorectal cancer incidence: Meta-analysis of prospective studies. *PLoS One* 6:1–3.

59. Bylsma LC, Alexander DD (2015) A review and meta-analysis of prospective studies of red and processed meat, meat cooking methods, heme iron, heterocyclic amines and prostate cancer. *Nutr J* 14:1–18.

60. Asif HM, Sultana S, Akhtar N, Rehman JU, Rehman RU (2014) Prevalence, risk factors and disease knowledge of breast cancer in Pakistan. *Asian Pac J Cancer Prev* 15:4411–4416.

61. Larsson SC, Wolk A (2006) Meat consumption and risk of colorectal cancer: A meta-analysis of prospective studies. *Int J cancer* 119:2657–2664.

62. Wu K, Spiegelman D, Hou T et al. (2016) Associations between unprocessed red and processed meat, poultry, seafood and egg intake and the risk of prostate cancer: A pooled analysis of 15 prospective cohort studies. *Int J Cancer* 138:2368–2382.

63. Neave N (2007) *Hormones and Behaviour: A Psychological Approach.* Cambridge University Press, London, UK.

64. Kumar VS, Rajan C, Divya P, Sasikumar S (2018) Adverse effects on consumer's health caused by hormones administered in cattle. *Int Food Res J* 25:1–10.

65. Epstein SS (1996) Unlabeled milk from cows treated with biosynthetic growth hormones: A case of regulatory abdication. *Int J Health Serv* 26:173–185.

66. Bohlke K, Cramer DW, Trichopoulos D, Mantzoros CS (1998) Insulin-like growth factor-I in relation to premenopausal ductal carcinoma in situ of the breast. *Epidemiology* 9:570–573.

67. Bauman DE, Eppard PJ, DeGeeter MJ, Lanza GM (1985) Responses of high-producing dairy cows to long-term treatment with pituitary somatotropin and recombinant somatotropin 1, 2. *J Dairy Sci* 68:1352–1362.

68. Elvinger F, Head HH, Wilcox CJ, Natzke RP, Eggert RG (1988) Effects of administration of bovine somatotropin on milk yield and composition. *J Dairy Sci* 71:1515–1525.

69. Khandwala HM, McCutcheon IE, Flyvbjerg A, Friend KE (2000) The effects of insulin-like growth factors on tumorigenesis and neoplastic growth. *Endocr Rev* 21:215–244.

70. Chan JM, Stampfer MJ, Giovannucci E, Gann PH, Ma J, Wilkinson P, Pollak M (1998) Plasma insulin-like growth factor-I and prostate cancer risk: A prospective study. *Science* 279:563–566.

71. Galbraith H (2002) Hormones in international meat production: Biological, sociological and consumer issues. *Nutr Res Rev* 15:293–314.

72. Juskevich JC, Guyer CG (1990) Bovine growth-hormone–human food safety evaluation. *Science* 249:875–884.

73. United States Food and Drug Administration (1993) Freedom of information summary: Posilac (Sterile Sometribove Zinc Suspension). Available at http://www.fda.gov/downloads/AnimalVeterinary/Products/ApprovedAnimalDrugProducts/FOIADrugSummaries/ucm050022.pdf. Accessed March 3, 2018.

74. Holmes MD, Pollak MN, Willett WC, Hankinson SE (2002) Dietary correlates of plasma insulin-like growth factor I and insulin-like growth factor binding protein 3 concentrations. *Cancer Epidemiol Biomarkers Prevent* 11:852–861.

75. Norat T, Dossus L, Rinaldi S et al. (2007) Diet, serum insulin-like growth factor-I and IGF-binding protein-3 in European women. *Eur J Clin Nutr* 61:91–98.

76. Missmer SA, Smith-Warner SA, Spiegelman D et al. (2002) Meat and dairy food consumption and breast cancer: A pooled analysis of cohort studies. *Int J Epidemiol* 31:78–85.

77. Mepham TB, Schofield PN, Zumkeller W, Cotterill AM (1994) Safety of milk from cows treated with bovine somatotropin. *Lancet* 344:1445–1446.

78. Ganmaa D, Sato A (2005) The possible role of female sex hormones in milk from pregnant cows in the development of breast, ovarian and corpus uteri cancers. *Med Hypotheses* 65:1028–1037.

79. Bouvard V, Loomis D, Guyton KZ, Grosse Y, El Ghissassi F, Benbrahim-Tallaa L, Straif K (2015) Carcinogenicity of consumption of red and processed meat. *Lancet Oncol* 16:1599–1600.

80. Samraj AN, Pearce OM, Läubli H et al. (2015) A red meat-derived glycan promotes inflammation and cancer progression. *Proc Natl Acad Sci* 112:542–547.

81. Fearon ER (2011) Molecular genetics of colorectal cancer. *Annu Rev Pathol* 6:479–507.

82. Sugimura T, Wakabayashi K, Nakagama H, Nagao M (2004) Heterocyclic amines: Mutagens/carcinogens produced during cooking of meat and fish. *Cancer Sci* 95:290–299.

83. Le Leu RK, Winter JM, Christophersen CT (2015) Butyrylated starch intake can prevent red meat-induced O 6-methyl-2-deoxyguanosine adducts in human rectal tissue: A randomised clinical trial. *Br J Nutr* 114:220–230.

84. Lewin MH, Bailey N, Bandaletova T (2006) Red meat enhances the colonic formation of the DNA adduct O6-carboxymethyl guanine: Implications for colorectal cancer risk. *Cancer Res* 66:1859–1865.

85. Platt K, Edenharder R, Aderhold S, Muckel E, Glatt H (2010) Fruits and vegetables protect against the genotoxicity of heterocyclic aromatic amines activated by human xenobiotic-metabolizing enzymes expressed in immortal mammalian cells. *Mutat Res Genet Toxicol Environ Mutagen* 703:90–98.

86. Bernstein AM, Song M, Zhang X (2015) Processed and unprocessed red meat and risk of colorectal cancer: Analysis by tumor location and modification by time. *PLoS One* 10:1–16.

87. Inoue-Choi M, Sinha R, Gierach GL, Ward MH (2016) Red and processed meat, nitrite, and heme iron intakes and postmenopausal breast cancer risk in the NIH-AARP Diet and Health Study. *Int J Cancer* 138:1609–1618.

88. IARC (2015) IARC Monographs evaluate consumption of red meat and processed meat. World Health Organization. https://www.iarc.fr/en/mediacentre/pr/2015/pdfs/pr240_E.pdf. Accessed February 29, 2018.

89. Steinfeld H, Gerber P, Wassenaar TD, Castel V, De Haan C (2006) *Livestock's Long Shadow: Environmental Issues and Options*. Food & Agriculture Organization of the United Nations (FAO), Rome, Italy, pp. 79–125.

90. Schader C, Muller A, Scialabba NE (2015) Impacts of feeding less food-competing feedstuffs to livestock on global food system sustainability. *J R Soc Interface* 12:1–12.

91. Cole JR, McCoskey S (2013) Does global meat consumption follow an environmental Kuznets curve? *Sustain Sci Pract Policy* 9:26–36.

92. Abbasi T, Abbasi SA (2016) Reducing the global environmental impact of livestock production: The minilivestock option. *J Clean Prod* 112:1754–1766.

93. Putaud JP, Van Dingenen R, Alastuey A et al. (2010) A European aerosol phenomenology–3: Physical and chemical characteristics of particulate matter from 60 rural, urban, and kerbside sites across Europe. *Atmos Environ* 44:1308–1320.

94. Gerber PJ, Steinfeld H, Henderson B et al. (2013) *Tackling Climate Change Through Livestock: A Global Assessment of Emissions and Mitigation Opportunities*. Food and Agriculture Organization of the United Nations (FAO), Rome, Italy.

95. Leip A, Billen G, Garnier J et al. (2015) Impacts of European livestock production: Nitrogen, sulphur, phosphorus and greenhouse gas emissions, land-use, water eutrophication and biodiversity. *Environ Res Lett* 10:1–13.

96. Reid RS, Bedelian C, Said MY et al. (2010) *Global Livestock Impacts on Biodiversity. Livestock in a Changing Landscape, 1st ed.* Island Press, Washington, DC.

97. Van Grinsven HJ, Rabl A, De Kok TM (2010) Estimation of incidence and social cost of colon cancer due to nitrate in drinking water in the EU: A tentative cost-benefit assessment. *Environ Health* 9:1–12.

98. Yılmaz F, Ozdemir N, Demirak A, Tuna AL (2007) Heavy metal levels in two fish species Leuciscus cephalus and Lepomis gibbosus. *Food Chem* 100:830–835.

99. Zhao S, Feng C, Quan W, Chen X, Niu J, Shen Z (2012) Role of living environments in the accumulation characteristics of heavy metals in fishes and crabs in the Yangtze River Estuary, China. *Mar Poll Bull* 64:1163–1171.

100. Monikh FA, Safahieh A, Savari A, Doraghi A (2013) Heavy metal concentration in sediment, benthic, benthopelagic, and pelagic fish species from Musa Estuary (Persian Gulf). *Environ Monit Assess* 185:215–222.

101. Authman MM, Zaki MS, Khallaf EA, Abbas HH (2015) Use of fish as bio-indicator of the effects of heavy metals pollution. *J Aquac Res Dev* 6:1–13.

102. Rashed MN (2001) Monitoring of environmental heavy metals in fish from Nasser Lake. *Environ Int* 27:27–33.

103. Mustafa C, Guluzar A (2003) The relationships between heavy metal (Cd, Cr, Cu, Fe, Pb, Zn) levels and the size of six Mediterranean fish species. *Environ Poll* 121:129–136.

104. El-Moselhy KM, Othman AI, El-Azem HA, El-Metwally MEA (2014) Bioaccumulation of heavy metals in some tissues of fish in the Red Sea, Egypt. *Egyptian J Basic Appl Sci* 1:97–105.

105. Castro-Gonzalez MI, Mendez-Armenta M (2008) Heavy metals: Implications associated to fish consumption. *Environ Toxicol Pharmacol* 26:263–271.

106. Al-Busaidi M, Yesudhason P, Al-Mughairi S, Al-Rahbi WAK, Al-Harthy KS, Al-Mazrooei NA, Al-Habsi SH (2011) Toxic metals in commercial marine fish in Oman with reference to national and international standards. *Chemosphere* 85:67–73.

107. Rahman MS, Molla AH, Saha N, Rahman A (2012) Study on heavy metals levels and its risk assessment in some edible fishes from Bangshi River, Savar, Dhaka, Bangladesh. *Food Chem* 134:1847–1854.

108. Meche A, Martins MC, Lofrano BE, Hardaway CJ, Merchant M, Verdade L (2010) Determination of heavy metals by inductively coupled plasma-optical emission spectrometry in fish from the Piracicaba River in Southern Brazil. *Microchem J* 94:171–174.

109. Demirak A, Yilmaz F, Tuna AL, Ozdemir N (2006) Heavy metals in water, sediment and tissues of Leuciscus cephalus from a stream in southwestern Turkey. *Chemosphere* 63:1451–1458.

110. Levy SB (1998) Multidrug resistance, a sign of the times. *New Engl J Med* 338:1376–1378.
111. American Society for Microbiology (1995) Report of the ASM task force on antibiotic resistance. *Antimicrob Agents Chemother* 1:1–23.
112. Gold HS, Moellering RC (1996) Antimicrobial drug resistance. *N Eng J Med* 335:1445–1453.
113. Piddock LJV (1995) Mechanisms of resistance to fluoroquinolones: State of the art 1992–1994. *Drugs* 49 Suppl 2:29–35.
114. Callaway TR, Edrington TS, Anderson RC et al. (2008) Probiotics, prebiotics and competitive exclusion for prophylaxis against bacterial disease. *Anim Health Res Rev* 9:217–225.
115. Gaggia F, Mattarelli P, Biavati B (2010) Probiotics and prebiotics in animal feeding for safe food production. *Int J Food Microbiol* 141:15–S28.
116. Seal BS, Lillehoj HS, Donovan DM, Gay CG (2013) Alternatives to antibiotics: A symposium on the challenges and solutions for animal production. *Anim Health Res Rev* 14:78–87.
117. Biliouris K, Babson D, Schmidt-Dannert C, Kaznessis YN (2012) Stochastic simulations of a synthetic bacteria-yeast ecosystem. *BMC Syst Biol* 6:1–13.
118. Kenny M, Smidt H, Mengheri E, Miller B (2011) Probiotics – do they have a role in the pig industry? *Animal* 5:462–470.
119. Huyghebaert G, Ducatelle R, Van Immerseel F (2011) An update on alternatives to antimicrobial growth promoters for broilers. *Vet J* 187:182–188.
120. Balogh B, Jones JB, Iriarte FB, Momol MT (2010) Phage therapy for plant disease control. *Curr Pharm Biotechnol* 11:48–57.
121. Goodridge LD, Bisha B (2011) Phage-based biocontrol strategies to reduce foodborne pathogens in foods. *Bacteriophage* 1:130–137.
122. Chan BK, Abedon ST, Loc-Carrillo C (2013) Phage cocktails and the future of phage therapy. *Future Microbiol* 8:769–783.
123. Koskella B, Meaden S (2013) Understanding bacteriophage specificity in natural microbial communities. *Viruses* 5:806–823.
124. Allen HK, Trachsel J, Looft T, Casey TA (2014) Finding alternatives to antibiotics. *Ann N Y Acad Sci* 1323:91–100.
125. Papagianni M, Anastasiadou S (2009) Pediocins: The bacteriocins of Pediococci. Sources, production, properties and applications. *Microb Cell Fact* 8:1–16.
126. Snyder AB, Worobo RW (2014) Chemical and genetic characterization of bacteriocins: Antimicrobial peptides for food safety. *J Sci Food Agric* 94:28–44.
127. Lou Y, Yousef AE (1997) Adaptation to sublethal environmental stresses protects Listeria monocytogenes against lethal preservation factors. *Appl Environ Microbiol* 63:1252–1255.
128. Lambert C, Sockett RE (2013) Nucleases in Bdellovibrio bacteriovorus contribute towards efficient self-biofilm formation and eradication of preformed prey biofilms. *FEMS Microbiol Lett* 340:109–116.
129. Kadouri DE, To K, Shanks RM, Doi Y (2013) Predatory bacteria: A potential ally against multidrug-resistant Gram-negative pathogens. *PLoS One* 8:1–4.
130. Chua LS, Rahaman NLA, Adnan NA, Tan E, Tjih T (2013) Antioxidant activity of three honey samples in relation with their biochemical components. *J Anal Methods Chem* 2013:1–8.
131. Charernsriwilaiwat N, Opanasopit P, Rojanarata T, Ngawhirunpat T (2012) In vitro antioxidant activity of chitosan aqueous solution: Effect of salt form. *Trop J Pharma Res* 11:235–242.
132. Barrett DM, Lloyd B (2012) Advanced preservation methods and nutrient retention in fruits and vegetables. *J Sci Food Agric* 92:7–22.
133. Kim YH, Huff-Lonergan E, Sebranek JG, Lonergan SM (2010) High-oxygen modified atmosphere packaging system induces lipid and myoglobin oxidation and protein polymerization. *Meat Sci* 85:759–67.
134. Nieto G, Jongberg S, Andersen ML, Skibsted LH (2013) Thiol oxidation and protein cross-link formation during chill storage of pork patties added essential oil of oregano, rosemary, or garlic. *Meat Sci* 95:177–84.
135. Babu RN, Ezhilvelan S (2014) Application of technologies in value addition of meat. Available at http://krishikosh.egranth.ac.in/bitstream/1/96278/1/TNV_Y2014-AMST_Pg121-130.pdf. Accessed February 9, 2018.
136. Scollan ND, Dannenberger D, Nuernberg K, Richardson I, MacKintosh S, Hocquette JF, Moloney AP (2014) Enhancing the nutritional and health value of beef lipids and their relationship with meat quality. *Meat Sci* 97:384–394.
137. Sultan A, Obaid H, Khan S, Rehman I, Shah MK, Khan RU (2015) Nutritional effect of flaxseeds on cholesterol profile and fatty acid composition in egg yolk. *Cereal Chem* 92:50–53.
138. Montgomery KS (2003) Soy protein. *J Perinat Educ* 12:42–45.

139. Bell JM, Keith MO (1991) A survey of variation in the chemical composition of commercial canola meal produced in Western Canadian crushing plants. *Can J Anim Sci* 71:469–480.
140. Deeth HC, Lewis MJ (2015) Practical consequences of calcium addition to and removal from milk and milk products. *Int J Dairy Technol* 68:1–10.
141. Apas AL, Arena ME, Colombo S, Gonzalez SN (2015) Probiotic administration modifies the milk fatty acid profile, intestinal morphology, and intestinal fatty acid profile of goats. *J Dairy Sci* 98:47–54.
142. United Nations Food and Agriculture Organization (FAO) (2013) The state of food insecurity in the world 2013. http://www.fao.org/publications/2013/sofi/en. Accessed November 30, 2013.
143. Ghosh S, Suri D, Uauy R (2012) Assessment of protein adequacy in developing countries: Quality matters. *Br J Nutr* 180:77–87.
144. Wu G (2013) *Amino Acids: Biochemistry and Nutrition*. CRC Press, Boca Raton, FL.
145. Wu G, Fanzo J, Miller DD, Pingali P, Post M, Steiner JL, Thalacker-Mercer AE (2014) Production and supply of high-quality food protein for human consumption: Sustainability, challenges, and innovations. *Ann NY Acad Sci* 1321:1–19.
146. Authman MM, Zaki MS, Khallaf EA, Abbas HH (2015) Use of fish as bio-indicator of the effects of heavy metals pollution. *J Aquac Res Dev* 6:1–7.

14 Animal-Source Foods in Human Nutrition

Aamir Shehzad, Asna Zahid, Sana Mehmood, and Sajeela Akram

CONTENTS

14.1   INTRODUCTION

Human beings require food and nutrients for essential growth and development. Variation in food consumption pattern exists in different parts of the world and it also varies from time to time. Fundamental sources of food and nutrients in human nutrition are plant and animals. Plant and animal foods provide essential nutrients for nourishment including macronutrients; which are carbohydrates, fats, and proteins, and micronutrients that include essential vitamin and mineral substances [1]. Animal foods play an important role in human nutrition. Animal food sources generally include meat, milk, eggs, hides, and feathers. These are also called livestock. Animal foods are an important source of good quality protein and essential vitamins and minerals; being rich in both macronutrients and micronutrients [2]. Furthermore, animal foods are more unique in texture and flavor and are often more appetizing than foods of plant origin. Consumption of animal-derived foods is high in developed countries and increase in consumption in developing countries is also being observed. Livestock is also important for non-food services like manure, income generation, cultural and religious services, and as a social symbol [3]. Animal foods are basically divided into two categories, namely meat and meat products and milk and milk products. Milk is secreted by the mammary gland of mammals to feed their offspring. Milk can be obtained from cows, sheep, goats, buffalos, yaks, horses, and camels. Milk is composed of mainly carbohydrates, lipids, and a range of essential vitamins and minerals. It is required for growth, reproduction, energy, maintenance, and repair. Babies are completely dependent upon milk for nourishment up to 6 months of life [4].

Meat is basically the flesh of animals that is used for edible purposes. Meat can usually be obtained from cattle, sheep, goats, deer, and poultry. Meat is rich in essential vitamins and minerals and is a source of high biological value protein. Meat, eggs, and milk account up to 13% of the energy and 28% of the protein consumed worldwide [5].

14.2   NUTRITIONAL IMPORTANCE OF FOODS OF ANIMAL ORIGIN

Animal sources are recognized for their nutritional profile. These are excellent sources of protein, essential fatty acids, vitamins, and minerals. These are crucial for nourishment and known as an important component of a balanced diet due to its nutritional profile [6,7].

Animal foods contain high biological value protein. Out of 20 amino acids, 9 are essential amino acids, namely isoleucine, leucine, lysine, methionine, tryptophan, threonine, valine, and phenylalanine, and they are not produced by human body [8]. Moreover, iron, zinc, magnesium, manganese, vitamin B12, and vitamin A are the primary micronutrients available in meat, while vitamin B12, riboflavin, calcium, conjugated linoleic acid, and medium chain triglycerides are prominent in milk [9]. Studies have shown that the bioavailability of nutrients in animal foods is high, in comparison to plant foods due to presence of highly bioavailable heme protein, and the absence of some antinutritional factors like fiber, phytates, and oxalates in foods of animal origin [10,11].

The following essential nutrients are present in animal foods and they play an imperative role in human health:

Iron is an important micronutrient that plays an essential role in the human body being a constituent of hemoglobin, a protein that is used to carry oxygen to all tissues and organs in the body while myoglobin, a protein that carries oxygen to muscles. It also participates in some enzyme activities, important for brain development and immune strength. Iron present in meat is highly bioavailable as compared to that in plant foods [12].

Zinc is an essential mineral present in animal meat in amounts required by the body. It plays a substantial role in cell differentiation and division, gene expression, and in synthesis of DNA and RNA. Zinc is crucial in the survival and health of pregnant and lactating mothers and infants [13].

Vitamin B12 is essential in the development of normal blood cells and also takes part in neurological functions. It plays an indispensable role in the synthesis of RNA and DNA components mainly pyrimidines and purine bases, transfer of methyl groups, synthesis of proteins from amino acids and carbohydrates, and fat metabolism. Deficiency of vitamin B12 is linked with decreased cognitive functions and anemia [14].

Vitamin A belongs to group of fat-soluble vitamins. It is present in considerable amounts in milk and meat [15]. It functions in promoting good vision and strengthening of the immune system. Deficiency of vitamin A causes impaired vision often leading to night blindness. Deficiency also compromises the immune system and causes stunting in children [14].

Vitamin D is a fat-soluble vitamin present in appropriate amounts in milk and functions in maintaining normal levels of calcium and phosphorous in body. Deficiency of vitamin D causes rickets in children and osteomalcia in adults [3].

Conjugated linoleic acid (CLA) is an extensive term for a combination of positional and geometrical isomers of C18:2 containing a conjugated double bond. These compound shows anticarcinogenic, antidiabetogenic, anti-atherogenic, and antiobesity possessions. They also support immunomodulation and modulation of bone growth [16].

14.3   MEAT AND MEAT PRODUCTS

The most valued product of livestock is meat. Meat can be consumed both as a kitchen-style food preparation and as a processed meat product. Over the past few decades, processed meat products have gained popularity in industrialized world [17].

Meat is usually defined as "the muscle tissue and internal organs of slaughtered animals."

14.3.1   THE PROCESSED AND SEMI-COOKED PRODUCTS

These include meat loaf, sausages, cutlet-mix, corn beef, curries, bacon, ham, and salami.

Cured meat cuts are entire pieces of muscle meat that can be divided into further categories.

Cured raw meat that do not undergo any heat treatment during manufacture. They are processed by fermentation in controlled conditions. Products are consumed raw or uncooked.

Cured cooked meat that undergo heat treatment to achieve desired palatability [18,19].

Raw-cooked meat products are meat products that are processed raw. After processing it is subjected to heat treatment [20].

Precooked-cooked meat products contain low grade trimmings. Two heat treatments are further involved that are precooking of raw meat materials and cooking of the finished product mix.

Dried meat products are made by simple dehydration or drying of lean meat. Nutritional properties of such products remain unchanged.

14.4   MILK AND MILK PRODUCTS

Among the animal derived foods which are major source of healthy and wholesome diet, the milk and dairy products are most important and wide group of animal foods. Milk or dairy products are defined as the liquid foods derived from animal milk such as goat, buffaloes, camels, and cows [21]. Milk is consumed in many parts of world as a nutritious commodity that is required for the health and growth of children and adults. There are many modified forms of dairy products available for people globally [1].

On the basis of fat content milk is divided into low fat or skim milk and whole milk containing about 90 or 120 kcal of calories per 240 mL, respectively. The consumption of dairy products is more than 150 kg/capita/year in Pakistan and many other Asian countries [22]. In India and South African regions, the per capita consumption is moderate, while there is low (less than 30 kg) intake of milk products in central Africa and East Asia. Some important and consumer friendly dairy products includes yogurt, cheese, butter, and ghee. These products are rich sources of all macronutrients and micronutrients needed by the human body [14].

14.4.1 YOGURT

Yogurt is a semi-solid fermented milk product. It is rich source of healthy and good bacteria to promote the health of large intestinal microflora. It is formed by the growth of lactic acid bacteria in milk through fermentation [23,24].

14.4.1.1 Consumption and Nutritional Profile of Yogurt

Yogurt is consumed in greater amounts in Pakistani culture in forms such as plain yogurt, fruit yogurt, and as a raita with various meals. The total nutritional composition and other functional perspectives of yogurt made it nature's most preferable food for all ages and gender groups [25]. As a functional product yogurt is used as potential source of live microorganisms called probiotics, and thus prevent against many gastrointestinal disorders [13,18]. Yogurt is made in a similar fashion as sour cream, but requires different conditions, such as temperature and bacteria growth, for formation.

14.4.1.2 Production of Yogurt

Different types of yogurts are prepared based on the total solids content such as low fat, fat free, and lactose digested yogurts. The procedure for yogurt formation requires the initial boiling of liquid milk at a temperature of 47°C, then the small portion of bacterial cultures including *Lactobacillus bulgaricus* and *Streptococcus thermophilus* is inoculated in milk [26]. Then it is kept overnight at a warm temperature. The product is then ready to use and is subjected to local markets for sale [27].

14.4.2 CHEESE

Cheese is a fermented milk product that is derived by the partial hydrolysis of whey protein. More than 2000 different types of cheeses have been discovered worldwide. No one knows exactly who invented cheese, but cheese was first discovered by passengers crossing the deserts [28]. In old times, the merchants preserved their milk in bags made of sheep's skin. Then, as result of sun exposure and pouch lining, rennin in the milk caused the milk to coagulate producing cheese [1,21,29].

14.4.2.1 Nutritional Profile of Cheese

It is a mixture of the milk components, chiefly casein, fat, and insoluble salts, along with water with a little amount of suspended particles of protein albumin, lactose, and other salts present. The oldest form of cheese that have been used for human consumption was originated from animals, mostly domestic [8,30].

14.4.2.2 Market and Consumption of Cheese

Cheese is widely used in processed food products as a taste enhancer. It also gives palatability to foods. Commercially, cheese is incorporated as a major ingredient in many foods, such as burgers, pizza, and sandwiches. The people of France consume more cheese than any other state in the world [31].

14.4.3 BUTTER

Butter is a product manufactured by the separation of milk liquid part from the solid portion or high fat part. It is also called a refined dairy product or anhydrous milk fat [16]. Butter is the most purified in terms that it contains a reduced amount of milk solid not fat content and moisture, which protects it from microbial attack and many other enzymatic processes. Butter is regarded as the most thick and concentrated type of liquid milk [11,23].

14.4.3.1 Nutritional Profile of Butter

Butter contains 80%–82% milk fat, 1%–2% solids other than fat, and 16%–17% water. Salt added to butter also counts in butter's nutritional value [26]. Unsalted butter is referred as "sweet butter." Another sort of butter includes reduced fat butter usually containing 40% milk fat.

14.4.3.2 Production of Butter

Butter is prepared when cream suspension in unhomogenized milk is destabilized by the act of churning or agitation. Emulsion or suspension breaks producing butterfat granules. The granules separate from the water phase or serum and mat together giving rise to buttermilk. The butterfat is washed with water and kneaded to separate buttermilk [10,32]. The process is continued until 16% of the water and milk solids remain. The formation of 1 kg of butter requires 20 L of whole milk. The process of butter formation also results in the production of buttermilk and skim milk, which are used for animal feeding or may be discarded. Nowadays, the value of skim milk is increased commercially. It is used as a major health promoting product for people on low fat diets [20].

14.4.4 GHEE

Ghee is hydrogenated form of vegetable oil obtained when the buttermilk is subjected to heat at a suitable temperature. Ghee is made in eastern tropical countries, usually from buffalo milk. Typical flavor comes from the burned milk in a process called hydrogenation [31]. Ghee is a more convenient product than butter in tropics because it is suitable in warm conditions. Ghee is used as a traditional and cultural product in Pakistan and many other countries for lubrication and smooth cooking of foods [32].

14.4.5 MARGARINE

It is a homogeneous milk emulsion termed as fat in water. It is widely used as a spread on numerous food products. It is available in many flavors, such as vegetable or chicken [11].

14.4.6 SOUR CREAM

Sour cream is manufactured by following the same culture and temperature processes as that for buttermilk. The major change is in culture media that is used for growth of bacteria [33].

14.4.7 FROZEN DESSERTS

Chief frozen desserts include ice cream, frozen custard, ice milk frozen yogurt, sherbet, and water ices. Frozen products have highly regulated temperatures [2].

14.4.8 ICE CREAM

Ice cream is widely consumed dairy product. Main ingredients of ice cream constitute flavor, color, sugar, and milk. Storage of ice cream at chilling temperatures is crucial for maintaining its properties and prevention from melting [25]. Ice cream comprises 10%–20% fat and refreezing of leftover portion can contribute to crystal formation. In order to create a low cost and consumer specific products, the cheaper ingredients including corn syrup, whey, and artificial flavoring agents can be employed as alternatives [34].

Frozen custard has almost same formula as that of ice cream but contains eggs or egg solids in addition, around 1.4% by weight.

Ice milk is normally referred as "reduced fat" or "light" ice cream. It comprises 11% total milk solids and between 2% and 7% fat [13].

Frozen yogurt is a cultured frozen product having ingredients similar to that of ice cream. It comprises 3.25% milk fat and 8.25% milk solids other than fat. Percentage of milk fat in **Low-fat frozen** is around 0.5% and 2%, whereas **Nonfat frozen yogurt** has less than 0.5% of milk fat [7].

14.4.9 SHERBETS

Sherbets are the milk beverages that are also used in many countries and consist of very little amount of milk. The major criteria for standardization of milk beverages is to have milk fat in a range of 1%–2%, while total milk solids as 2%–5%. From a nutritional point of view, these contain more calories per serving and also have more sugar leading to empty calories for consumers [35].

14.5 PROCESSING OF ANIMAL FOODS

14.5.1 MEAT PROCESSING

The potential hazards associated with consumption of meat products make them unfit for consumption since meat products are perishable commodities and contaminated through bacterial growth, autolysis and destruction by endotoxic enzymes [36].

Meat processing techniques, like salting and smoking, have been performed for decades before the invention of refrigeration. Both preserving tactics protect the meat from harmful physiological changes in organoleptic properties like color, taste, and appearance leading to preservation and making the meat edible for longer periods of time [34].

There are many other approaches to process meat for improving consumption in both developed and industrialized world. The major objective of processing is to develop healthy and nutritious products adding good mouth feel and texture to diet. The processed meat products such as sausages, salami, beef, and mutton are traditionally important in many parts of the world [37].

The process of canning has been used since the nineteenth century for the handling of meat that is preventive against contamination and a sterilized method. Freezing is a modern processing technique for meat with storage temperature of 4°C for few days [18]. Under hygienic conditions and suitable handling practices, these techniques can prolong the storage life to about 1 month. Chilling for meat products is also advantageous for inactivating bacterial pathogens and enzyme activity at a temperature range of −15°C, while growth of many harmful microorganisms stops at −10°C [38].

14.5.2 MILK PROCESSING

From nutritional point of view, milk is nature's most perfect and wholesome food and is full of all essential nutrients that are required to fulfill the basic needs for growth and development. It is the chief source of important macronutrients, such as calcium, vitamin D, and phosphorous, and necessary for the healthy teeth and bones development [24].

There has been extensive research on milk and dairy products used worldwide as a source of balance diet. As a valuable food commodity, milk requires careful processing and handling. In addition to use as complete food, milk is a food product that has less storage time and can be easily exposed to microbial growth leading to damage and various fatal diseases in human [25]. The processing of milk requires the maintenance of milk properties for hours, days, weeks, or months and prevents many illnesses caused by harmful pathogenic microorganisms. Milk processing is beneficial in terms of providing healthy nutrition, more profits rather than selling raw milk, means of income, and overall improvement in safety and quality of milk products consumed by human [39].

The techniques that are important from processing point of view for improving the shelf life of dairy products includes refrigeration for enhancing the raw milk attributes, fermentation and pasteurization. Pasteurization and UHT techniques prolong the shelf life of milk and other dairy products by lowering the risk of contamination from life threatening microorganisms to prevent health maladies [36]. Furthermore, for high quality and easily manageable products with longer shelf life, milk can be further processed into products like cheese, butter, and ghee. Seasonal changes are better managed due to availability of processed milk products in local and urban markets. The modification of fresh milk into various products is also beneficial for the whole society by providing the opportunities in collection of milk from various sources as well as marketing the products [22].

14.6 ANIMAL PRODUCTS CONSUMPTION PATTERN

14.6.1 MILK CONSUMPTION

For majority of people who are residents of developing countries, the consumption of milk and other dairy products is estimated at more than 6 billion people. Since the early 1960s, per capita milk consumption in developing countries has increased almost two-fold [9]. However, the consumption of milk has grown more slowly than that of other livestock products, like meat.

14.6.2 MEAT CONSUMPTION

The consumption rate of meat and egg has increased three and five folds, respectively due to high quality protein content. Over the last two decades, per capita milk consumption decreased in sub-Saharan Africa. In India, about 50% of milk is consumed on-farm [17,30]. Milk provides 3% of dietary energy supply in Asia and Africa, compared with 8%–9% in Europe, whereas dietary protein supply in Asia and Africa is 6%–7% compared to 19% in Europe and for dietary fat percentage is 6%–8% compared with 11%–14% in Europe, Oceania, and America.

It is possible to sum up the profile of meat consumption during human evolution in four periods: the first could be characterized by opportunist hunting; while in the second, hunting had grown to a bigger scale and lasted 2–3 million years; in the third period, men started to domesticate animals and plants, which began 10,000 years ago; during the fourth and last period studies determined that meat contained compounds that could increase disease risk [8]. Eaton and Konner (1997) stated that human genes had not changed since the Paleolithic period. Human beings are animals, submitted to the same environmental pressures as other animals and living species [21].

14.6.3 INSPECTION AND LABELING

Meat and poultry products are inspected by the US Department of Agriculture's Food Safety and Inspection Service (FSIS) every day. Inspectors monitor plant sanitation, proper processing, and cooking, when applicable. As part of their duties, inspectors also check to ensure that labels accurately reflect product ingredients. The exact amount and tolerable upper intake level of any ingredient used in processed meat and poultry product must be written on product label [40].

14.6.4 Safety and Preparation

Processed meat and poultry products have an excellent safety record. Some processed meats, like a marinated chicken breast, require additional cooking. Consumers should follow instructions on packages carefully and use an instant read thermometer to ensure that the product has reached the proper internal temperature [7,18].

14.7 POTENTIAL NEGATIVE EFFECTS OF FOODS OF ANIMAL ORIGIN ON HUMAN NUTRITION AND HEALTH OUTCOMES

The sections above have highlighted the positive impacts of consuming foods of animal origin on human and nutrition outcomes. However, there are also potential risks that need to be considered, indicating the need to devise strategies for their alleviation.

14.7.1 Overconsumption of Animal-Sourced Foods

Overconsumption of animal-sourced foods can harm human health and well-being, impacting whole societies, as well as individual households. Overconsumption of fatty red meat and hard cheeses, which have increased concentrations of saturated fats, can lead to cardiovascular disease, while overconsumption of processed meats, such as bacon and ham, has been associated with some cancers [26]. Increased consumption of energy-dense meat, milk, and eggs also contributes to the global obesity epidemic. This is not an issue confined to developed countries, and it is multi-faceted, with differences within a single household, and a diversity of views on "how much is too much" and how to influence [34].

14.7.2 Foodborne Diseases

Foods of animal origin are rich in nutrient content, so they are susceptible to microbial contamination progressing towards foodborne diseases. Major microbial contaminants comprising bacteria, viruses, fungi, or parasites ultimately lead to more than 3 million premature deaths across the world per year. To improve the access to foods of animal origin food safety education is required in parallel. Studies have shown that nutritional status of household has increased due to increased animal production along with nutritional education [33].

14.7.3 Zoonotic Diseases

Zoonotic diseases are the diseases that are transmittable from animals to humans. In recent years, zoonotic diseases, such as avian influenza, bovine, tuberculosis, Rift Valley fever, and foot-and mouth-disease, have been increasing tremendously [6]. Risks of such outbreaks can be increased by keeping livestock, which also increases access of vulnerable household to foods of animal origin by amplifying the number of animals or increasing production. It means that it is the necessity of time to control zoonoses, which will also include participation of communities, who own the animals, along with the participation of veterinary and health professionals [12].

14.7.4 Chronic Diseases

Chronic disease risks can be increased due to the consumption of foods of animal origin because there is a claimed association between saturated fats in animal origin foods and incidences of type 2 diabetes and cardiovascular diseases [24]. Many studies related to overconsumption of foods of animal origin have shown this association very well [19]. However, the consumption of foods related to animal origin is low in developing countries. Recent findings about fat quality have inappropriately given the relationship of fat consumption and chronic diseases [29].

The polyunsaturated fatty acids (CLAs and sphingolipids) found mostly in foods of animal origin play indispensable roles in the human body [37]. These polyunsaturated fatty acids are unable to be synthesized by humans and plants, so these are complementary to be supplied in diet which are provided by consumption of foods of animal origin. Consequently, several efforts have been made to increase the content of these polyunsaturated in milk and meat. Lock and Bauman reported strategies focused on increasing milk fatty acids that have proved advantageous to human health through nutritional management of dairy cows [14]. In the same way, Givens and Shingfield reported that by managing nutrition, amounts of CLA in both meat and milk can be enhanced [16]. Another researcher reviewed dietary manipulations that were aimed mostly at enhancing CLA content in beef and concluded that the best option is fresh forage diet. In most of the developing countries, ruminants are fed on fresh forage mostly, especially in wet season, which results in beneficial fatty acids profiles. Recent studies suggest that there is strong association between foods of animal origin and cancer [16,28]. Colorectal cancer is the third most prevalent malignancy, also contributed by the overconsumption of meat [39]. Thus, in developing communities the risk of chronic diseases because of low to moderate level of foods of animal origin is extremely limited [36].

14.8   CONCLUSION

Foods of animal origin have been consumed by man since prehistoric times. Animal foods are crucial for human consumption owing to their nutritional value. With changing trends and increases in processing and preservation of foods, consumption of animal foods is enhancing. Although animal products are an indispensable source of protein and other nutrients, increased consumption has led to many degenerative diseases. Animal products are high in saturated fat that pose risk factors for cardiovascular and other chronic diseases. Increased consumption of meat in the developed world has given rise to obesity, diabetes, hyperlipidemia, hypertension, and other health disorder. Furthermore, animals also serve as a source of various communicable and foodborne diseases.

REFERENCES

1. Aune D, Norat T, Romundstad P, Vatten LJ (2013) Dairy products and the risk of type 2 diabetes: A systematic review and dose-response meta-analysis of cohort studies. *Am J Clin Nutr* 98:1066–1083.
2. Fairweather TSJ, Collings R, Hurst R (2010) Selenium bioavailability: Current knowledge and future research. *Am J Clin Nutr* 91:1484–1491.
3. Olmedilla AB, Jiménez-CF, Sánchez MFJ (2013) Development and assessment of healthy properties of meat and meat products designed as functional foods. *Meat Sci* 95:919–930.
4. Bender AE (2012) *Meat and Meat Products in Human Nutrition in Developing Countries.* FAO, Rome, Italy.
5. Damez JL, Clerjon S (2013) Quantifying and predicting meat and meat products quality attributes using electromagnetic waves: An overview. *Meat Sci* 95:879–896.
6. Decker EA, Park Y (2010) Healthier meat products as functional foods. *Meat Sci* 86:49–55.
7. Lock AL, Dale EB (2004) Modifying milk fat composition of dairy cows to enhance fatty acids beneficial to human health. *Lipids* 12:1197–1206.
8. Givens DI, Shingfield KJ (2004) Foods derived from animals: The impact of animal nutrition on their nutritive value and ability to sustain long-term health. *J Anim Nutr* 29:325–332.
9. Andrée F, Jira W, Schwind KH, Wagner H, Schwägele F (2010) Chemical safety of meat and meat products. *Meat Sci* 86:38–48.
10. Aune D, Lau R, Chan D, Vieira R, Greenwood D, Kampman E, Norat T (2012) Dairy products and colorectal cancer risk: A systematic review and meta-analysis of cohort studies. *Ann Oncol* 23:37–45.
11. Stefani D, Boffetta EP, Ronco AL, Deneo PH, Mendilaharsu M, Silva C (2016) Meat consumption and risk of colorectal cancer: A case-control study in Uruguay emphasizing the role of gender. *Cancer Res Oncol* 2:015.
12. McAfee A, McSorley JEM, Cuskelly GJ, Moss BW, Wallace JM, Bonham MP, Fearon AM (2010) Red meat consumption: An overview of the risks and benefits. *Meat Sci* 84:1–13.

13. Larsen CS (2003) Animal source foods to improve micronutrient nutrition and human function in developing countries animal source foods and human health during evolution. *J Nutr* 1:3893–3897.

14. Eaton SB, Konner MJ (1997) Review paleolithic nutrition revisited: A twelve-year retrospective on its nature and implications. *Eur J Clin Nutr* 51:207–216.

15. Bradbear N (2009) Bees and their role in forest livelihoods: A guide to the services provided by bees and the sustainable harvesting, processing and marketing of their products. *Meat Sci* 42:51–63.

16. Herrero M, Thornton PK, Notenbaert AM, Wood S, Msangi S, Freeman HA et al. 2010. Smart investments in sustainable food production: Revisiting mixed crop–livestock systems. *Science* 327:822–825.

17. Campus M (2010) High pressure processing of meat, meat products and seafood. *Food Engr Rev* 2:256–273.

18. Baba Y, Kallas Z, Costa FM, Gill JM, Realini CE (2016) Impact of hedonic evaluation on consumers' preferences for beef attributes including its enrichment with n-3 and CLA fatty acids. *Meat Sci* 111:9–17.

19. Kratz M, Baars T, Guyenet S (2013) The relationship between high-fat dairy consumption and obesity, cardiovascular, and metabolic disease. *Eur J Nutr* 52:1–24.

20. Leroy JL, Frongillo EA (2007) Can interventions to promote animal production ameliorate undernutrition? *J Nutr* 137:2311–2316.

21. Micha RS, Wallace K, Mozaffarian D (2010) Red and processed meat consumption and risk of incident coronary heart disease, stroke, and diabetes mellitus. A systematic review and meta-analysis. *Am J Clinc Nutr* 121:2271–2283.

22. Panesar PS (2011) Fermented dairy products: Starter cultures and potential nutritional benefits. *Food Nutr Sci* 2:47.

23. Larsson SC, Wolk A (2012) Red and processed meat consumption and risk of pancreatic cancer: Meta-analysis of prospective studies. *Br J Cancer* 106:603–607.

24. Leroy JL, Edward AF (2007) Can interventions to promote animal production ameliorate undernutrition? *J Nutr* 137:2311–2316.

25. Martin J, Woerner D, Delmore R, Belk K, Tatum J (2016) Beef's role in a healthy diet. *J Anim Sci* 94:436–437.

26. McEvoy C, Temple TN, Woodside JV (2012) Vegetarian diets, low-meat diets and health: A review. *Public Health Nutr* 15:2287–2294.

27. D'Evoli L, Salvatore P, Lucarini M, Nicoli S, Aguzzi A, Gabrielli P et al. (2009) Nutritional value of traditional Italian meat-based dishes: Influence of cooking methods and recipe formulation. *Int J Food Sci Nutr* 60:38–49.

28. Pires SM, Evers EG, Van PW, Ayers T, Scallan E, Angulo FJ, Havelaar A, Hald T (2009) Attributing the human disease burden of foodborne infections to specific sources. *Foodborne Pathog Dis* 6:417–424.

29. O'Mara FP (2011) The significance of livestock as a contributor to global greenhouse gas emissions today and in the near future. *Anim Feed Sci Technol* 166–167:7–15.

30. Pearson AM, Gillett TA (2012) *Processed Meats.* Springer-Verlag, New York, pp. 324–327.

31. Granato D, Branco GF, Cruz AG, Faria JDAF, Shah NP (2010) Probiotic dairy products as functional foods. *Compr Rev Food Sci Food Saf* 9:455–470.

32. Ndlovu LR (2010) The role of foods of animal origin in human nutrition and health. In: Swanepoel F, Stroebel A, Moyo S (Eds.) *The Role of Livestock in Developing Communities: Enhancing Multifunctionality*, National University of Science and Technology, Bulawayo, Zimbabwe. Technical Centre for Agricultural and Rural Cooperation, Wageningen, the Netherlands, pp. 67–111.

33. Ballin NZ (2010) Authentication of meat and meat products. *Meat Sci* 86:577–587.

34. Verma AK, Banerjee R (2010) Dietary fibre as functional ingredient in meat products: A novel approach for healthy living-a review. *J Food Sci Technol* 47:247–257.

35. Pugliese C, Sirtori F (2012) Quality of meat and meat products produced from southern European pig breeds. *Meat Sci* 90:511–518.

36. Valbuena D, Erenstein O, Tui SH, Abdoulaye T, Claessens L, Duncan AJ, Gérard B (2012) Conservation agriculture in mixed crop–livestock systems: Scoping crop residue trade-offs in sub-Saharan Africa and South Asia. *Field Crops Res* 132:175–184.

37. Robinson RK (2012) *Modern Dairy Technology: Advances in Milk Products*, 2nd ed. Chapman & Hall, London, UK, pp. 1121–1125.

38. Smith J, Sones K, Grace S, Macmillan TS, Herrero M (2013) Beyond milk, meat, and eggs: Role of livestock in food and nutrition security. *Anim Front* 3:6–13.

39. Zucoloto F (2011) Evolution of the human feeding behavior. *Psychol Neurosci* 4:131–141.

40. Yildiz F (2016) *Development and Manufacture of Yogurt and Other Functional Dairy Products.* CRC Press, New York, pp. 117–215.

15 Nutritional and Safety Aspects of Animal-Based Irradiated Foods

Muhammad Yasin, Aurang Zeb, and Ihsan Ullah

CONTENTS

15.1 INTRODUCTION

Animal-based foods are prone to a high chance of contamination with microorganisms due to their higher moisture content along with dense nutrients, such as protein, fat, and carbohydrates that are essential for the growth and development of the microbes. Multiple hurdle technologies, such as thermal and non-thermal treatments, are currently used to immunize the microbial load in highly perishable food, such as meat from various animals, like chicken, beef, and fish. [1]. These hurdle treatments are responsible for preventing the reproduction of microorganisms and inactivate or kill of these microorganisms [2]. Among the non-thermal preservation treatments of foods, γ-radiation, electron beam (EB), and X-ray irradiation are prominent along with other technologies to minimize the initial microbial load in the food commodities [3]. For the reduction of initial microbial load in the food, non-thermal techniques are used but antimicrobial agents are responsible for inhibiting the growth of microorganisms during the storage [4].

Presently, consumers demand the ready-to-cook or ready-to-eat food products. Therefore, demand of marinated meat products is increasing dramatically in the both developed and developing countries. Thus, the shelf life of the seasoned meat product improved by using cost effective irradiation technology without affecting the hedonic characteristics of the products [5].

Irradiation treatment has the potential to improve the safety, enhance the shelf life, and quality of the food with better nutritional value than that of thermal processed food commodities. In this context, various countries now permit food irradiation and about a million tons of food is irradiated per annum [6]. Additionally, restricted doses of irradiation, such as 1.5 and 3 kGy, were approved for raw and packaged poultry meat, whereas higher doses as 4.5 and 7 kGy were allowed for fresh and frozen red meat, respectively. The purpose of these irradiation treatments was to eliminate the pathogens with a minimum irradiation dose that has non-significant variations in the hedonic characteristics of the food. Moreover, the quality parameters along with a hedonic response were affected badly depending upon the dose [7,8]. Gamma irradiation below a 10 kGy dose rate destroys almost all the pathogens without deteriorating the food nutritional quality parameters.

Gamma irradiation reduces or eliminates the bacterial population by destroying their nucleic acid and has a potential to enhance the shelf life of food products [9]. However, irradiation treatment produces the highly reactive radicals, such as hydrogen and hydroxyl radicals, from water molecules when the dose is higher than the specific food requirement. The highly reactive radicals can interact with other organic and inorganic compounds, dissolved oxygen in water and produce the numerous radicals that negatively affect food quality [10].

Irradiation is one of the most prominent preservation technological processes for the destruction of microbial pathogens in food. This technology has a potential to enhance the safety aspects of food with extended shelf live [11]. Thus, for better results, a combination of hurdles will be used to ensure oxidative stability, pathogen safety, and hedonic profile of food. The most important hurdle technologies that are used with irradiation are preservatives (natural or synthetic), high or low temperature, water activity, and redox potential [12].

15.2 MEAT

15.2.1 Chicken Meat

Irradiation techniques along with other non-thermal technologies, like high pressure (HP) processing, are used with or without the natural antioxidant in the marinated chicken meat to lower the initial microbial load. Alahakoon et al. [5] reported that the breast chicken meat has 3.16 log CFU/g after electron beam (2 kGy) treatment, whereas no viable cells were observed after the same treatment with citrus peel extract (2%). Furthermore, electron beam application has a non-momentous effect on the sensory profile of the marinated chicken breast meat. Moreover, the addition of citrus peel may affect the hedonic properties of the chicken.

Earlier, Javanmard et al. [11] delineated that the use of γ-irradiation at the dose rate of 0.75, 3.0, and 5.0 kGy had momentous effects on microbial reduction in frozen chicken at −18°C during 9 months of storage. Moreover, there were non-significant differences observed in nutritional, microbial, and sensory characteristics of control, as well as irradiated chicken meat. The combination of irradiation and frozen storage has greater impact to maintain the nutritional quality, extension of shelf life, and reduction of microbial load in the chicken meat.

Irradiation process reduced the initial bacterial load in a dose-dependent manner in the chicken carcass. A higher bacterial population along with coliform (5.0×10^7 and 1.0×10^7 CFU/g) was observed in the non-irradiated chicken meat. Previously, it was reported that the 2.0 kGy or higher irradiation dose, almost 99%, inactivated microbial population in chicken meat [13].

Poultry meat is contaminated with *Salmonella* during slaughtering and other related processes. It was completely eliminated with the low dose of irradiation, such as 2 and 3 kGy, due to a very low concentration of *Salmonella* immediately after the slaughtering of the poultry birds. Similarly, another group of researchers, Lamulka et al. [14] also concluded that the 2.5 kGy is an effective dose for the complete removal of *Salmonella* from the freshly processed chicken meat. Moreover, *E. coli* was also destroyed in the poultry meat after irradiation at the dose rate of 3–5 kGy. There were no recovery and growth of the irradiation damaged microbes at this dose. However, a lower dose (0.75 kGy) indicated that about 46% samples were *E. coli* positive. Therefore, it may be suggested that the amount of irradiation was high enough to eliminate the pathogenic microorganisms [15].

Sensory response of seasoned breast chicken meat processed with electron beam (1 and 2 kGy) and high pressure (300 and 400 MPa) showed non-significant differences as compared to control [5]. However, irradiation can persuade oxidative deterioration in the fatty acids of the food product and, consequently, generate the off-flavors and odors that lower the score of consumer acceptability [16]. Currently, various methods such as low temperature irradiation, modified atmosphere packaging, and incorporation of antioxidant are applied to inhibit the synthesis of off-flavor in meat products especially meat [17]. Likewise, chicken breast meat treated with an electron beam also has non-significant differences in the sensory profile of the marinated chicken meat [5].

Freeze irradiation of chicken meat at the doses of 0.75, 3.0, and 5.0 kGy revealed to have non-significant differences in all sensory characteristics, which are evaluated by using the 4-point hedonic score to the preliminary sensory score of the fresh meat. Additionally, an irradiation dose at 5 kGy or less along with frozen storage conditions after 9 months did not impart any deterioration in the organoleptic profile of the chicken meat [11].

Cooked minced chicken meat, irradiated at 2.5 or 4.0 kGy, showed the non-momentous variations in tocopherol content. Irradiation accelerated the thiobarbituric acid-reacting substances (TBARS) developed during storage, but this was hampered by the addition of α-tocopheryl acetate at 200 mg /kg in the feed of the chicken. Irradiation tended to increase cholesterol oxidation products (COPS) during storage, although no consistent effects were observed [18]. Complete elimination of the *K. pneumoniae* that was initially $3.17 \pm 1.8 \times 10^5$ CFU/g present in fish and poultry food after the treatment of radiation at 1.5 kGy was observed. *K. pneumoniae* was not recovered in the treated samples stored at 4°C up to 12 days [19].

15.2.2 BEEF MEAT

Gamma irradiation at the dose of 0, 1, 2, 3, and 4 kGy improved the shelf life of the luncheon meat 14 weeks by destroying the population of microorganisms compared to control, which only had 10 weeks of storage life. Volatile basic nitrogen, acidity, and lipid oxidation content were enhanced within 2 weeks of irradiation process of the luncheon meat. However, these traits have lesser values in irradiated meat than that of non-irradiated luncheon meat after 10 weeks. Taste and flavor of luncheon meat exhibited non-significant variations between irradiated and non-irradiated samples. However, volatile basic nitrogen concentration was decreased during storage, whereas irradiation had non-momentous effect [20].

Clostridium botulinum spore in the beef meat enriched with pork fat was significantly decreased by the application of γ-radiation combination with nitrite concentration. The nitrite level (150 ppm) was effective at inhibiting the growth or germination of *C. botulinum* in non-irradiated cooked beef meat after 48 hours of processing. However, a higher dose of γ-irradiation (410 kGy) has the potential to inactivate the *C. botulinum* in meat products, without the application of sodium nitrite level. Furthermore, for commercial sterilization of meat products, the addition of NaCl and curing salts, such as nitrite/nitrate, were used to minimize the dose of irradiation. Similarly, NaCl in combination with 5–10 kGy irradiation treatment is sufficient to impede the growth of botulinum toxin in meat. Likewise, in bacon, the addition of 40 mg/kg of NaCl along with 15 kGy radiation is considered the effective dose to prevent the formation of botulinum toxin after 2 months storage at ambient temperature 27°C [21].

Earlier, Shamsuzzaman et al. [22] reported that the irradiation (10 kGy) exposure had non-momentous effect on the flavor in both vacuum packed and cured meat. One of their peers, Oztasiran et al. [23] explicated that the dose of 1, 2, and 4 kGy of γ-irradiation reduced the load of microbes in the Turkish beef-based fermented sausage to the levels lesser than the community health concern. Later, Robert and Wees [24] depicted that the fresh ground beef exposed to 3 kGy was acceptable up to 42 days when stored at 4°C, whereas the non-irradiated control ground beef spoiled within 7 days. Earlier, Diehl [25] delineated that the irradiation treatment may modify genetic materials of the microbes, especially deoxyribonucleic acid (DNA) in various microorganisms. These changes occurred during alignment of replication and repairing of enzymes that carry out the DNA degradation or synthesis. Microbes may eliminate the damaged sequence of nucleotides and resynthesize the absent sequence.

Beef patties with soy sauce did not produce the sulfur containing volatile compounds after irradiation. Both irradiated and non-irradiated beef patties containing soy sauce had volatile compounds, such as 3-hydroxy-2-butanone, acetic acid, 2-methyl-1-butanol, and 3-methyl-1-butanol. Nonetheless, aldehyde volatile compounds, like hexanal, declined after irradiation in soy sauce beef patties compared with patties prepared with NaCl after 5 days. Additionally, a combination of other technologies, like soy sauce supplementation and vacuum packaging, inhibit the synthesis of TBARS in the beef patties during storage [26]. Further, Kwon et al. [27] expounded that prior to irradiation treatment (5 kGy), cooking significantly minimized the synthesis of dimethyl disulfide and dimethyl trisulfide in chicken, beef, and pork. In cooked meat, important volatile compounds responsible for the off-flavor and off-odor are aldehydes, especially hexanal, heptanal, octanal, and nonanal. Furthermore, these hexanal compounds are positively associated with lipid oxidation in beef patties irrespective of the concentration of brine solution and packaging method. Earlier, Nam et al. [28] reported that the sulfur volatile compounds were extinct by the supplementation of antioxidants prior to irradiation under aerobic conditions.

15.2.3 LAMB MEAT

Lamb meat, enriched with mint extract (0.05% and 0.1%), showed better total phenolic and flavonoid contents. Moreover, mint extract-enriched lamb meat possesses excellent antioxidant activity measured in terms of 1,1-diphenyl-2-picrylhydrazyl (DPPH) and beta-carotene bleaching assays. The tested meat also exhibited the better superoxide- and hydroxyl-scavenging activity but has low iron-chelating ability. Additionally, the antioxidant capacity of mint extract is equivalent to the synthetic antioxidant, such as butylated hydroxytoluene (BHT). Mint extract is suitable as a natural antioxidant for the lamb meat during the irradiation treatment, which retarded the lipid oxidation after irradiation technology. Moreover, TBARS values of mint-enriched lamb meat were momentously less than control when stored at chilled temperatures. Instantaneously, after irradiation 0.05% and 0.1% mint-enriched lamb meat had 18% and 34% less TBARS values, respectively. The antioxidant activity of irradiated at the dose level 2.5 kGy mint enriched lamb meat (0.1%) was non-significantly varied from 0.02% BHT enriched lamb meat [29]. Earlier, Murcia et al. [30] reported that the irradiated spices did not exhibit momentous variations in antioxidant potential compared with non-irradiated spices. Mint extract supplementation in the lamb meat prior to irradiation has potential to minimize the lipid peroxidation and also imparts the pleasant flavor and taste to the meat. The combination of irradiation treatments and natural antioxidant supplement significantly minimized the losses due to spoilage and also allows the products to reach new and distant markets [29].

15.2.4 Camel Meat

Camel meat is known to be one of the toughest meats and differed from beef in terms of content of connective tissues. Microbial load in the camel meat is high and originates from various sources. Also, several approaches of food processing have been proposed to minimize the initial microbial load and prolong the shelf life of the camel meat. A suggested, alternative method is the use of a medium dose of irradiation (1–10 kGy) to lower the microbiological load in the camel meat and to extend the shelf life [31].

Nutritional quality, in terms of proximate composition and total volatile nitrogen, was unaffected momentously after the irradiation dose of 1.5 and 3.0 kGy of aerobic packaged fresh camel meat, whereas lipid peroxidation content, like TBARS, increased. Moreover, during storage of irradiated and non-irradiated camel meat, the meat exhibited an increase in TBARS, TVN, and cooking loss. Structural changes in myofibrils and increases in the size of sarcomere length of camel meat were noticed after irradiation than that of control [32].

Camel meat that was irradiated at 2, 4, and 6 kGy with γ-irradiation and stored in a refrigerator (1°C–4°C) showed less numbers of total coliforms and total mesophilic aerobic load that prolonged the shelf life up to 6 weeks than that of control, which had just 2 weeks of storage life. Non-significant variations were observed in moisture, protein, fat, thiobarbituric acid (TBA) values, total acidity, and fatty acids after the irradiation treatment. However, a slight increment was noticed in the total volatile basic nitrogen content and lipid oxidation of camel meat after the irradiation treatment. Sensory evaluation exhibited non-momentous variations between non-irradiated and irradiated camel meat. There are non-significant differences noticed in saturated fatty acids, such as myristic acid (C14:0), palmitic acid (C16:0), margarine acid (C17:0) and stearic acid (C18:0). Similarly, unsaturated fatty acids, like oleic acid (C18:1) and linoleic acid (C18:2) concentrations, also varied non-significantly in both irradiated and non-irradiated camel meat [32]. Gamma irradiation did not impart any deterioration in the nutritional quality characteristics and sensory profile of camel meat within two days of irradiation [33]. Later, Fallah et al. [34] expounded that the irradiated camel meat with the dose level 1.5 and 3.0 kGy showed a significant decline in the load of lactic acid bacteria (LAB), psychophilic bacteria, *Listeria monocytogenes*, *Staphylococcus aureus*, *E. coli*, *Pseudomonas,* and coliforms. Moreover, irradiation dose is positively associated with the storage period of camel meat at refrigeration temperature.

15.2.5 Rabbit Meat

Raw rabbit meat is initially contaminated with relatively high amounts of microorganisms, such as psychrophilic and aerobic mesophilic bacteria, enterobacteriaceae, and yeasts and molds. Irradiation (1.5 kGy) treated rabbit meat indicated that these microbes are eliminated by 96%, 94%, 98%, and 84%, respectively; however, after a higher dose of irradiation (3 kGy) the reductions were relatively more at 99.7%, 99.3%, and 94%, respectively. Thus, the irradiation dose of 3 kGy is effective to curtail the load of harmful bacteria with extending shelf life without any significant effects on the sensory quality of the meat in refrigeration. Proximate composition of rabbit meat showed nonmomentous variations due to the irradiation treatment at the dose rate 1.5 or 3 kGy [35].

Rabbit meat is also irradiated with various irradiation techniques, such as gamma irradiation and electron beam, to lower the population of foodborne pathogenic bacteria and improve the refrigerated storage shelf life. In this context, rabbit meat at γ-irradiated at 0, 1.5, and 3 kGy followed by storage at refrigeration temperature. Moreover, irradiation treatment at 1.5 kGy momentously reduced the population of *Staphylococcus aureus*, *Listeria monocytogenes*, enterobacteriaceae, and *Enterococcus faecalis* but this dose was not enough to complete eliminate of *Salmonella*. However, higher doses of γ-irradiation, such as 3 kGy, momentously decreased the load of psychrophilic and aerobic mesophilic bacteria, yeast, and molds. The resultant product had a shelf life of up to 21 days of refrigeration, respectively, compared to that of non-irradiated meat, which only had 6 days of shelf life. Irradiation treatment in rabbit meat increased the concentration of TBARS but did not significantly effect the total volatile nitrogen (TVN) contents. However, during storage TBARS and TVN content were increased for both non-irradiated and irradiated rabbit meat. TBARS content has positive association with the applied dose of irradiation and storage time.

Sensory characteristics of rabbit meat did not vary significantly by the γ-irradiation treatments. Moreover, an irradiated fried rabbit meat burger showed better sensory acceptability compared with non-irradiated meat fried burger [35].

15.2.6 PORK MEAT

The pork meat irradiated with an X-ray accelerator (15 kW, 5 MeV) showed the higher total protein solubility, myofibrillar protein solubility, apparent viscosity, and lightness. However, expressible fluid separation, hardness, and cooking loss were decreased. Whereas other parameters, such as cohesiveness, springiness, sarcoplasmic protein solubility, and fat separation were varied and non-momentous. Moreover, physico-chemical characteristics of irradiated pork meat were also affected [36]. Earlier, Shin et al. [37] explicated that the X-ray treatment did not affect the cooking loss of bologna sausage prepared from lean pork meat. Additionally, irradiated and non-irradiated carboxymethyl cellulose (CMC) emulsified meat has similar characteristics of emulsion stability and fat separation. Moreover, color was varied non-momentously with different doses of irradiation compared to control. Nevertheless, the solubility of myofibrillar proteins is increased with X-rays in a dose dependent manner. Later, Choi et al. [36] reported that the similar behavior of cohesiveness and springiness of the CMC emulsified meat irradiated treated or non-treated meat. However, the viscosity of irradiated meat is positively associated with the dose rate of irradiation. Likewise, Heath et al. [38] delineated that the low dose (1 kGy) of the electron beam (EB) dose is effective at reducing the total number of aerobic bacteria by 2–3 logs in both chicken breast and thigh meats. Aerobic plate bacteria in boneless pork chops were 4–5 log reduced after the treatment of the EB dose at the dose rate of 2.5 kGy [39]. Similarly, Lewis et al. [40] did not observe the microbial populations in chicken breast meat after 1.8 kGy irradiation treatment. EB irradiation at the dose rate of 1 and 2 kGy enhanced the shelf life of marinated loin slices from 7 to 16, respectively [41].

The pork jerky was EB irradiated at the dose of 0.5, 1, 2, 3, and 4 kGy with the combination of antioxidant-rich extract of leek (*Allium tuberosum* R.) and exhibited the momentous decline in count of *E. coli, Salmonella Typhimurium,* and *Listeria monocytogenes*. They inferred that irradiation treatment has a synergistic effect with leek extract to eliminate the population of *L. monocytogenes* in jerky. However, both gram-negative and gram-positive bacteria behave differently in a combination treatment of leek extract and electron-beam treatments [42].

Marinated and low dose of γ-irradiation (1.5 kGy) ready-to-cook meat has a synergistic effect to eliminate the pathogenic bacteria, such as *S. typhimurium, E. coli O157:H7,* and *Clostridium sporogenes* and enhanced the shelf life without affecting its sensory and nutritional characteristics [1]. Moreover, irradiation application at 1 kGy significantly decreased *E. coli* under the detectable level after 28 days. Furthermore, at 0.5 kGy and 1 kGy, irradiation doses have the potential to minimize *E. coli* up to 1.6 and 3.3 log CFU/g, respectively. Marinated pork meat was acceptable for 21 days, compared with un-marinated meat with only 17 days shelf life. Moreover, irradiation treatment at dose level 1.5 kGy has increased the 29 days shelf life. The same dose of irradiation without marinating increased the lag phase of lactic acid bacteria (LAB bacteria) up to 5 days; however, LAB bacteria were not increased to 29 days storage. The irradiation exposure at the dose of 1 kGy to the meat packed in vacuum showed the sufficient reduction in *S. typhimurium* below the limit of detection, and no colony forming unit (CFU) was noticed after the treatment. Moreover, similar results were also observed when the meat was packed under air in polyethylene bag [43].

Gamma irradiation also reduces the concentration of ochratoxin A in the meat of pork that was fed on ochratoxin-enriched feed. The ochratoxin was reduced about 8.5%, 13.9%, and 22.5% with the dose rate of 3, 7, and 10 kGy, respectively. However, no further reduction in ochratoxin A in meat products such as bacon and smoked ham were found during refrigeration storage at +4°C after irradiation. They also inferred that the ochratoxin is linked with fat content of the meat therefore, ochratoxin content was decreased up to limited extent in the dry-cured meat products due to the complexity of the food matrix. Moreover, at the dose rate of 10 kGy, the maximum reduction was noted as 33.7% of ochratoxin in dry-cured meat products. Furthermore, researchers have suggested eliminating the ochratoxin from meat products by using the ionizing radiations application combination with other chemicals or hurdle technologies [44].

Consumer acceptability is a major aspect of product development. Therefore, irradiated animal-based products are evaluated for their hedonic response to the consumers. In sensory evaluation, color, odor, flavor, texture, and overall acceptability is determined by using trained, semi-trained, or untrained personnel. Pork loin irradiated meat at the dose of 1.5 kGy is evaluated for its sensory characteristics using a 9-point hedonic scale and found that there were non-significant variations between irradiated marinated meat and non-irradiated marinated meat. The mean hedonic score was 7, "Like moderately," was observed and no negative effect was given by any panelist on overall organoleptic properties [1]. Similarly, a higher dose of irradiation as 3 kGy to beef, pork, and turkey meat under vacuum also showed non-momentous differences in the hedonic profile [45]. Conversely, irradiation odor was developed after the treatment of 5 kGy of irradiation treatment with same conditions. Moreover, during storage the intensity of the characteristics order of irradiation treatment declined and showed no negative effect on overall acceptance of the meat [46]. Earlier, Lebepe et al. [47] expounded that after the irradiated treatment (3 kGy) to the pork loins, shelf life was prolonged up to 91 days and stored at refrigeration (2°C–4°C) under vacuum packaging. Later, Nam et al. [48] reported that supplementation of rosemary and onion, as an antioxidant, momentously reduced the content of hexanal in the irradiated cooked pork patties.

15.2.6.1 Cooked Ham Read-to-Eat Products

Temperature vaporizer and subsequent thermal desorption of multidimensional chromatographic analysis is recommended for the analysis of volatile compounds produced during irradiation in the food commodities. Non-irradiated cooked ham exhibited the flour peaks of ethyl acetate, mixture of ethyl propanoate and octanol, (R,R)-2,3-butanediol and nonanoic acid. However, both (R,R) and (S,S)-2,3-butanediol were also noticed in the irradiated (8 kGy) cooked ham that possibly suggests that irradiation may induce isomerization in the beef products [49].

15.2.6.2 Chemical Quality Characteristics of Irradiated Meat

The γ-irradiation had non-significant effects on the peroxide value of chicken meat, compared with control. Additionally, peroxide value was varied non-momentously with the increased dose level of irradiation. However, total volatile nitrogen formation was decreased by the reduction in the preliminary concentration of spoilage bacteria of the foods [11]. The thiamin content was negative associated with the dose level of irradiation. Moreover, about 6%, 15%, 27%, and 47% thiamin level was decreased by the application of γ-radiation at 1, 1.5, 3, and 6 kGy, respectively. However, riboflavin is radio-resistant and has non-momentous differences at 1 and 1.5 kGy with control. The riboflavin was deceased by 11% when the 3 kGy dose was applied to the meat [1].

Generally, the irradiation may cause variations in the structure and molecular weight of some meat proteins. Five proteins disappeared in *pectoralis major* chicken meat after the irradiation at 6 kGy, whereas six new proteins were synthesis during irradiation process. Progressively increased in the dose of irradiation (at 10–20 kGy) positively associated with the synthesis of new fractions of proteins and about 25 new protein fractions were recorded during in the SDS-polyacrylamide electrophoresis analysis (SDS-PAGE). Furthermore, the number of contemporary fractions of proteins were also increased from 48 to 61 by the application of irradiation dose 0 to 20 kGy at the end of shelf-life [50].

Alpha-macroglobulin, as the heaviest protein, is present in un-irradiated meat and completely disappears in irradiated meat. Among the other polypeptides, plasminogen and pyruvate kinase were totally absent in the irradiated meat irrespective of dose level. However, transferrin is a radio-stable polypeptide chain in the meat and it may degrade at the dose rate of 20 kGy, which is commonly not recommended for the poultry meat irradiation purpose. Fragmentation of proteins and polypeptides, such as actin, myosin, phosphorylase, carboxypeptidase, pepsin, and carbonic anhydrase, occurred during irradiation process (6 kGy) in meat; however, at a higher dose rate, slow repolymerization of these proteins was carried out increasing the molecular weight [50].

15.2.6.3 Lipid Oxidation

Irradiated meat exhibited lipid oxidation, which is measured in terms of the malondialdehyde content in the treated meat. The concentration of malondialdehyde was enhanced significantly as 10.14 and 11.62 µg MDA/g in fresh meat after the application of 1.5 and 3 kGy dose of ionizing radiation, respectively. However, the malondialdehyde level was changed non-momentously after 14 days storage in irradiated meat subsequently the concentration of malondialdehyde compounds (measure in term of TBARS value) was decreased as 6.56, 6.46. 6.56, and 6.21 µg MDA/g 10 g meat by the treatment of irradiation at the dose rate 0, 1, 1.5, and 3 kGy, respectively, due to the interaction of malondialdehyde with amino acids, protein (myosin), and glycogen [51]. Later, Gomes et al. [52] explicated that the non-significant variations were founds in irradiated mechanically-deboned chicken meat at the dose 4 and 5 kGy, compared with non-irradiated meat. Therefore, irradiation is considered one of the promising technology to maintain the fresh frozen meat pathogen free during transportation and storage where some problems of temperature fluctuations occurred. Moreover, they also inferred that refrigeration or freeze transportation of mechanically-deboned irradiated meat had the same impact on lipid peroxidation of the meat.

15.2.6.4 Flavor of Irradiated Meat

In organoleptic characteristics, aroma (odor and flavor) was the most affected parameter after irradiation in the meat and meat-based products. Off-odor and off-flavor, which is produced after irradiation in the meat, is characterized as rotten egg, fishy, burnt, barbecued corn, bloody, alcohol, sulfur, and acetic acid. The variations were noticed in the flavor according to type of meat, irradiation dose, and product temperature during the irradiation process, exposure of oxygen during and after irradiation, type of packaging, and presence of antioxidants. By the irradiation application, iso-octane-soluble carbonyls ware generated from the lipid and protein fractions of meat. Irradiation has positive associations with the formation of these compounds, whereas the cooking process has the ability to lower the off-odor compounds produced after irradiation. Volatile and water soluble compounds could generate the off-odor and flavor during irradiation with the basic taste of sweet, bitter, salt, sour, and umami [17]. The precursor of these off-odor and off-flavor compounds in the meat are aldehydes, alcohols, acids, esters, aromatic compounds, ethers, hydrocarbons, furans, ketones, pyrazines, lactones, pyrroles, pyridines, oxazoles, thiazoles, thiophenes, and sulfides. Approximately seven of the volatile compounds mentioned are synthesized from the hydrocarbons in the irradiated thermally processed or unprocessed foods. Among the volatile compounds, 1-nonene and 1-heptene are the most affected by irradiation doses; however, aldehydes compounds, such as propanal, pentanal, and hexanal, were affected by packaging types (i.e. vacuum or aerobic). Sulfur-containing amino acids are responsible for the synthesis of sulfur-containing volatiles along with irradiation dose. Free radical species, such as H_3O^+, H^+, and OH^-, were produced by the radiolysis of water during irradiation process that might be responsible for the breakdown of lipid oxidation products and sulfur-containing volatile compounds [53,54].

15.3 FISHES

Biogenic amines are determined due to their toxicity and as a quality indicator of fishes. Bacteria existing in water, which may have contaminated the fish during handling, has the capability to synthesis the histidine decarboxylase enzyme, which converts the histidine to histamine. The formation of histamine is augmented if fish are not stored in frozen or chilled temperature [55].

Biogenic amines, such as putrescine, spermidine, cadaverine, spermine, histamine, tryptamine, and tyramine, are naturally present at low concentrations in fresh fish tissue, whereas their higher amount was observed after the decomposition of fish muscles. During the spoilage of fish, biogenic amines are synthesized from free amino acids that liberate from peptides and proteins by the action of bacterial decaroxylases rather than endogenous enzymes activity. The higher amount of protein in fish meat has a potential risk to produce prompt biogenic amines [56–58].

Irradiated or non-irradiated fish fillets (*Oncorhynchus mykiss*) are identified using real-time PCR technique. Molecular weight of damaged DNA was notably decreased with the increase of the irradiation dose from 0.25, 0.50, 1, 3, 5, 7, and 9 kGy, and indicated the fish meat quality after a specific storage interval. However, DNA of 1000-bp was promising and present in the non-irradiated fish meat [59]. Later, it was considered that the DNA Comet Assay EN 13,784 (CEN, 2001) is one of the most promising detection methods, mostly used for irradiated foods and is related to DNA damage caused by ionizing radiation. This method is not appropriate for freeze-thawed or stored for a long time foods. It is a screening method only to identify foods that have been irradiated, but not dose applied [60,61].

15.3.1 RAINBOW TROUT

Rainbow trout (*Oncorhynchus mykiss*) was treated with high energy EB at doses of 0.25, 0.50, 0.75, 1.0, and 2.0 kGy and has shelf life up to 98 days when it was stored at 3.5°C in vacuum. The biogenic amines, such as putrescine, tyramine and cadaverine, exhibited the better response with irradiation dose and organoleptic profile. Good quality trout fish had less than 10 mg/kg of individual amines concentration. Polyamines, such as spermine and spermidine, non-significantly varied with the irradiation dose and storage time. They inferred that irradiated trout at the dose of 0.25 kGy did not exhibit the indication of deterioration on the twenty-eighth day of the treatment. However, slight spoilage was noticed after 42 days. Finally the trout were hedonically unsuitable after 70 days due to exceeding the amount putrescine from 20 mg/kg and cadaverine content was also increased [62].

Comparatively, γ-irradiation (1, 3 and 5 kGy) treatment to rainbow trout fillet with a combination of frozen temperature at −20°C for 5 months showed significant effect on peroxide value, TBARS, total volatile nitrogen contents, and pH. The concentration of these parameters was enhanced with increasing the frozen storage time. However, color, odor and texture of irradiated rainbow fillet at the dose level 3 kGy showed better consumer acceptance up to 5 months at frozen temperature [63]. Rainbow trout fillet irradiated with 0.75, 1.5, 2.25, 3, 3.75, and 4.5 kGy showed that the total saturated fatty acids were amplified; however, total polyunsaturated fatty acids were less than that of non-irradiated trout fillet. Likewise, total monounsaturated content was higher than control [64].

15.3.2 AUSTRIAN FISH

Austrian marine fish (i.e. Black Bream and Redfish), having very low lipid content (1.02% and 1.37%), showed non-significant affects in fatty acid composition after the γ-irradiation. However, vitamin E content was decreased in the fish fillet but did not have an association with dose of irradiation treatment. Nevertheless, vacuum packed Austrian marine fish showed some pink discoloration in all treatment, which was corrected by air-packed fillets. Moreover, vitamin E content in the Austrian fish was above the level required for human consumption accompanying with polyunsaturated fatty acids after irradiation. Generally, it is recommended that the oxygen-free environment prevents the lipid oxidation, but it did not necessarily for very lean fish meat or actually undesirable in some cases. Irradiated fish fillet showed non-significant differences in phospholipid fatty acid chromatograms of irradiated or control [65].

15.3.3 CHUB MACKEREL

A combination of γ-irradiation and vacuum packaging significantly delays the deterioration of the chub mackerel (*Scomber japonicus*) during 14 days of refrigerated storage. The combination of low dose γ-irradiation (1.5 kGy) and vacuum packaging showed a 4 log reduction in mesophiles, coliforms, staphylococci, and pseudomonas species and alleviated chemical changes in TBARS and biogenic amines, especially histamine. The consumers appreciated the irradiated chub mackerel up to 7 days [66].

15.3.4 CLAMS (*RUDITAPES DECUSSATUS*)

Biochemical and microbiological quality of clams (*Ruditapes decussatus*) irradiated at 0.5 and 1 kGy revealed less ammonia content than control. A one to three log reduction was noticed after 1 kGy irradiation in *faecal streptococcus*, *E. coli*, total mesophiles, coliforms, and staphylococcus count. Irradiation treatment (up to 1 kGy) did not show instant effect on fatty acids profile. Moreover, lipid profile was better in irradiated clams, whereas polyunsaturated fatty acid content was stable throughout storage period at 5°C. Slight modification was noticed in proteins bands after irradiation detected by sodium dodecyl sulfate-polyacrylamide gel electrophoresis [67].

15.3.5 SHRIMP

Shrimp was γ-irradiated with the dose of 1, 3, 6, 9 kGy and observed that, at the 6 kGy, maximum of spoilage microorganisms were eliminated without affecting the sensory response. Color parameters, such as L* value, was higher, while a* value was lower as the dose of irradiation was increased. Additionally, texture properties changed non-significantly after the treatment of irradiation. However, at 9 kGy dose level volatile compounds, like furans, oxides, aldehydes, ketones, and alcohols, were increased momentously. Overall, appearance and flavor of the shrimp was adequate to the sensory panelists up to the dose of 6 kGy. Therefore, it was suggested that the γ-irradiation treatment <6 kGy significantly enhanced the shelf life of fried shrimp [68]. Moreover, irradiated shrimp are identified by using the multispectral imaging system with 100% prediction accuracy when using 10 kGy dose or above.

15.3.6 ATLANTIC SALMON

Astaxanthin (mg/kg muscle) and redness in color were decreased with the increase of e-beam irradiation doses (0, 1, 1.5, 2, and 3 kGy) for both the fresh light and dark muscles of Atlantic salmon. There was a positive association between redness in color and astaxanthin level with irradiation dose. The change in color, which is indicated by a decrease in a* value of Atlantic salmon during irradiation, might be due to the destruction of astaxanthin. The a* value and astaxanthin content were non-significantly differed at 1 kGy irradiation treatment of salmon fillets compared with control but momentously varied with other irradiation doses. Conclusively, irradiating salmon fillets at 1 kGy, can be successfully used and leads to no significant change in color and amount of astaxanthin [69].

15.3.7 GRASS CARP SURIMI

Grass carp surimi was treated with a 10-MeV E-beam at 1, 3, 5, and 7 kGy and stored in vacuum packaging at 4°C. The treated carp surimi had lesser amounts of total base nitrogen and variable load than that of control. Moreover, irradiation significantly inhibits the production of biogenic amines, such as putrescine, tyramine, histamine, and cadaverine concentrations. However, these parameters were amplified during prolong storage period. After irradiation, carp showed more lightness and lower the values of a* and b* along with hardness and chewiness. Hedonic analysis revealed unfavorable "metal odor" or "irradiated odor" in surimi irradiated with the dose of 5 and 7 kGy [70].

15.4 MILK AND DAIRY PRODUCTS

The prevalence of foodborne pathogens in food commodities, such as raw and processed dairy products, may be responsible for the spread of diseases among the population and may cause huge economic losses in developing countries.

15.4.1 LIQUID MILK

In dairy products, raw milk and milk-based foods are the prime source of foodborne illness. Mesophilic, psychrotrophic, coliforms, and Lactic acid bacteria (LAB) are the most common pathogenic and spoilage microorganisms existing in milk-based products. The sources of these pathogenic microorganisms are teats and udders, which may contaminate the milk and cause possible threat for public health and deteriorate the food by declining the shelf life [71].

Raw whole milk treated with gamma irradiation, mainly 2 and 3 kGy, exhibited a lesser bacterial count than the non-irradiated milk. Moreover, mesophilic load and acidity did not increase significantly during storage. Consumers identified the all irradiated raw milk sample from control due to browning products developed by the Millard reaction of lactose and amino acids. They inferred that 2 kGy irradiation dose reduced the bacteriological load of raw whole milk and did not impart any negative effects on the sensory score up to 60 days of refrigerator storage at 4°C [72].

The mesophilic growth revealed persistent behavior in irradiated milk during storage. Different susceptibility of the microorganisms was noticed against the gamma irradiation depending on the surrounding environment condition. Some damaged bacteria have a capability to recover and restart their growth under boosting conditions [73].

Milk is a rich source of amino acids and sugars, especially lactose. During the γ-irradiation, Maillard reaction was initiated among amino acids and sugars and produced brown pigments. In this context, Chawla et al. [74] reported that the development of brown pigments during irradiation treatment of whey protein powder is positively associated with irradiation dose. Additionally, the higher the brown pigments exhibited the better antioxidant ability as compared with non-irradiated whey protein powder. Consequently the amount of free amino acids and lactose content were reduced due to the formation of glycated crosslinked proteins during irradiation treatments.

The rancid flavors and odors are produced by gamma irradiation treatment to the liquid milk, which generates the free radicals that affected the lipid fraction of milk, primarily fatty acid composition. The carbonyl group of unsaturated fatty acid having electron-deficient carbon–carbon double bonds are mainly vulnerable to free radical attack [17]. Moreover, the irradiation treatment has a dose dependent effect on the degree of change of lipid fraction, whereas higher irradiation dose leads toward intense fat changes [75]. This change is detected by almost all panelists, whereas 19% panelists have positive attributes for irradiation and 21% panelists observed the rancid odors and flavors, especially at 3 kGy treatment.

Earlier, studies confirmed that the higher dose of γ-irradiation may cause the lipid peroxidation. The use of 15, 30, and 45 kGy cause the forceful modification in the fat structure [76]. With a low dose rate at 1–2 kGy, minor alterations ware noticed in the molecular structure of milk fat and at 3–4 kGy degradation of lipid is occurred [77]. Earlier it was reported that the application of the UV light to the aflatoxin M1 contaminated raw whole milk reduces the 60% toxin by the destruction of double bone in the terminal furan ring of aflatoxin M1 at room temperature [78].

15.4.2 Yogurt

Sterilization of nonfat dry milk, yogurt bars, and ice cream by γ-irradiation with 40 kGy and stored at $-78°C$ showed significant decreases in overall acceptance [83]. Similarly, irradiation of liquid milk also exhibited the objectionable flavor. Lactose was involved for the production of off-flavors and browning during the irradiation. However, plain yogurt after the gamma irradiation (1 kGy) showed 18 days stability at incubation, whereas, at room temperature, the population of microbes reached 109 CFU/g after 6 days in non-irradiated samples and was found unacceptable. Additionally, irradiation treatment with refrigeration storage of yogurt prolonged the shelf life up to 30 days, compared with only refrigerated non-irradiated yogurt with only 15 days shelf life [79].

Similarly, Silva et al. [72] delineated that milk treated with 1 and 2 kGy irradiation exhibited a slight modification in lipid structure, and the total degradation of lipids was observed at 3 kGy. Generally, dairy products treated with gamma irradiation up to 10 kGy had non-significant effect on color, odor, taste, and over all acceptance of plain yogurt after 2 hours of irradiation [80]. However, appearance of irradiated plain yogurt at 5 and 10 kGy attained the lesser score when stored at 20°C, compared with 3 kGy. Earlier, Mortensen et al. [81] expounded that the light exposed yogurts had more reddish color and lesser yellow, compared to the yogurts stored in dark. Moreover, beta carotene and riboflavin contents of yogurt were also degraded.

15.4.3 Cheeses

Irradiation treatment with 2 kGy is considered to be sufficient for the total inactivation of *Mycobacterium tuberculosis, Mycobacterium paratuberculosis*, and *Mycobacterium bovis* in fresh soft cheese. Irradiation cheese showed non-significant variations in niacin pantothenic acid and riboflavin contents, whereas vitamin A and thiamin concentrations were decreased significantly. Moreover, pH and nitrogen fractions of fresh soft cheese varied non-momentously after irradiation treatment; however, ammonia content increased significantly without alterations in the sensory properties. The irradiation treatment with 2 kGy has the potential to minimize the mycobacteria count for safety concerns without alterations on their hedonic properties. Irradiation treatments can cause a momentous increase in lipid oxidation, but this proliferation is relatively low [82].

A minor dose of irradiation (0.2 kGy) did not produce the off-flavor in the cheddar cheese; however, when the dose was increased up to 0.5 kGy, the off-flavor developed. Subsequently, an increase of the irradiation dose more than 1.5 kGy to Turkish Kashar cheese also showed non-momentous differences in the flavor, whereas color scores were affected and indicated some deteriorations [83]. Nonetheless, cheddar cheese turned light yellow after the exposure of γ-irradiation, compared to the non-irradiated cheese sample with an orange color. After irradiation of the cheddar cheese with the dose of 4.0 kGy, higher concentration of TBARS and water-soluble nitrogen/total nitrogen was observed. Moreover, the sensory score of cheddar cheese was unaffected by the irradiation treatment compared to that of the non-irradiated cheddar cheese samples. Irradiated cheddar cheese with a dose of 4.0 kGy showed non-momentous variations between the irradiated or non-irradiated ones. After 3–4 days, irradiated cheese (2 and 4 kGy) developed the unpleasant odor and taste, which diminished after the seventh day of storage at 4°C [84].

Sensory problems were mitigated by reducing the dose of irradiation to 1.2 kGy and mold-free shelf life was enhanced up to 15 days compared with non-irradiated cheese at room temperature, which became moldy within 3–5 days. A fivefold increment was observed by the use of a combination of irradiation and refrigeration treatments. However, taste was unaffected by the application of irradiation (3.3 kGy) to Gouda cheese compared to that of non-irradiated cheese [85]. In contrast, the sensory profile of irradiated Mozzarella cheese had less scores. The relatively high-dose treatment showed slight changes in color.

Earlier Hashisaka et al. [86] reported that a burnt or musty flavor was produced in Camembert cheese when it was treated with 0.30 kGy. They also inferred that the dose of 2.0 kGy is required to prevent the additional growth of *Penicillium roqueforti*. Later, Chincholle [87] delineated that the irradiation dose up to 3 kGy is required to eliminate the microorganism population in full-fat Camembert cheese without changes in flavor.

In contrast, Jones and Jelen [83] reported that irradiated cottage cheese with the dose of 0.75 kGy clearly had noticeable changes in flavor. The cottage cheese had a cooked, slightly bitter or foreign taste. Psychrotrophic bacteria count declined by 3 logs when the irradiation dose was 1.5 kGy. The irradiated cottage cheese had a burnt off-flavor. Nevertheless, electron beam irradiated cheddar cheese with the dose of 0.21 and 0.52 kGy prolonged the shelf life about 42 and 52 days, respectively, at 10°C and having 101 CFU/cm^2 *Aspergillus ochraceus* spores initially under vacuum packaging. However, *Penicillium cyclopium* spores contaminate cheese under the same conditions and only have 3 and 5.5 days shelf life, respectively. Prolonged in a post-irradiation storage temperature from 10°C to 15°C and significantly delinked the keeping quality of the cheese contaminated with mesophilic fungi [88].

Feta is white cheese, which is contaminated with *Listeria monocytogenes,* either pre-process or post process. Pre-process contaminated cheese had 103 CFU/ml that was increased 105 CFU/g after two months. None of the irradiation doses (1.0, 2.5, and 4.7 kGy) had potential to completely eliminate the count of *L. monocytogenes*; however, the highest dose (4.7 kGy) declined the viable count up to the compliance of EC regulation. Nonetheless, in post-process, contaminated cheese did not show the count of *L. monocytogenes* at the dose level of 2.5 and 4.7 kGy. The texture of Feta cheese was unaffected with the application of irradiation. Moreover, at a higher dose (4.7 kGy), hedonic characteristics were affected temporarily and restored after 30 days of cold storage. Likewise, redness increased after the irradiation treatment, while yellowness and lightness were decreased [89]. In Feta cheese, pH, moisture, salt, and fat contents were varied non-significantly after the irradiation treatment [90]. By the application of irradiation, Feta cheese turned its color more towards redness and became the brown. This browning might be due to either enzymatic or non-enzymatic. However, later the Millard reaction was started among the amino groups (proteins, peptides, amino acids, amines) for reducing sugars, vitamin C, or oxidized lipids. Non-enzymatic browning might be due to a Millard reaction or as a consequence of lipid oxidation, or both. During the irradiated of cheese, the Millard reaction may happen between milk amino acids or proteins with lactose. Moreover, lipid oxidation moieties were polymerized, and brown-colored oxy-polymers products were also synthesized in the existence of milk proteins and/or antioxidants. The sensory panelists were unable to detect the variations in the textural profile of the irradiated cheese. Moreover, taste and odor of irradiated cheese at the rate of 1.0 and 2.5 kGy were affected badly. Moreover, irradiation treatment on the Feta cheese did not affect the texture and might be due to the fact that the cheese was already ripened and comparatively stabilized condition [89].

Irradiation with doses of 4.0 kGy did not eliminate the *Listeria monocytogenes* population in the soft whey cheese, Anthotyros, and caused slight reversible hedonic scores [90]. Frozen dairy food products, such as ice cream, yogurt, cheddar, and Mozzarella cheese, were irradiated and they were all sterilized except cheeses [86]. Oxidized flavor was detected in cheese, namely "Res," which was prepared by irradiated milk; however, after one month this characterized odor disappeared. Moreover, organoleptic profile of the cheese irradiated at 1–3 kGy is better than that of cheese irradiated with 5.0 kGy. Moreover, Anthotyros, a traditional fresh cheese, had brighter color than that of non-irradiated one [90].

During irradiation, free-radical species are generated that triggered the oxidation phenomena among the lipids and protein content of the food product. These free radicals are the predecessors of lipid hydroperoxides and are considered primary oxidation products, such as oxidation progresses that have the ability to produce the secondary oxidation products, such as alcohols, aldehydes, alkanes, alkenes, acids, and ketones. These secondary oxidation products have been hedonically designated as rancid, metallic, fishy, and oxidized flavor. These compounds further degraded in to volatile molecules and/or undergo polymerization, cyclization, and isomerization [54,91].

After a few days of irradiation, the secondary oxidation compounds are volatile and off-flavor in the milk-based food product, especially in cheese, are detectable. After the few weeks, cheese off-flavor disappeared due to the further possible polymerization or isomerization of secondary moieties of oxidation products that were less volatile in nature and below in sensorial threshold level even at 4°C storage. Later, Ahn and Lee [92] delineated that the decline in volatile compounds of PUFA emulsion after irradiation was due to higher rates of radiolytic moieties of secondary lipid oxidation products that lead towards the non-volatile or less volatile compounds formation.

15.4.4 Whey Protein

Sterilization of dairy products for longer shelf life through irradiation treatment is less acceptable due to the development of radiolytic compounds particularly in high lipid-based foods and production of objectionable off-odors and flavors through oxidation. Therefore, in combination with other complementary preservation techniques, like chemical preservatives that include sorbic acid, low temperatures should be used [93].

DPPH free radical-scavenging activity is 33.8% enhanced by the application of gamma irradiation @ 40 kGy in the whey protein dispersion and higher dose of irradiation (80 kGy) non-significant increased the free radical scavenging activity [94]. Later, Chawla et al. [95] explicated that after the irradiation of whey protein dispersion, new compounds were formulated that inhibited the beta-carotene bleaching, indicating the strong antioxidant potential. However, at higher irradiation doses, β-carotene bleaching activity, DPPH radical-scavenging of superoxide, and hydroxyl anion is not stabilized [74]. Irradiation treatment at a dose of 60 kGy enhances the polypeptides of higher molecular weight and are incapable of passing through gel due to dose-dependent polymerization of whey proteins. These higher molecular weight proteins are formed during heat-induced Maillard reactions in porcine plasma protein/glucose and beta-lactoglobulin model [96,97].

15.4.5 Irradiated Egg

Irradiated egg yolk powder showed higher oxidation in the polyunsaturated fatty acids, such as linolenic, arachidonic, and docosahexaenoic acid, along with cholesterol. The total cholesterol oxidation content was increased to 467 µg/g from 11 µg/g, whereas arachidonic acid concentration was decreased from 4.58 g/100 g to 3.07 g/100 after a 5 kGy irradiation dose. Cholesterol oxidation products were varied non-significantly by the used of antioxidants during and after irradiation process although vacuum packaging momentously lowered these oxidation products in the egg. Moreover, color was also affected by irradiation; that is, redness (a value) was decreased after irradiation, whereas the b value reduced during storage [98]. Earlier, Ferreira and Mastro [99] reported that the rheological behavior of the egg white, yolk, and whole egg was affected by the application of γ-irradiation at the dose rate of 25 kGy. Although, for the decontamination of the bacterial load, a 5 kGy dose is sufficient without affecting the rheological properties of the respective powder. Rheological characteristics were positively associated with irradiation dose, and polymerization and degradation were the most affected parameters.

Fresh shell eggs subjected to gamma irradiation (0.97, 2.37, and 2.98 kGy) showed a noticeable decline in internal quality as exhibited by the loss in Haugh values and yolk color. Sensory evaluation revealed a momentous difference between irradiated and non-irradiated eggs. Irradiation caused a decrease in apparent viscosity of liquid egg white and whole egg, but the viscosity of egg yolk was increased. Polyacrylamide gel electrophoresis of the egg white proteins revealed the appearance of some minor bands in the irradiated samples. Differential scanning calorimetry of albumen from irradiated eggs showed no significant changes in temperature and enthalpy of denaturation.

Irradiation at 2.37 and 2.98 kGy led to increases in emulsification activity, whipping power, and foam stability of egg white, and the gel rigidity was increased. Angel cake showed higher cake volume and better density when prepared by using the irradiated egg white [100].

15.5 CONCLUSION

Multiple hurdle technologies, like thermal and non-thermal technologies, are used to control the deterioration of animal-based food, such as meat from various animals, like chicken, beef, and fish. Among the non-thermal preservation treatments of foods, γ-radiation, X-rays, and electron beam (EB) irradiation are prominent along with other technologies for reducing the initial microbial level in the food. The radiation treatments have a non-significant effect on the production of toxic compounds in the foods. Therefore, the limitation of the irradiation treatment is defined for each category of the animal-based food and food products. Gamma irradiation below 10 kGy destroys almost all the pathogen without deteriorating the food quality. Thus, for better results, a combination of food preservation techniques will be used to ensure oxidative stability, pathogen safety, and hedonic profile of food.

ACKNOWLEDGMENTS

Authors are highly thankful to the Pakistan Atomic Energy Commission (PAEC), Islamabad for providing the generous support and facilities to complete this manuscript.

REFERENCES

1. Fadhel, Y.B., V. Leroy, D. Dussault et al. 2016. Combined effects of marinating and γ-irradiation in ensuring safety, protection of nutritional value and increase in shelf-life of ready-to-cook meat for immunocompromised patients. *Meat Sci.* doi:10.1016/j.meatsci.2016.03.020.
2. Corbo, M.R., A. Bevilacqua, D. Campaniello, D. D'amato, B. Speranza and M. Sinigaglia. 2009. Prolonging microbial shelf life of foods through the use of natural compounds and non-thermal approaches—A review. *Int. J. Food Sci. Technol.* 44: 223–241.
3. Dincer, A.H. and T. Baysal. 2004. Decontamination techniques of pathogen bacteria in meat and poultry. *Crit. Rev. Microbiol.* 30: 197–204.
4. Hugas, M., M. Garriga and J.M. Monfort. 2002. New mild technologies in meat processing: High pressure as a model technology. *Meat Sci.* 62: 359–371.
5. Alahakoon, A.U., D. Jayasena, S. Jung, S.H. Kim, H.J. Kim and J. Cheorun. 2015. Effects of electron beam irradiation and high pressure treatment combined with citrus peel extract on seasoned chicken breast meat. *J. Food Process. Pres.* doi:10.1111/jfpp.12480.
6. Eustice, R.F. and C.M. Bruhn. 2013. Consumer acceptance and marketing of irradiated foods. In *Food Irradiation Research and Technology* (Eds.) X. Fan and C.H. Sommers, pp. 173–195, Blackwell Publishing, Hoboken, NJ.
7. Sommers, C.H. 2004. Food irradiation is already here. *Food Technol.* 58: 22–27.
8. Kang, M., H.J. Kim, D.D. Jayasena et al. 2012. Effects of combined treatments of electron-beam irradiation and addition of leek (*Allium tuberosum*) extract on reduction of pathogens in pork jerky. *Foodborne Pathog. Dis.* 9: 1083–1087.
9. Monteiro, M.L.G., E.T. Mársico, S.B. Mano et al. 2013. Influence of good manufacturing practices on the shelf life of refrigerated fillets of tilapia (*Oreochromis niloticus*) packed in modified atmosphere and gamma-irradiated. *Food Sci. Nutr.* 1: 298–306.
10. Vital, H.C. and M.J.R. Freire. 2008. Tecnologia de alimentose inovação: Tendências e perspectivas. *Embrapa Informação Tecnológica*, Brasília, Brazil. pp. 149–164.
11. Javanmard, M., N. Rokni, S. Bokaie and G. Shahhosseini. 2006. Effects of gamma irradiation and frozen storage on microbial, chemical and sensory quality of chicken meat in Iran. *Food Control* 17: 469–473.
12. Leistner, L. 2000. Basics aspects of food preservation by hurdle technology. *Int. J. Food Microbiol.* 55: 89–96.
13. Katta, S.R., D.R. Rao, G.R. Sunki and C.B. Chawan. 1991. Effect of irradiation of whole chicken carcasses on bacterial loads and fatty acids. *J. Food Sci.* 56: 371–372.

14. Lamulka, P.O., G.R. Sunki, D.R. Chawan, D.R. Rao and L.A. Shacckelford. 1992. Bacteriological quality of freshly processed broiler chickens as affected by carcass pretreatment and gamma irradiation. *J. Food Sci.* 57: 330–332.

15. Thayer, D.W., G. Boyd, J.R. Fox, L. Lakritz and J.W. Hamson. 1995. Variations in radiation sensitivity of food borne pathogens associated with the suspending meat. *J. Food Sci.* 60: 63–67.

16. Carrasco, A., R. Tarrega, M.R. Ramirez, F.J. Mingoarranz and R. Cava. 2005. Color and lipid oxidation changes in dry-cured loins from free-range reared and intensively reared pigs as affected by ionizing radiation dose level. *Meat Sci.* 69: 609–615.

17. Brewer, M.S. 2009. Irradiation effects on meat flavor: A review. *Meat Sci.* 81: 1–14.

18. Galvin, K., P.A. Morrissey and D.J. Buckley. 1998. Effect of dietary α-tocopherol supplementation and gamma-irradiation on α-tocopherol retention and lipid oxidation in cooked minced chicken. *Food Chem.* 62(2): 185–190.

19. Gautam R.K., V. Nagar and R. Shashidhar. 2015. Effect of radiation processing in elimination of *Klebsiella pneumoniae* from food. *Radiat. Phys. Chem.* 115: 107–111.

20. Al-Bachira, M. and A. Mehiob. 2001. Irradiated luncheon meat: Microbiological, chemical and sensory characteristics during storage. *Food Chem.* 75: 169–175.

21. Dutra, M.P., G.C. Aleixo, A.L.S. Ramos et al. 2016. Use of gamma radiation on control of *Clostridium botulinum* in mortadella formulated with different nitrite levels. *Radiat. Phys. Chem.* 119: 125–129.

22. Shamsuzzaman, K., N. Chuaqui-Offermann, L. Lucht, T. McDougall and J. Borsa. 1992. Microbial and other characteristics of chicken breast meat following electron-beam and sous-vide treatments. *J. Food Prot.* 55: 528–533.

23. Oztasiran, I., S. Akin, S. Ersen, H. Cerci and B. Dincer. 1993. Effect of ionizing radiation on the hygienic quality and shelf-life of Turkish fermented sausage. *Proceedings of the Final Research Co-ordination Meeting Held in Cadarache*, France, March 8–12, 1993, pp. 97–120.

24. Robert, W.T. and J.O. Wees. 1998. Shelf-life of ground beef patties treated by gamma radiation. *J. Food Prot.* 61(10): 1387–1398.

25. Diehl, J.F. 1990. *Safety of Irradiated Foods*. New York: Marcel Dekker.

26. Kim, H.W., S.Y. Lee, K.E. Hwang et al. 2014. Effects of soy sauce and packaging method on volatile compounds and lipid oxidation of cooked irradiated beef patties. *Radiat. Phys. Chem.* 103: 209–212.

27. Kwon, J.H., Y. Kwon, T. Kausar et al. 2012. Effect of cooking on radiation-induced chemical markers in beef and pork during storage. *J. Food Sci.* 77(2): C211–C215.

28. Nam, K.C., E.J. Lee, D.U. Ahn, and J.H. Kwon. 2011. Dose-dependent changes of chemical attributes in irradiated sausages. *Meat Sci.* 88: 184–188.

29. Kanatt S.R., R. Chander and A. Sharma. 2007. Antioxidant potential of mint (*Mentha spicata* L.) in radiation-processed lamb meat. *Food Chem.* 100: 451–458.

30. Murcia, M.A., I. Egea, F. Romogaro, P. Parras, M. Jimenez and M. Martinez-Tome. 2004. Antioxidant evaluation in dessert spices compared with common food additives, influence of irradiation procedure. *J. Agric. Food Chem.* 52: 1872–1881.

31. Chomanov, U. and G. Humaliyeva. 1999. Sausage products from camel meat. *Food Proc. Indu. Kazakhstan* 3: 28–30.

32. Al-Bachir, M. and R. Zeinou. 2009. Effect of gamma irradiation on microbial load and quality characteristics of minced camel meat. *Meat Sci.* 82: 119–124.

33. Fallah, A.A., H. Tajik and A.A. Farshid. 2010. Chemical quality, sensory attributes and ultrastructural changes of gamma-irradiated camel meat. *J. Muscle Foods* 21(3): 597–613.

34. Fallah, A.A., H. Tajik, M.R. Rohani and M. Rahnama. 2008. Microbial and sensory characteristics of camel meat during refrigerated storage as affected by gamma irradiation. *Pak. J. Biol. Sci.* 11: 894–899.

35. Badr, H.M. 2004. Use of irradiation to control foodborne pathogens and extend the refrigerated market life of rabbit meat. *Meat Sci.* 67: 541–548.

36. Choi, Y.S., J.M. Sung, T.J. Jeong et al. 2016. Effect of irradiated pork on physicochemical properties of meat emulsions. *Radiat. Phys. Chem.* 119: 279–281.

37. Shin, M.H., J.W. Lee, Y.M. Yoon et al. 2014. Comparison of quality of bologna sausage manufactured by electron beam or X-ray irradiated ground pork. *Korean J. Food Sci. Anim. Resour.* 34: 464–471.

38. Heath, J.L., S.L. Owens, S. Tesch and K.W. Hannah. 1990. Effect of high-energy electron irradiation of chicken meat on thiobarbituric acid values, shear values, odor, and cooked yield. *Poultry Sci.* 69: 313–319.

39. Luchsinger, S.E., D.H. Kropf, C.M.G. Zepeda et al. 1996. Color and oxidative rancidity of gamma and electron beam-irradiated boneless pork chops. *J. Food Sci.* 61: 1000–1006.

40. Lewis, S.J., A. Velasquez, S.L. Cuppett and S.R. Mckee. 2002. Effect of electron beam irradiation on poultry meat safety and quality. *Poultry Sci.* 81: 896–903.

41. García-Márquez, I., J.A. Ordóñez, M.I. Cambero and M.C. Cabeza. 2012. Use of e-beam for shelf-life extension and sanitizing of marinated pork loin. *Int. J. Microbiol.* 12

42. Kang M, H.J. Kim, D.D. Jayasena, Y.S. Bae, H.I. Yong, M. Lee and C. Jo. 2012. Effects of Combined Treatments of Electron-Beam Irradiation and Addition of Leek (*Allium tuberosum*) Extract on Reduction of Pathogens in Pork Jerky. *Foodborne Pathog. Dis.* 9(12): 1083–1087.

43. Clavero, M.R.S., J.D. Monk, L.R. Beuchat, M.P. Doyle and R.E. Brackett. 1994. Inactivation of *Escherichia coli* O157:H7, *Salmonella*, and *Campylobacter jejuni* in raw ground beef by γ-irradiation. *Appl. Environ. Microbiol.* 60: 2069–2075.

44. Domijan, A.M., J. Pleadin, B. Mihaljevi, N. Vahčić, J. Freced and K. Markov. 2015. Reduction of ochratoxin A in dry-cured meat products using gamma irradiation. *Food Addit. Contam. Part A.* doi:10.1080/19440049.2015.1049219.

45. Kim, Y., K. Nam and D. Ahn. 2002. Volatile profiles, lipid oxidation and sensory characteristics of irradiated meat from different animal species. *Meat Sci.* 61(3): 257–265.

46. Ahn, D.U., C. Jo and D. Olson. 2000. Analysis of volatile components and the sensory characteristics of irradiated raw pork. *Meat Sci.* 54(3): 209–215.

47. Lebepe, S., R.A. Molins, S.P. Charoen, H. Farrar IV and R.P. Skowronsdi. 1990. Changes in microflora and other characteristics of vacuum-packaged pork loins irradiated at 3.0 kGy. *J. Food Sci.* 55: 918–924.

48. Nam, K.C., K.Y. Ko, B.R. Min, H. Ismail, E.J. Lee, J. Cordray and D.U. Ahn. 2007. Effects of oleoresin–tocopherol combinations on lipid oxidation, off-odor, and color of irradiated raw and cooked pork patties. *Meat Sci.* 75: 61–70.

49. Barba, C., G. Santa-María and M.M. Calvo. 2013. Analysis of irradiated cooked ham by direct introduction into the programmable temperature vaporizer of a multidimensional gas chromatography system. *Food Chem.* 139: 241–245.

50. Hassan, I.M. 1990. Electrophoretic analysis of proteins from chicken after irradiation and during cold storage. *Food Chem.* 35: 263–276.

51. Fernández, J., J. Pérez-Álvarez and J. Fernández-López. 1997. Thiobarbituric acid test for monitoring lipid oxidation in meat. *Food Chem.* 59(3): 345–353.

52. Gomes, H.A., E.N. da Silva, M.R.L. do Nascimento and H.T. Fukuma. 2003. Evaluation of the 2-thiobarbituric acid method for the measurement of lipid oxidation in mechanically deboned gamma irradiated chicken meat. *Food Chem.* 80: 433–437.

53. Shahidi, F. 1994. Flavor of meat and meat products—An overview. In F. Shahidi (Ed.), *Flavor of Meat and Meat Products* (pp. 1–3). London, UK: Blackie Academic and Professional.

54. Nawar, W.W., R. Zhu and Y. Yoo. 1990. Radiolytic products of lipids as markers for the detection of irradiated foods. In D.E. Johnson and M.H. Stevenson (Eds.), *Food Irradiation and the Chemist* (pp. 13–24). Cambridge, UK: Springer.

55. Lehane, L. 2000. Update on histamine fish poisoning. *Med. J. Australia* 173(3): 149–152.

56. Brink, B., C. Damink, H.M.L.J. Joosten and J.H.J. Veld. 1990. Occurrence and formation of biologically active amines in foods. *Int. J. Food Microbiol.* 11(1): 73–84.

57. Krízek, M., F. Vácha, L. Vorlová, J. Lukášová and S. Cupáková. 2004. Biogenic amines in vacuum-packed and non-vacuum-packed fl 20 of carp (*Cyprinus carpio*) stored at different temperatures. *Food Chem.* 88(2): 185–191.

58. Ozogul, F., E. Kuley and M. Kenar. 2011. Effects of rosemary and sage tea extract on biogenic amines formation of sardine (*Sardina pilchardus*) fillets. *Int. J. Food Sci. Technol.* 46(4): 761–766.

59. Şakalar, E. and S. Mol. 2015. Determination of irradiation dose and distinguishing between irradiated and non-irradiated fish meat by real-time PCR. *Food Chem.* doi:10.1016/j.foodchem.2015.02.143.

60. Erel, Y., N. Yazici, S. Ozvatan, D. Ercin and N. Cetinkaya. 2009. Detection of irradiated quail meat by using DNA comet assay and evaluation of comets by image analysis. *Radiat. Phys. Chem.* 78: 776–781.

61. Villavicencio, A.L.C.H., M.M. Araujo, N.S. Marín-Huachaca, J. Mancini-Fiho and H. Delincée. 2004. Identification of irradiated refrigerated poultry with the DNA comet assay. *Radiat Phys. Chem.* 71: 189–191.

62. Krízek, M., K. Matejková, F. Vácha and E. Dadáková. 2012. Effect of low-dose irradiation on biogenic amines formation in vacuum-packed trout fl 20 (*Oncorhynchus mykiss*). *Food Chem.* 132: 367–372.

63. Oraei, M., A. Motallebi, E. Hoseini and S. Javan. 2012. Effect of gamma irradiation and frozen storage on chemical and sensory characteristics of rainbow trout (*Oncorhynchus mykiss*) fillet. *Int. J. Food Sci. Technol.* 47(5): 977–984 1–8.

64. Javan, S. and A.A. Motallebi. 2015. Changes of fatty acid profile during gamma irradiation on of rainbow trout (*Oncorhynchus mykiss*) fillet. *Biol. Forum—Int. J.* 7(1): 165–170.

65. Armstrong, S.G., S.G. Wyme and D.N. Leach. 1994. Effects of preservation by gamma-irradiation on the nutritional quality of Australian fish. *Food Chem.* 50: 351–357.

66. Mbarki, R., N.B. Miloud, S. Selmi, S. Dhib and S. Sadok. 2009a. Effect of vacuum packaging and low-dose irradiation on the microbial, chemical and sensory characteristics of chub mackerel (*Scomber japonicus*). *Food Microbiol.* 26: 821–826.

67. Mbarki, R., H. Nahdi, I. Barkallah and S. Sadok. 2009b. The potential use of irradiation to extend the shelf-life of clams (*Ruditapes decussatus*) during live storage: Effect on bacterial and biochemical profiles. *Int. J. Food Sci. Technol.* 44: 1229–1234.

68. Wang, H., R. Yang, Y. Liu et al. 2010. Effects of low dose gamma irradiation on microbial inactivation and physicochemical properties of fried shrimp (*Penaeus vannamei*). *Int. J. Food Sci. Technol.* 45: 1088–1096.

69. Yagiz, Y., H.G. Kristinsson, M.O. Balaban, B.A. Welt, S. Raghavan and M.R. Marshall. 2010. Correlation between astaxanthin amount and a* value in fresh Atlantic salmon (*Salmo salar*) muscle during different irradiation doses. *Food Chem.* 120: 121–127.

70. Zhang, H., W. Wang, S. Zhang, H. Wang and Q. Ye. 2016. Influence of 10-MeV E-beam irradiation and vacuum packaging on the shelf-life of grass carp surimi. *Food Bioprocess Tech.* doi:10.1007/s11947-016-1675-4.

71. Mathusa, E.C., Y. Chen, E. Enache and L. Hontz. 2010. Non-O157 Shiga toxin producing *Escherichia coli* in foods. *J. Food Prot.* 73: 1721–1736.

72. Silva, A.C.D.O., L.A.T. De Oliveira, E.F.O. De Jesus et al. 2015. Effect of gamma irradiation on the bacteriological and sensory analysis of raw whole milk under refrigeration. *J. Food Process. Preserv.* 1–8. doi:10.1111/jfpp.12490.

73. Smigic, N., A. Rajkovic, E. Antal et al. 2009. Treatment of *Escherichia coli* O157:H7 with lactic acid, neutralized electrolysed oxidizing water and chlorine dioxide followed by growth under sub-optimal conditions of temperature, pH and modified atmosphere. *Food Microbiol.* 26: 629–637.

74. Chawla, S.P., R. Chander and A. Sharma. 2009. Antioxidant properties of Maillard reaction products obtained by gamma-irradiation of whey proteins. *Food Chem.* 116: 122–128.

75. Stefanova, R., S. Toshkov, N.V. Vasilev, N.G. Vassilev and I.N. Marekov. 2011. Effect of gamma-ray irradiation on the fatty acid profile of irradiated beef meat. *Food Chem.* 127: 461–466.

76. Day, E.A. and S.E. Papaioannou. 1963. Irradiation-induced changes in milk fat. *J. Dairy Sci.* 46: 1201–1206.

77. Guimarães, C.F.M., A.O.C. Silva, F.M. Costa, E.F.O. Jesus and E.T. Mársico. 2005. Efeito da radiação gama sobre os componentes sólidos do leite cru. In C.F.M. Guimarães (Ed.), *II Congresso Latino Americano de Higienistas de Alimentos – VII Congresso Brasileiro de Higienistas de Alimentos* pp. 1–3. Rio de Janeiro, Brazil: CBMVHA.

78. Yousef, A.E. and E.H. Marth. 1987. Kinetics of interaction of aflatoxin Ml in aqueous solutions irradiated with ultraviolet energy. *J. Agri. Food Chem.* 35: 785–789.

79. Kunstadt, P. 2001. Economic and technical considerations in food irradiation. In R.A. Molins (Ed.), *Food Irradiation: Principles and Applications*. New York: Wiley-Interscience, pp. 415–442.

80. Ham, J.S., S.G. Jeong, S.G. Lee et al. 2009. Quality of irradiated plain yogurt during storage at different temperatures. *Asian Aust. J. Anim.* 22: 289–295.

81. Holm, V.K. and G. Mortensen. 2004. Food packaging performance of polylactate (PLA). In *14th IAPRI World Conference on Packaging*. Stockholm, Sweden June 13–16.

82. Badr, H.M. 2011. Inactivation of *Mycobacterium paratuberculosis* and *Mycobacterium tuberculosis* in fresh soft cheese by gamma radiation. *Radiat. Phys. Chem.* 80: 1250–1257.

83. Jones, T.H. and P. Jelen. 1988. Low dose gamma irradiation of camembert, cottage cheese and cottage cheese whey. *Milchwissenschaft* 43: 233.

84. Seisa, D., G. Osthoff, C. Hugo, A. Hugo, C. Bothma and J. Van der Merwe. 2004. The effect of low-dose gamma irradiation and temperature on the microbiological and chemical changes during ripening of cheddar cheese. *Radiat. Phys. Chem.* 69: 419–431.

85. Rosenthal, I., M. Martinot, P. Linder and B.J. Juven. 1983. A study of ionizing radiation of dairy products. *Milchwissenschaft* 38: 467.

86. Hashisaka, A.E., J.R. Matches, Y. Batters, F.P. Hungate and F.M. Dong. 1990. Effects of gamma irradiation at −78°C on microbial populations in dairy products. *J. Food Sci.* 55: 1284–1289.
87. Chincholle, R.C. 1991. Action of the ionization treatment on the soft cheeses made from unpasteurized milk. *CR. Acad. Agric. Fr.* 77: 26.
88. Blank, G., K. Shamsuzzaman and S. Sohal. 1992. Use of electron beam irradiation for mold decontamination on Cheddar cheese. *J. Dairy Sci.* 75: 13.
89. Konteles, S., V.J. Sinanoglou, A. Batrinou and K. Sflomos. 2009. Effects of γ-irradiation on *Listeria monocytogenes* population, colour, texture and sensory properties of Feta cheese during cold storage. *Food Microbiol.* 26: 157–165.
90. Tsiotsias, A., I. Savvaidis, A. Vassila, M. Kontominas and P. Kotzekidou. 2002. Control of *Listeria monocytogenes* by low-dose irradiation in combination with refrigeration in the soft whey cheese "Anthotyros". *Food Microbiol.* 19: 117–126.
91. Kochhar, S.P. 1996. Oxidation pathways to the formulation of off-flavours. In *Food Taints and Off-flavours*, 2nd eds. London, UK: Balckie Academic and Professional. pp. 168–225.
92. Ahn, D.U and W.J. Lee. 2004. Mechanisms and prevention of off-odor production and color changes in irradiated meat. Irradiation of food and packaging: Recent developments. *Am. Chem. Soc. Symp. Ser.* 875: 43–76.
93. Patel, B.K., J.P. Prajapati and S.V. Pinto. 2005. Potentiality of use of irradiation for dairy products. *National Seminar on Indian Dairy Industry - Opportunities and Challenges*. Gujarat, India, pp. 223–227.
94. Benjakul, S., W. Lertittikul and F. Bauer. 2005. Antioxidant activity of Maillard reaction products from a porcine plasma protein–sugar model system. *Food Chem.* 93: 189–196.
95. Chawla, S.P., R. Chander and A. Sharma. 2007. Antioxidant formation by γ-irradiation of glucose–amino acid model system. *Food Chem.* 103: 1297–1304.
96. Miralles, B., A. Martinez-Rodriguez, A. Santiago, J. Lagemaat and A. Heras. 2007. The occurrence of a Maillard type protein–polysaccharide reaction between of b-lactoglobulin and chitosan. *Food Chem.* 100: 1071–1075.
97. Lertittikul, W., S. Benjakul and M. Tanaka. 2007. Characteristics and antioxidant activity of Maillard reaction products from a porcine plasma protein–glucose model system as influenced by pH. *Food Chem.* 100: 669–677.
98. Du, M. and D.U. Ahn. 2010. Effects of antioxidants and packaging on lipid and cholesterol oxidation and color changes of irradiated egg yolk powder. *J. Food Sci.* 65(4): 625–629.
99. Ferreira, L.F.S. and N.L.D. Mastro. 1998. Rheological changes in irradiated chicken eggs. *Rad. Phys. Chem.* 52: 59–62.
100. Ma, C.Y., M.R. Sahasrabudhe, V.R. Poste and J.R. Harwalkar. 1990. Chambers. gamma irradiation of shell eggs. Internal and sensory quality, physicochemical characteristics, and functional properties. *Can Inst. Food Sci. Technol. J.* 23(4/5): 226–232.

16 Poultry and Livestock Production for Foods

Shaihid-ur-Rehman and Salim-ur-Rehman

CONTENTS

16.1   INTRODUCTION

Livestock and poultry production is the backbone of the Pakistan agriculture sector and its share in the Gross Domestic Product (GDP) is about 11.4% and 1.4%, respectively. The share in agriculture value addition is 58.3% and 7.1%, respectively, by livestock and poultry production, while the share of the poultry sector in livestock value added is 12.2%. The growth rates of livestock and poultry sectors in 2016 and 2017 were 3.7% and 7.7%, respectively. Approximately 8 million families and about 1.5 million people are directly or indirectly involved in livestock and poultry farming operations, respectively [1].

Livestock farming, in particular, and poultry farming, in general, are the major sources of income of the rural poor of the country. It is estimated that more than 35% of the income is derived from livestock activities in rural areas in Pakistan. Poultry farming was probably the easiest business with a minimum investment a decade ago. Recent developments in the poultry sector, especially the transformation of poultry farming from open-sided poultry houses to controlled-environment houses, has eliminated the small farmers [2].

Livestock is the insurance package of the poor farmers in the rural areas. The agriculture sector in Pakistan is mainly run by the landless farmers or farmers having land holdings less than 12.5 acres. For emergency needs, these farmers rely on the livestock, mainly the sheep and goat, and less commonly cattle, buffalo, and camels, as a cash income source. This sector is not only a source of poverty alleviation, but it is also a source of foreign exchange for the country and way of improving the nutritional status of resource-poor families. Goat is still considered a poor man's cow in rural areas and helps to elevate the nutritional status of the poor families in rural areas. Sheep and goat are the rural reserves of the highest quality of animal protein that is available to the families of farmers at the time of emergencies, both health and economic related issues [3].

Poultry sector is probably the savior of the Pakistani nation, about 31% of the total meat produced is contributed by poultry meat. It is envisaged that if poultry farming had not been commercialized in Pakistan, mutton and beef would have been out of the purchasing power of people. Poultry farming sector provides probably the finest quality of animal protein by consuming the industrial wastes.

It is estimated that the poultry sector consumes more than 7 million metric tons of agricultural wastes (direct or indirect industrial residues). Commercial poultry consists of the breeder, broiler, and layer farming setups, which showed 5%, 10%, and 7% growth. Broiler farming has resulted in about 7 kg poultry meat per capita per year in 2018 from 0.3 kg in 1965, similarly egg consumption has increased to about 90 eggs in the same period. As far a milk production is concerned, about 20% of the total milk produced in the country is either wasted or fed to calves (about 15%). During 2017–2018, about 45,227 thousand tons of milk was consumed by humans with a major share produced by the buffalos (60%) followed by cattle milk (36%), while the remaining is contributed by camel, goat, and sheep milk. Similarly, major shares in meat is contributed by beef (cattle, buffalo, and camel meat), which is about 51% followed by poultry meat (31%), while rest, 18%, is contributed by mutton (sheep and goat meat). Layer farming is contributing 12,900 million eggs/year with a total number of 49 million layers, which is about 76% of the total egg produced, and rest, 24%, is contributed by rural birds [1].

Animal production for milk, meat, or egg production supplements the human food system with not only high-quality protein, but it also helps to utilize poor quality land. The animal sector does not directly compete with the crop sector for human food and it also improves the soil fertility by producing organic fertilizer. Furthermore, an efficient utilization of resources can help to increase per animal production of milk, meat, and eggs to be integrated into human food by processing of products in carefully designed meat, milk, or egg processing plants. Processing of the products requires storage, preservation transport, and marketing operations.

16.2   NUTRITIONAL SIGNIFICANCE

Milk, meat, and eggs are essential products and probably the costliest part of the human diet. They provide almost all of the essential amino acids, making high quality and complete animal protein source. These are nutrient-dense foods because these contain more amounts of protein per unit of energy. Consumption of 8 oz of whole milk (227 g) is considered a standard serving size of milk as stated by the US Food and Drug Administration (FDA) and provides about 135 calories and 8 g protein [4], while one serving of cooked lean beef, about 3 oz (85 g) provides about 195 calories and 25 g of protein [5]. Similarly, one standard grade A egg (53 g) provides 70 calories and 6 g of high quality protein [6]. Hence, each gram of whole milk protein gains only about 17 calories, while cooked lean beef provides 7.8 calories per gram of protein. As such, about 11.6 calories are furnished by the consumption of 1 g of egg protein. Milk is considered the most important and nutritious food source because it is an excellent source of almost all the nutrients with very high digestibility for growing children, teens, seniors, adults, and even athletes. It would not be wrong to say that milk contains all the nutrients, except iron, which are essential to human body. One serving of milk contributes 30% Calcium, 25% Riboflavin, 25% Phosphorus, 25% Vitamin D, 22% Vitamin B, 11% Potassium, 10% Vitamin A, and 10% Niacin of daily nutritional value as recommended by FDA [4].

However, milk can be a source of infections if an animal from which the milk is obtained carries the disease-causing microorganisms. This situation is further aggravated when milk from multiple animals is mixed, as is the case with commercially packaged milk brands. To overcome this problem, milk is pasteurized, or ultra-heat treated. People are becoming more diet conscious, especially when they are having disease problems like diabetes, heart problems, or obesity. Dairy industry while processing the milk, also standardizes the milk fat and produces various milk products based on fat percentage (Table 16.1). These milk percentages do not change the other health benefits obtained by the milk consumption [7].

Another important problem associated with milk is allergic responses to the milk constituents that are mainly associated with lactose digestion, and people with lactase insufficiency may develop digestive disturbances. Lactose-free milk is also available that is produced by the milk processor by adding lactase enzyme in the milk, which digests the lactose in the milk so that people with lactase

TABLE 16.1

Various Types of Milk with Their Caloric Intake per 8 Ounce Serving

Type of Milk	Fat %	Fat g/Serving	Calories/Serving
Whole milk	3.5	8	150
Two percent milk	2	5	120
One percent milk	1	2.5	100
Skim milk	0	0	80

insufficiency can consume it without digestive trouble. Similarly, people with a1 beta casein hypersensitivity can consume a2 milk, which is from cows that contain only a2 casein so it can reduce the chances of digestive disturbance with milk [7].

Meat in any form is a very good supplement of dietary essential amino acids, which are mostly deficient in any stable food. Furthermore, meat is an excellent source of iron, which is deficient in milk. Also, about 60% of the meat's iron is in the form of heme iron, which is the form that is highly digestible in human body. One serving of cooked beef can provide 25 g protein, 9 g fat, one-third the daily requirement of zinc, and 15% of daily requirement of iron. Like milk, meat also contains proteins, B complex vitamins (thiamine, riboflavin, niacin, B6, and Vitamin B12), iron and zinc [5].

Comparison of various sources of meat reveals that beef is the most nutritious followed by mutton, and poultry meat is the least nutritious in terms of the coverage of nutrients. As far as the protein quantity and quality is concerned, the ranking is reversed with the highest quality and quantity obtained from poultry meat, followed by mutton and beef obtained from identical serving size. Poultry meat, especially broiler meat, is the highest in protein percentage as inter and intra muscular fat is at a minimum in broiler meat in comparison with mutton and beef, where inter and intra muscular fat is present and cannot be trimmed off from the meat. Moreover, the protein quality is also the highest in the case of broiler meat as the least amount of collagen fibers are present in broiler meat as broiler muscles are the least used and collagen protein cannot be digested by the human stomach because collagenase enzyme is not produced in human body. Low level of collagen protein makes the broiler meat furnish the highest biological value of broiler meat as compared to beef and mutton. Biological value is defined as the ability of the protein to be digested, metabolized, and become the part of the body of a consumer [5].

An egg is the purest and safest gift of God, it is a complete food on this earth. An egg contains all of the nutrients, except Vitamin C. An egg enclosed in a hard-calcareous shell, which is about 10% of its weight. Internally double layer of selectively permeable membrane is present, which not only restrict the microbial entry to the contents, but it also acts a container of the contents. Among the contents, two distinct liquid parts of egg are present; the translucent albumen that is about 58% of the egg and yellow ball enclosed in a membrane—the yolk—which is 32% of the egg. Egg shells may have different colors ranging from dark brown to white, which is purely a breed characteristic and it does not have any influence on nutritive quality of the egg. Similarly, yolk can also have light yellow to reddish yellow color that is due to the xanthophyll color pigments present in the diet, and yolk color does not affect the nutritive value of the egg [6].

An average egg having 53 g weight contributes 70 calories, 6 g protein, 5 g fat, which is about 8% of daily value, of which 1.5 g is in saturated form and no trans fats are present. It also contains 195 mg cholesterol in which high- and low-density lipoproteins (HDL and LDL) are present in equal amounts. The protein and fats present in the egg are of the highest quality and are easily digestible. Eggs are very low in carbohydrates (1%) of which about 40% is in free and rest is in conjugated form. An egg contains 6% iron, 2% calcium and 65 mg sodium, which is only 3% of daily requirement. Vitamin A is present about 10%, Vitamin D 15%, Riboflavin 15%, Vitamin B12 50%, Niacin 8%, and folate 15% of the daily value. It contains iodine, copper, manganese, magnesium, zinc, potassium, sulphur, and chloride [8]. It also contains cholesterol, which gives a bad name to the egg especially for heart patients. The findings of the American Heart Association reveal that consumption of one egg per day does not affect the heart attack risk. The levels of HDL and LDL in eggs are in equal amount that neither increase nor decrease the coronary heart disease risk. It is further reported that egg yolk contains lutein that protects against heart disease. Additionally, eggs can be enriched with nutrients, which are deficient in human diet, and designer egg can fulfil the requirements of deficient nutrients by diet (designer eggs). For example, feed layers with flaxseed can enrich eggs with omega-3 fatty acids [9].

16.3 INSPECTION, GRADING, AND COMPOSITION OF POULTRY MEAT

Poultry inspection can be defined as the process of detecting and eliminating the meat, which is not suitable for human consumption. Either the poultry has some disease-causing organism contamination, or it may carry chemical (drug) residues that can pose a threat to public health. There are about six types of inspections that are taken care of by the inspectors. Firstly, birds should be inspected before slaughtering for any abnormal/disease conditions, which is called antemortem inspection. Secondly, after slaughtering, each carcass should be inspected before processing, and that is called postmortem inspection. Thirdly, processing plant facilities should also be inspected to make sure that the birds are being slaughtered/processed in sanitary conditions. Fourthly, all of the operations performed on the birds at the processing plant should be inspected. A fifth type of inspection can be done at any time at the processing plant, during transportation of the product, at the wholesaler's facilities, or at the retailer's display to verify the accuracy of the label on the product. The sixth or last type of inspection is performed at the point of entry of the processed product in the country to assess the wholesomeness of the product being imported.

The main objective of inspection can be that the poultry being processed in sanitary conditions in the approved facility and is wholesome, not adulterated, and properly labelled. To fulfill these objectives, the inspectors have to perform various responsibilities that include the ante and postmortem inspections of animals to be used as human food and processing. Through finding out disease conditions and to decide and declare the carcasses and products unfit due to infections, diseases, extraneous materials, chemical and drug residues or any adulteration. Inspectors are responsible for making emergency decisions regarding adulterated products to retain, detain, or recall the product. Inspectors are responsible to investigate foodborne disease outbreaks. Monitoring the effectiveness inspection program, also comes under the responsibilities of the inspectors. Inspectors also have the responsibility to develop and implement strategies to control animal production practices related to food safety hazards. The inspectors are also responsible to monitor facilities and inspection systems of foreign countries from where meat or its products are being imported. Last, but not the least, the re-inspection of the imported meat and products at the point of entry and destination also comes under the responsibilities of the inspectors. Public awareness regarding safe handling of meat and products by handlers and consumers is also included in the responsibilities list [10].

16.3.1 Step by Step Process of Inspection Services at Processing Plants

16.3.1.1 Antemortem Inspection

The main aim for antemortem inspection is to decide for the batch/flock/truck and segregate the healthy animals from suspect animals. Prior to slaughter, the animals are examined for any abnormal or diseased conditions. Suspect animals are slaughtered separately, either in a different facility or in the same facility, after the healthy animals are slaughtered. Antemortem inspection prevents slaughter of dead and dying animals.

16.3.1.2 Postmortem Inspection

Postmortem inspection is the discretionary operation, but it is mandatory by law that all slaughtered animal carcasses should be inspected individually. It requires the inspection of not only the internal organs, but also the external and internal surfaces of the carcasses for contamination and disease conditions and decide to declare unfit the whole or part of the carcass for human consumption. Various types of post-mortem inspection systems namely Streamlined Inspection System, New Enhanced Line Speed, New Turkey Inspection System and New Poultry Inspection Systems by utilizing 2, 3, 4 and 5 inspector per line allow to process 70, 91, 50 and 140 birds per minute line speeds. It is mandatory for all these systems that carcasses and respective viscera be exposed to the inspector so that all the internal and external surfaces and organs can easily be and thoroughly inspected. Hock joints must be cut so that tendons and synovial membranes can be examined. For this purpose, in traditional methods, viscera are left attached to carcass, while in new systems, a separate line with viscera along with the carcass run to reduce the chances of contamination of carcass with digestive contents [10,11].

16.3.1.3 Condemnation and Final Disposition

After the postmortem inspection, the carcasses are classified into four categories: inspection passed, trimmed/salvaged/washed and passed, retained for disposition by the veterinarian, and condemned as whole carcasses. The wholesome carcasses without any visible symptoms of disease remain on the line and may require a little trimming before chilling are termed as inspection passed. Local and distinct lesions due to disease or contaminated with extraneous material are marked and separated on the salvage line for trimming and washing, which is called trimmed/salvaged/washed and passed. Carcasses with doubtful lesions are retained for inspector in-charge/veterinarian. Carcasses with unrecoverable conditions are condemned as whole carcasses and recorded on the inspection tally sheet and categorized as field/farm- or plant-related condemnation. Various disease conditions due to which whole carcass is condemned include tuberculosis, leucosis, septicemia/toxemia, airsacculitis, synovitis, cellulitis, tumors, and bruises are categorized as field/farm-related condemnation. Condemnations of whole carcasses related to plant are cadavers, contamination/mutilation, and over scalding. Death of bird from reason other than blood loss due to slaughter, usually has cherry red color viscera, and carcass with or without foul odor are called cadavers. Contaminated carcasses with extraneous materials like oil, paint, or grease may be inspected due to excessive contamination with feces or damaged carcasses due to the equipment or falls in drain are called contamination/mutilation. Cooked carcasses having white color in pectoral muscles are called over-scald [10,12].

16.3.1.4 Sanitary Slaughtering and Dressing

One of the important objectives of the inspection in poultry processing is prevention of fecal contamination in carcasses, either from digestive tract contents spillage or fecal material smearing on meat surfaces. To achieve sanitary slaughtering and dressing regulation aims, contaminated carcasses are removed from the evisceration line by the inspectors and sent for reprocessing at a separate station. Reprocessing involves single or any combination of trimming, vacuuming, or washing with chlorinated water (20 ppm), reprocessed carcasses are presented for reinspection before allowing for chilling. The target of sanitary slaughtering and dressing step is not to allow any carcass to enter the chiller, contaminated with fecal contents with the motto of Zero Fecal Tolerance [12].

16.3.1.5 Poultry Meat Chilling

The monitoring of chiller and chilling operation is also under the jurisdiction of the inspectors. A flow of 3 and 2 gallon per bird entering in the chiller and scalder must be maintained along with monitoring of temperatures of chiller water and carcass which regulate the moisture uptake by the carcasses. The inspection passed carcasses after trimming and giblet removal are called as ready-to-cook (RTC) and require chilling to reduce temperature for inhibition of microbial growth preferably in immersion chillers.

The objectives of chilling operations are that the temperature of the carcasses must be reduced to 4.4°C below within 4 hours for 4 pounds broilers, 6 hours for 4–8 pounds broilers, and 8 hours for 8 pounds broilers or turkeys. Similarly, giblets (liver, gizzard, heart and necks) need to be chilled within 2 hours separately from carcasses in immersion chillers.

16.3.1.6 Plant Sanitation

Monitoring of plant facilities and equipment also comes under the responsibilities of the inspectors. The structures of the processing plant and premises like supply of water, drainage and waste handling, processing and slaughtering equipment, dry and ice storage rooms, chillers and freezers, personnel facilities and practices, pest control operations and hygiene features of plant structure, and environment are monitored. Sanitation standard operating procedures (SSOPs) for pathogen reduction and Hazard Analysis and Critical Control Points (HACCP) for each processing plant should be developed and implemented covering preoperational and establishment of sanitary conditions during processing and slaughtering. Record keeping of these operations, like written sanitation protocols, usage frequency, assignment of responsibilities and development of any hazard and corrective actions, are necessary to take [10].

16.3.1.7 Carcass Reinspection

Poultry inspectors and quality control personnel reinspect the carcasses after postmortem inspection and salvage/trim operations. Carcasses having defects related with processing operation like excess feathers, ingesta, bile stain, remnants of viscera, trimming defects, or extraneous materials like grease or metal particles need to be evaluated again and inspected on a separate line. As with any other operation, record keeping of defective on time scale is done which is later evaluated on the basis of cumulative sum system or acceptable quality level standards. Samples of carcasses, both before and after chilling operations, are also examined for fecal contamination and achievement of proper chilling temperatures and water uptake, respectively. However, salvage products are reprocessed in inspected for fecal contamination prior to chilling.

16.3.1.8 Residue Monitoring

Inspection activities are also required to monitor chemical and drug residues in carcasses and processed products or any indiscriminate or accidental exposure of birds/carcasses to herbicides, pesticides, therapeutic drugs, feed additives, especially antibiotic growth promoters, or any large-scale accidental contaminating of animal feeds or environment.

The minimal residue levels of poultry and poultry products are defined for various drugs and chemicals by different regulatory bodies like the Food and Drug Administration Authority, Environment Protection Agency, or any other food authority. It is the responsibility of the inspectors to take random samples of tissues to test for various drugs and chemicals to be below their minimum residue levels and record their persistence levels, toxicity, and exposure.

16.3.1.9 Microbial Contamination Testing

The main focus of the inspection services is to reduce microbial contamination in the processed poultry products. In this regard, the inspector along with the visual inspection requires the laboratory testing for fecal contamination and screening for pathogenic bacteria species. Pathogen Reduction/Hazard Analysis Critical Control Points (HACCP) protocol requires that at least two bacterial species must be tested at each inspected processing plant, namely *E. coli* for monitoring of process control (i.e. fecal contamination of the products) and *Salmonella* for performance standards (i.e. pathogen control) [10].

16.3.1.9.1 Testing for E. coli

E. coli genetic strain Biotype I testing is done at processing plants to check that chilled processed carcasses were successful in removing fecal contamination to have an estimation of processing activities in reducing fecal contamination. For the generic strain of *E. coli,* it is necessary to apply the test on fecal contamination. This is a cheap and easy test to culture and count the genetic *E. coli. E. coli* testing is not a regulatory binding; however, this test provides an objective estimation of process control. Written protocols for sampling and testing of *E. coli* must be available at the processing plants. The record keeping of the testing procedures, approved method to detect 5 cfu/mL, culture, shipping conditions, sampling location, responsibility, handling, randomization, collection, and sample integrity are the requirements of HACCP. After chilling and drip one whole carcass randomly out of 22,000 broilers and 3000 turkeys is rinsed in a bag, then *E. coli* is counted in this fluid by applying an approved method. The results are recorded on process control tables and 13 recent tests are displayed. If *E. coli* count in no test out of 13 displayed tests is more than 1000 cfu/mL and less than three tests are between the higher and low limit (i.e. 100 cfu/mL) then performance of the processing plant is in an acceptable range [10].

16.3.1.9.2   Testing for Salmonella

Salmonella testing is done and recoded in a similar fashion by the inspections. Moreover, it is a mandatory requirement of the processing plant that they should constantly and routinely test for *Salmonella*. The performance standard for *Salmonella* is that out of 51 samples a maximum of 12 *Salmonella* positive samples are acceptable. In contrary to *E. coli* performance criteria, *Salmonella* standard must be maintained at plant level not on batch by batch level and corrective actions must be taken by the plants failing to achieve the performance standards otherwise the particular product of the plant is withdrawn from the market [10].

16.3.1.10   Grading of Poultry Products

Grading is the sorting of products, like poultry meat and egg, into different categories based upon conditions and characteristics. Wholesomeness is the pre-requisite of grading; that is, any carcass having inspection defects cannot be graded until those defects are removed and the carcass is reinspected and passed. All of the ready-to-cook poultry products starting from whole carcass, cut-up parts, or further process should be graded. Processing defects in ready-to-cook poultry, like bruises to be trimmed, protruding feathers, remains of trachea, lungs, or any other visceral organs or foreign materials or having any off-quality parameters like slippery, slimy, sour, or putrid smells, are not graded until the off condition is removed [13].

16.3.2   Ready-to-Cook Carcasses and Parts: Standards of Quality

16.3.2.1   Conformation

The distribution of meat on various bones is affected by the deformities in the bones. Crooked, twisted, broken, or V-shaped breasts, wedge shaped frame of body, and deformed wings and legs are the defects that change the normal conformation of the carcass and parts.

16.3.2.2   Fleshing

Proportion of meat and bones on various parts and carcasses is called fleshing. Typically, most of the meat is present on the breast, drumsticks, and thighs. Fleshing is affected by the sex; that is, there is more amount of meat on the back of females than in males.

16.3.2.3   Fat Covering

Normally most of the fat in the chicken is present under the skin, mainly neat the feather tracks along with hips and back.

16.3.2.4   Feathers

Hair-like small extended feathers in chickens and down feathers on the carcasses of geese and ducks affect the normal look of the carcass. These feathers must be removed to fulfill the ready-to-cook requirement of carcass and make the meat ready for grading.

16.3.2.5 Exposed Flesh

Tearing of skin due to trimming, cuts and exposes the meat on the carcass. Exposed flesh lowers the visual as well as cooking and eating qualities of the meat as the meat becomes dry during chilling, freezing, and cooking operations.

16.3.2.6 Discolorations

Change in color of carcasses, as a whole or in patches due to hemorrhages or improper and partial bleeding, may result in different light and dark color areas on the skin. Such red, green, blue, or dark red areas must be trimmed to make the carcass fit for grading.

16.3.2.7 Disjointed or Broken Bones and Missing Parts

Dislocated joints and bones that are broken or a carcass with some major part missing are not considered fit for grading, such carcasses are used for cut-up parts.

16.3.2.8 Freezing Defects

Dehydrated and darkened parts of the carcass and skin and freeze burns on exposed flesh are also a defect in the carcass.

16.3.2.9 Accuracy of Cut

In cut-up parts of the carcass, the parts are cut at the joints, which are equally cut. Moreover, the part should have only the required bones, which are present in the standard cut.

16.3.3 COMMON PARTS OF A READY TO COOK CHICKEN CARCASS

16.3.3.1 Half Carcass

The whole carcass of chicken cut from spine into right and left halves [14].

16.3.3.2 Breast Quarter

Front quarter or the breast (left or right) having half spine, ribs, major and minor pectoral muscles and respective wing is called breast quarter [14].

16.3.3.3 Leg Quarter

Lower part of the carcass (left or right) having half spine, thigh and drumstick is called the leg quarter [14].

16.3.3.4 Wing

The part of the carcass containing the scapula, humer, radious, and ulna bones forming three bone parts of the wing with some breast meat is considered as wing [14].

16.3.3.5 Breast

The pectoral muscles (major and minor) with sternum and skin, it may also have ribs is called breast [14].

16.3.3.6 Thigh

The part of leg having the femur bone is called the thigh [14].

16.3.3.7 Drumstick

The leg portion containing the tibia fibula is called the drumstick [14].

16.3.3.8 Drumette

Inner part of wing is termed the drumette [14].

16.3.3.9 Wing Portion

The central part of the wing having radious and ulna bones with or without attached wing tip is called the wing portion [14].

16.3.3.10 Whole Breast

Front half of the carcass having both the breast parts connected together without wings, with or without spine connecting them in back is called the whole breast [14].

16.3.3.11 Keel Piece

Tip of the breast having the cartilage part of sternum cut from the whole breast and almost one third part of the breast [14].

16.3.3.12 Breast Piece

The whole breast cut into halves (left and right) after cutting the keel piece is called the breast piece [14].

16.3.3.13 Whole Leg

The leg with thigh and drum stick part (i.e. femur, tibia, and fibula) without spine is called the whole leg [14].

16.3.3.14 Back or Strip Back

Pelvis and spine part of the back is called back or strip back (if without skin); however, in case of quarter parts, this portion goes with the respective quarters [14].

16.3.3.15 Breast Half or Front Half

The entire front half of the carcass is called the breast half [14].

16.3.3.16 Leg Half, Back Half, or Saddle

The intact rear half of the carcass is called the leg half or saddle [14].

16.3.4 COMPOSITION OF POULTRY MEAT

Chicken meat has the highest protein content. This is mainly due to its comparatively low-fat content compared with beef, mutton, and other sources of meat. Like other sources of protein, it is a balanced source of protein as it contains nine dietary essential amino acids. About a 0.25 kg piece of chicken meat provides more than 60 g of protein. Skinless chicken meat is free from carbohydrates; it provides the lowest amount of fat (3 g), calories (143), and saturated fat (1 g) from a 95 g breast piece. Leg meat contains relatively high content of fat compared with breast meat so comparatively more total fat (8 g), calories (165), and saturated fat (3 g) are produced from 86 g piece of skinless leg meat. Vitamin B6 and B3 are present in higher amounts, 16% and 40% of the recommended daily allowance. Being low in fat content, chicken meat does not contain Vitamin A and it is also deficient in Vitamin C. Moreover, chicken meat is also rich with two important minerals, like selenium and phosphorus with 30% and 16% of recommended daily allowance. Sodium is about 2% while potassium is 3% of the daily value for a normal human. The iron content of chicken meat is 4% and calcium is 3% of the daily value. Chicken meat contains comparatively less amounts of cholesterol, which is about 18% of the recommended daily allowance; moreover, breast meat does not contain cholesterol and most of the cholesterol is present in the leg portion of meat [15].

16.3.5 POULTRY PROCESSING TECHNIQUES

Poultry processing is defined as slaughtering the live birds, remove the offal/non-edible organs, inspect, and convert poultry to ready-to-cook safe products to be consumed by humans. The processing plant is the place where mechanical equipment is used in a systemized and coordinated manner to slaughter, process, pack, preserve, and market/distribute the safe and healthy poultry and products to the consumers. Various operations performed in poultry processing facilities are discussed in logical pattern in the following section [16].

16.3.5.1 Unloading of Birds

Finished broilers are transported to the processing facilities, and the first step in the processing plant is unloading. Sometimes at the processing plant the transport carriage is temporarily retained or held before unloading, waiting for the turn. The birds kept in transportation coops are shifted to the conveyor manually, or the dumper machine automatically dump the coops to the conveyor. This can be source of downgrading of carcass if not properly handled due to broken and displaced bones/joints, bruising, and cuts/tears in birds as the dumper throws the coops on a conveyor from a height of more than one meter. Decrease in this distance can help to reduce the downgrading. On the other hand, manual unloading can be more variable in terms of damage to the birds as workers may vary their handling. To reduce damage to the birds at this step, training of the staff engaged for this purpose is required regarding humane handling of live poultry. In case of manual unloading operation, the birds are directly shackled rather than shifted to the conveyor.

16.3.5.2 Stunning of Birds

Knocking birds out of consciousness before killing is required for humane slaughter. This is called stunning. The birds can be stunned either by electric shock or by exposing the birds to a higher concentration of carbon dioxide in the stunning chamber. Electric stunning is more popular method in which the shackled birds' heads are dipped in a 1% salt solution where electric current is flowing for about 90–60 seconds. The strength of the current is variable depending upon the regulatory bodies, 10–20 mA in United States, while 90 mA in European countries. The exposure time to electric shock is dependent upon current flow, the higher the strength of current flow the lower the time required to be exposed; for example, about 4–6 seconds in Europe while 10–12 seconds exposure time per broiler is required in United States. The other method for stunning is exposure to a higher concentration of carbon dioxide, and according to this method either 40%–10% carbon dioxide mixed with 90%–60% air or a mixture of 30% carbon dioxide, 0%–15% nitrogen, and 55%–70% argon is used. In the earlier mixture, less time is required, about 30–45 seconds compared with 2–3 minutes in the later mixture. Improper stunning, for example, more stunning can result in bursting blood vessels and broken bones, while insufficient stunning may result in inadequate bleeding in birds.

In Islamic communities, stunning is not allowed so for Halal method of slaughtering the stunning step is not done.

16.3.5.3 Slaughtering of Birds

In the case of humane slaughtering, the shackle is moved after stunning chamber to the killing operation, while in Islamic slaughtering after shackling, the birds are moved for slaughtering.

Slaughtering can either be automatic or manual in most of Islamic slaughter facilities, manual slaughtering is practiced after recitation of Takbeer. However, a recording of Takbeer is played in case of automatic slaughtering operation for each broiler to be slaughtered. The neck cutting machine grasps the lower neck skin and wattles and guides the bird's head in the machine for sharp rotating blades, which cut the carotid arteries and jugular veins. Birds are kept for about 2–3 minutes in the bleeding section for proper bleeding time, 30%–50% blood is lost during this time, and results in death of the bird. If the bird is insufficiently slaughtered or not slaughtered at this step and the live bird enters the next section; the scalder. A bright red color in meat and skin indicates that the bird died due to scalding heat water rather than slaughtering.

16.3.5.4   Scalding of Birds

In order to loosen the feather follicles, the slaughtered birds are dipped in the hot water to denature the proteins holding the feather shafts. Two different temperatures are used for this purpose, named as soft and hard scalding. When the scalding water temperature is kept higher 145°F–148°F, it is called hard scalding while at comparatively low scalding temperature of 128°F, soft scalding is done. However, the time required for scalding is more with soft scalding, around 120 seconds compared with 45 seconds for hard scalding.

16.3.5.5   Feather Picking

The feather removing machine performs the task of feather removal, and this process is called picking. Flexible rubber fingers are attached to rotating holders in different rows, these ribbed fingers by their abrasive action removes the loosened feathers from the skin. There are five clusters of these rotating fingers focused in different regions of the body so that the whole carcass is cleared of feathers. Improper picking may result in downgrading of carcasses. Too distant adjustment of finger clusters may not be able to remove the feathers while too close fingers may result in tearing of skin or broken bones in leg wing or breast regions. This operation is however, not very efficient as it leaves the pin feathers on the skin.

16.3.5.6   Feather Singeing of Carcass

The small pin feather left on the skin of carcasses pose a dirty appearance and may offend the customers. To remove these hair-like feathers, the singeing of carcasses is performed. In the singeing operation, carcasses are conveyed over the burning flames to burn these pin feathers left on the skin after picking. The heads and feet are also removed during this process, and the carcasses are shifted to the evisceration shackle line, manually or mechanically.

16.3.5.7   Evisceration of Carcass

The splitting of inedible offals from the edible portion of the carcass is called evisceration. It is a step-by-step process of automatically removing the visceral organs from the carcass, but the design of this machine may vary with brand. The evisceration operation in broilers is focused on three basic aims. Firstly, the opening of the body cavity in which a cut is made between cloaca to the tip of breast bone. Secondly, the intestines, reproductive tract, and attached parts, like heart, liver, gizzard, and lugs, are pulled out of the body cavity. Thirdly, the visceral organs, which are edible namely liver, heart, and gizzard, are removed from the inedible parts and washed. Sometimes the neck is included in the giblets (liver, heart, and gizzard) and sometimes it is sold separately; however, necks are removed after the inspection of carcass. The equipment used for evisceration is shown sequentially in Figure 16.1.

16.3.5.8   Chilling of Carcass

The carcasses that are passed by the inspection operation are chilled; that is, their temperature is reduced below 4°C as early as possible. The aim of the chilling operation is to minimize, or more precisely, slow down the microbial growth and enhance the shelf life of the products by keeping the food safe. The focus of chilling is to reduce the temperature of carcass within 1–2 hours after evisceration below 4°C. The chilling of carcasses can be done by dipping the carcass in the chilled water (usually in United States) or by circulating chilled air (usually in Europe) on the carcasses. Multiple water tanks having chilled water temperature 7°C–12°C in pre-chiller where carcasses are kept for about 15 minutes. Then the carcasses are shifted to the chiller tank having about 1°C at exit and 4°C at entrance chiller tank, which is larger than pre-chiller, and the carcasses are kept here for about 45–60 minutes. However, the water intake by carcasses is reduced by dripping of carcasses on the drip line for about 15 minutes. While in air chilling, carcasses are hung on shackle lines and a cold wind blast with a temperature about 2°C–7°C for 1–3 hours is applied. Cold water can be sprayed

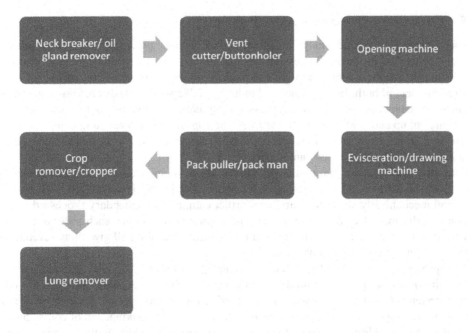

FIGURE 16.1 Typical sequence and common names for evisceration equipment.

on the carcasses to speed-up the cooling process. To enhance evaporative efficiency of chilled air, humidity can be reduced to enhance air's ability to retain evaporated water along with heat from the carcasses. Air chilling results in drier carcasses compared with water chilled carcasses. The drying effect of air chilled carcasses is compensated by the packaging operation. Water chilled carcasses are relatively higher in weight compared with air chilled carcasses.

16.3.6 Determination of Yield in Poultry Processing

The yield of meat measures the efficiency of any production setup, measured in percentage of output per unit of input is the appraisal of efficiency. The processing operation yield can be measured by using different types of indices with their significance from different aspects. Ready-to-cook yield, for example, determines the first processing efficiency; that is, the amount of carcass produced per unit of live body weight of the broilers. It assesses the efficiency of the processing plant crew or machines (in case of automated operation) in various activities of unloading, evisceration, and trimming, as well as preprocessing efficiency of catching crew and transportation conditions. Ready-to-cook yield becomes important in cases of vertically integrated companies, where the farming and processing operations are owned by the same company. Ready-to-cook yield can be further categorized as a little higher yield when the giblets are sold with carcass compared with carcasses without giblets, where the giblets are sold separately. On an average, 70%–75% ready-to-cook yield is recorded. Feed conversion ratio of ready-to-cook poultry can be used to estimate the combined efficiency of both production and processing operations in case of a bigger enterprise, where both operations are owned by the same owner. In case of without giblets, ready-to-cook yield is 40% bone and the rest is 60% meat, of which 40% consists of leg meat and 60% breast meat. These are variable values, which are affected by bird age, strain, and even by processing plant. However, these values can be helpful in estimating the meat to be produced in case of further processing activities, like minced meat or deboned meat production or value-added production like nuggets or burger patties. Similarly, in cases of cut up poultry production, the yield in case of breast is higher (25%), than wings (14%), legs (33%), back and neck (17%), and giblets (11%), which can be used for estimation purpose.

16.3.7 Overview of Processed Poultry Products

The processed poultry products may be categorized as primary processed, secondary processed, and further processed products. Processing has main objective of consumer likeness and convenience. Primarily, the most common product of poultry processing is whole carcass but cut-up parts are the requirement of both the consumer and industry. Salvage or carcasses having some trimmed anatomical part cannot be sold as whole carcass, it is a great economic loss to the processor, so such carcasses are cut up and sold as parts. Sometimes, the consumer is interested in some specific part of the carcass. However, in such cases, it is not feasible economically for the consumer to purchase the whole carcass and dump the unwanted part.

Cut-up, packaged parts of the poultry carcasses are also considered as secondary processed poultry products. Various cut-up parts are discussed earlier in this chapter. Deboned, portioned, ground, and mechanically separated parts are further examples of secondary processed products. It is economically more feasible for processor and consumer to produce such processed products as cutting, deboning, portioning, grinding, and mechanical separation all give more revenue to the processor and convenience to the consumer.

Further processed poultry products include marinated, coated, cooked, glazed, and frozen products. The aim of further processed products is the same as that of secondary processed products; consumer preference and convenience. Provision of ready-to-cook recipe products may require marinated products that may provide a branded look, save time in cooking, and of course money to the consumer. Value addition increases the return of processor by addition of sometimes inexpensive ingredients or treatments with greater economic return. Coating of carcass, parts, and cooked products add safety features to the processed products. Coating of the product is mostly done to reduce the bacterial growth and contamination. Nowadays, edible coatings are extensively used for various poultry products to facilitate the provision of safe and healthy products to the consumers. Cooking, glazing, and freezing facilitate provision of ready-to-eat poultry products to the consumer, which may require heating or in some cases frying or mild cooking of the product before serving. Moreover, this value addition fetches many times more economic returns to the processor compared with raw or primary processed poultry products. It provides the greatest convenience to the working ladies and single men living in highly populated cities to use ready-to-eat products with not only saving time but also certified as the safe products.

16.3.8 Poultry Products Marketing Trend in Developing Countries

Marketing of poultry products in developing countries like Pakistan is mostly as a live bird sale. However, this trend is changing in the previous decade; the pandemic out breaks of various zoonotic diseases like bird flu has provided a paradigm shift. The consumers in developing countries are becoming more conscious of safe food products. Moreover, the Governments are also taking initiatives in developing and implementing the rules and regulations to produce safe food for their populace. International organizations like Food and Agriculture Organization of United Nations are also facilitating the governments of developing countries in provision of safe food to their community.

Pakistan is also affected with this paradigm shift and in the last decade, primary poultry processing plants has been installed by private companies. Currently, four fully functional primary processing plants are operating in Pakistan and more companies are either in planning or erection phases. However, more than half dozen companies are involved in the value addition of poultry and poultry products. The government of Pakistan has developed and implemented the rules and regulations regarding food safety and processed products. The consumers in Pakistan are also shifting towards processed and further processed poultry meat products. The consumption of processed and value-added poultry products is increasing at an increasing rate.

16.3.9 POULTRY BY-PRODUCTS AND WASTE

By-products of the poultry industry include two types of waste products, namely edible and inedible waste products. Major amount of waste produced by poultry industry includes litter and droppings, feathers, dead, dying or culled birds, and poultry processing industry wastes. Poultry litter and hatchery waste is inedible and utilized in animal feeds by utilizing various types of processing treatments or can be used as a bio-fertilizer by agriculture land applications. Processing industry waste includes 7%–8% feathers, 2.5%–3.0% heads, 3.2%–3.7% blood, 3.5%–4.2% proventiculus and gizzards, 3.5%–4.0% feet, and 8.5%–9.0% gastrointestinal tract, as percent of live body weight. Heads, blood (in some countries), gizzards, feet, skin, and intestines (sausage industry) are edible waste of poultry industry.

Waste water is probably the most abundant waste of poultry processing industry. Although, waste water production is highly variable among processing plants, it is estimated that about 9.3 gallons water is required to process one bird with a range of 4.2–23 gallon/bird. To reduce the treatment cost of waste water, the management of processing plants is focusing on the minimization of waste water production. Water is utilized in washing of birds or carcasses before and after evisceration and chilling, scalding, and washing, as well as sanitization of machines, rooms, floors, and conveyors. Mechanical equipment like pumps, trucks, coops, and compressors also require water. Moreover, over flow water from chilling and scalding tanks is also included in this category. The waste water contains soluble proteins, vitamins, minerals as well as fat in the form of suspension giving translucent appearance. This water contains blood, viscera, feathers, and soft tissues, bones, dirt, and litter from soiled feathers along with fat in the form of suspension. The appearance and organic contents of poultry processing waste water requires it to be treated before disposal. Various techniques like reverse osmosis and ultrafiltration are used to treat this water. Poultry by-products like feathers, intestines, blood, bones, fat and meat trimmings, and hatchery wastes are subjected to high temperature and pressure (rendered) to produce various types of products to be used in industrial and agricultural operations [17].

16.4 CONCLUSION

Poultry and livestock are the richest source of high quality of animal protein sources in the form of milk, eggs, and meat. Despite the zoonotic pandemics, careful processing and food safety measures, animal products are the best sources of food.

REFERENCES

1. Anonymous (2017) *Economic Survey of Pakistan*. Government of Pakistan, Islamabad, Pakistan.
2. Thornton PK, Steeg JV, Notenbaert A, Herrero A (2009) The impacts of climate change on livestock and livestock systems in developing countries: A review of what we know and what we need to know. *Agr Syst* 101:113–127.
3. Ali A, Khan MA (2013) Livestock ownership in ensuring rural household food security in Pakistan. *J Anim Plant Sci* 23:313–318.
4. Anonymous (2013) The Nutritional Composition of Dairy products. The Dairy Council. http://ilrestoealtrove.altervista.org/wp-content/uploads/2013/05/Composition_of_Dairy.pdf. Accessed June 7, 2018.
5. Boyle E (1994) The Nutritive Value of Meat. https://www.asi.k-state.edu/doc/meat-science/the-nutritive-value-of-meat.pdf. Accessed September 7, 2018.
6. Frey M (2018) Egg Health Benefits and Nutritional Information. https://www.verywellfit.com/hard-boiled-egg-calories-and-fat-3495628. Accessed September 7, 2018.
7. Anonymous (2018) The Health Benefits of Dairy. http://thedairyalliance.com/health-benefits-of-dairy. Accessed June 7, 2018.
8. Anonymous (2018) Egg Nutrition & Calories. http://eggs.ab.ca/eggs/egg-nutrition. Accessed June 7, 2018.

9. Zelman KM (2018) Good Eggs: For Nutrition, They're Hard to Beat – The egg is no Longer a Nutritional no-no. https://www.webmd.com/diet/features/good-eggs-for-nutrition-theyre-hard-to-beat#1. Accessed June 7, 2018.

10. Bilgili SF (2010) Poultry meat inspection and grading. In: Owens CM, Alvarado CZ, Sams AR (Eds.) *Poultry Meat Processing*, 2nd ed. CRC Press, Taylor & Francis Group, Boca Raton, FL.

11. Still WS (2015) Impacts and potential impacts of the new poultry inspection system. In *Proceedings of the AMSA 68th Reciprocal Meat Conference (RMC)*, June 14–17, 2015, University of Nebraska, Lincoln, NE.

12. Barbut S (2015) *The Science of Poultry and Meat Processing*. University of Guelph, Guelph, Canada.

13. Anonymous (1998) *Poultry Grading Manual*. U.S. Department of Agriculture, Washington, DC.

14. Alvarado CZ (2006) Poultry processing quality. In: Hui YH (Ed.) *Handbook of Food Science*. Taylor & Francis Group, Boca Raton, FL, Volume 1, 33:1–33:13.

15. Oliveira J, Avanço SV, Garcia-Neto M, Ponsano EGH (2016) Composition of broilers meat. *J Appl Poult Res* 25:173–181.

16. Clark S, Jung S, Lamsal B (2014) *Food Processing: Principles and Applications*. Wiley and Blackwell, Chichester, UK.

17. Jayathilakan K, Sultana K, Radhakrishna K, Bawa AS (2012) Utilization of by-products and waste materials from meat, poultry and fish processing industries: A review. *J Food Sci Technol* 49:278–293.

Index

Note: Page numbers in italic and bold refer to figures and tables respectively.

Printed in the United States
by Baker & Taylor Publisher Services